The Essential Pocket Guide for Clinical Nutrition

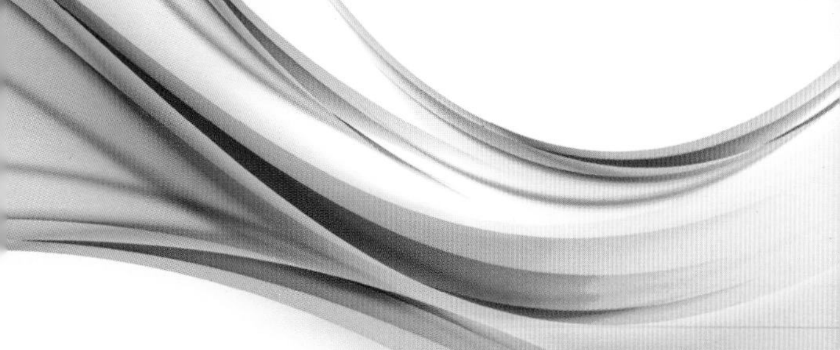

The Essential Pocket Guide for Clinical Nutrition

Second Edition

Mary Width, MS, RD
Director
Coordinated Program in Dietetics
Department of Nutrition and Food Science
Course Director
Clinical Nutrition, School of Medicine
Wayne State University
Detroit, Michigan

Tonia Reinhard, MS, RD, FAND
Senior Lecturer
Coordinated Program in Dietetics
Department of Nutrition and Food Science
Course Director
Clinical Nutrition, School of Medicine
Wayne State University
Detroit, Michigan

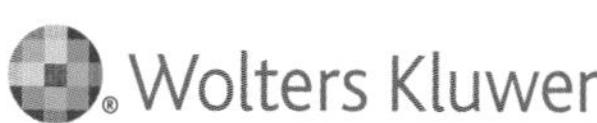

Philadelphia • Baltimore • New York • London
Buenos Aires • Hong Kong • Sydney • Tokyo

Acquisitions Editor: Jonathan Joyce
Product Development Editor: John Larkin
Editorial Coordinator: Emily Buccieri
Editorial Assistant: Tish Rogers
Marketing Manager: Leah Thomson
Production Project Manager: David Orzechowski
Design Coordinator: Teresa Mallon
Manufacturing Coordinator: Margie Orzech
Prepress Vendor: S4Carlisle Publishing Services

Second edition

9 8 7 6 5 4

Printed in China

Library of Congress Cataloging-in-Publication Data

Names: Width, Mary, author. | Reinhard, Tonia, author.
Title: The essential pocket guide for clinical nutrition/Mary Width and Tonia Reinhard.
Other titles: Clinical dietitian's essential pocket guide
Description: Second edition. | Philadelphia: Wolters Kluwer Health, [2018] |
Preceded by: The clinical dietitian's essential pocket guide/Mary Width,
Tonia Reinhard. c2009. | Includes bibliographical references and index.
Identifiers: LCCN 2016029106 | ISBN 9781496339164
Subjects: | MESH: Nutrition Assessment | Dietetics—methods | Nutrition Therapy—methods | Handbooks
Classification: LCC RM217.2 | NLM QU 39 | DDC 615.8/54—dc23 LC record available at https://lccn.loc.gov/2016029106

LWW.com

"In loving memory of my sweet friend and esteemed colleague, Lisa Ventrella Lucente, PhD, RD. You are forever in my heart."

Mary Width

"This book is dedicated to the Reinhard Clan, John Francis, Faye and Jeff, Brendan and Karen, and the upcoming crew of Claire, Zoe, Gea, and Anthony."

Tonia Reinhard

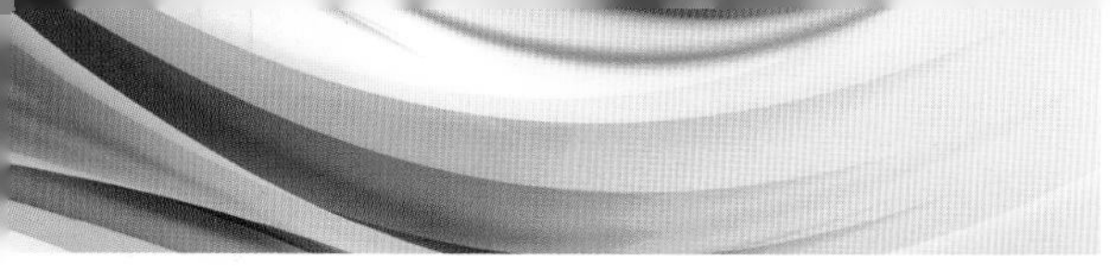

Contributors

Lindsey Battistelli, RDN
Metabolic and Bariatric Surgery Program Coordinator
Henry Ford Wyandotte Hospital
Wyandotte, Michigan

Sheri Betz, RD
Clinical Dietitian
St. John Hospital and Medical Center
Detroit, Michigan

Damien H. Buchkowski, RD, CSO
East-Region Outpatient Oncology Dietitian
St. John Providence Health System
Grosse Pointe Woods, Michigan

Katherine Hilbrecht, RD
Renal Dietitian
DaVita HealthCare Partners Inc.
Dearborn, Michigan

Brenda Howell, RD, CNSC
Nutrition Support Team Clinician
Genesys Regional Medical Center
Grand Blanc, Michigan

Tilakavati Karupaiah, PhD, APD, AN
Associate Professor
Dietetics Program, Faculty of Health Sciences
National University of Malaysia
Kuala Lumpur, Malaysia

Lynn Kuligowski, RD
WIC Program Coordinator
Downriver Community Services North Macomb WIC
Mt. Clemens, Michigan

Vikki Lasota, RDN
Consultant Dietitian
TouchPoint Support Services
Sandy Springs, Georgia

Ellen McCloy, MS, RD
Clinical Dietitian II
Children's Hospital Los Angeles
Los Angeles, California

Thomas Pietrowsky, MS, RD
Dietitian
Henry Ford Transplant Institute
Henry Ford Hospital
Detroit, Michigan

Kelly Sanna-Gouin, RD, CNSC
Clinical Dietitian
Food and Nutrition Services
Detroit Receiving Hospital
Detroit, Michigan

Maria Segovia, MD
Medical Director
Intestine and Multivisceral Transplant Program
Henry Ford Hospital
Detroit, Michigan

Virginia Uhley, PhD, RDN
Assistant Professor, Biomedical Sciences and Nutrition
Discipline Director
Co-Course Director
Endocrinology and Promotion and Maintenance of Health
Oakland University William Beaumont School of Medicine
Rochester, Michigan

Melanie Wierda, RD, CSR
Renal Dietitian
DaVita HealthCare Partners Inc.
Detroit, Michigan

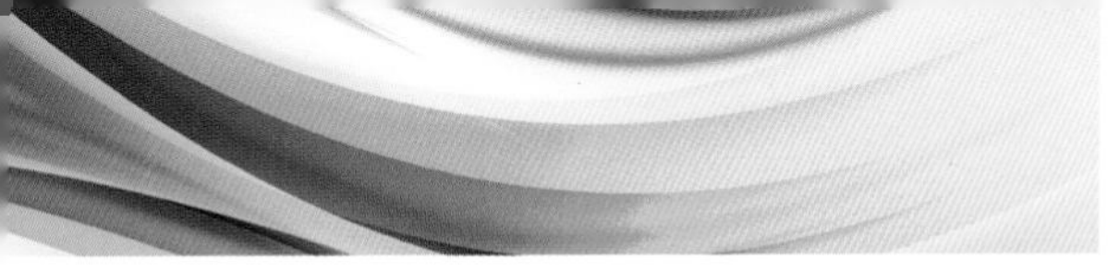

Reviewers

Dorothy Chen-Maynard, PhD, RDN, FAND
DPD Director
Department of Health Science and Human Ecology
CSU San Bernardino
San Bernardino, California

Jill Comess, MS, RD
Food Science & Nutrition Program Director, Instructor
Department of Nursing and Allied Health
Norfolk State University
Norfolk, Virginia

Matthew Durant, PhD, MEd, PDt, CDE, FDC
Associate Professor
School of Nutrition and Dietetics
Acadia University
Wolfville, Nova Scotia

Elizabeth Z. Emery, MS, RD, CNSC, LDN
Director and Assistant Professor
Coordinated Program in Dietetics
Department of Urban Public Health and Nutrition
La Salle University
Philadelphia, Pennsylvania

Rubina Haque, PhD, RD
Associate Professor
Department of Nutrition and Dietetics
Eastern Michigan University
Ypsilanti, Michigan

Joyce T. Price, MS, RDN, LDN
Faculty Preceptor, Dietetic Internship
Department of Human Sciences
North Carolina Central University
Durham, North Carolina

Alessandra Sarcona, EdD, RD
Assistant Professor
Department of Nutrition
West Chester University
West Chester, Pennsylvania

Louise E. Schneider, DrPH, RD
Associate Professor
Department of Nutrition and Dietetics
Loma Linda University
Loma Linda, California

Emily Shupe, PhD, RD, LDN
Assistant Professor
Dietetics, Fashion Merchandising, and Hospitality
Western Illinois University
Macomb, Illinois

Preface

The Essential Pocket Guide for Clinical Nutrition is a concise pocket-sized reference that health care professionals can tailor to their own practice. As practitioners, we both had our own pocket clinical books—homemade productions consisting of small tabbed binders stuffed with snippets of information that we collected on an ongoing basis. Initially, we couldn't find the ideal guide to meet all the needs of dietitians and other health care practitioners engaged in clinical nutrition, which inspired us to develop this book for our students to use. And in this digital age, we still see that even the most technologically savvy practitioners cram their lab coat pockets with notes they can pull out in seconds. In this edition, we struggled to update the information with the latest research, add new content areas and sections, and yet keep the book pocket-sized. We believe we've achieved our goal, and we hope that you do, too. The following is a list of features we kept from the first edition and new features:

- The compact size fits into any lab coat pocket.
- The colored tabs enable quick, easy searching of contents.
- The latest research is incorporated into all chapters, and so the busy clinician doesn't have to spend valuable time searching textbooks or the Internet for the most updated information.
- Blank pages in each chapter allow the clinicians to customize their book by adding their own resources and references. Writing in a formula, cutting and pasting an article, or stapling a hospital formulary card can be done with ease.
- Use of the Nutrition Assessment-Diagnosis-Intervention-Monitoring and Evaluation (ADIME) format for quick

synopses of all major nutritionally relevant diseases, including sample nutrition diagnosis statements in Problem-Etiology-Signs and Symptoms (PES) format.
- Addition of new chapters and sections, including Bariatric Surgery, Intestinal Transplant, Nutrition-Focused Physical Exam, Herbs and Dietary Supplements, Essential Minerals, and tables for Dietary Reference Intakes.

The audience for this book is health professionals, students, and interns from all disciplines who are interested in and actively engaged in clinical nutrition, and working in hospitals, nursing homes, and clinics. However, we also believe that the book will be a handy resource for practitioners in a wide range of venues, including community programs, nutrition education, and wellness programs, who need a quick reference for nutrition screening and assessment. Part I contains chapters covering nutritional assessment, life stage assessment, and nutrition support. Part II includes chapters on the major nutritionally relevant diseases. The book includes appendices on food and drug interactions, laboratory assessment, herbs and dietary supplements, and a miscellaneous appendix of useful reference materials, such as conversion tables, and food sources of vitamins and minerals.

This book could not have been developed without the help of our expert contributors, and we thank them for their hard work and valuable contributions to the book. In addition, we thank all the countless colleagues and preceptors who offered constant encouragement and excellent suggestions during the writing process.

Mary Width, MS, RD
Tonia Reinhard, MS, RD, FAND

Contents

PART 1

Nutrition Assessment and Support

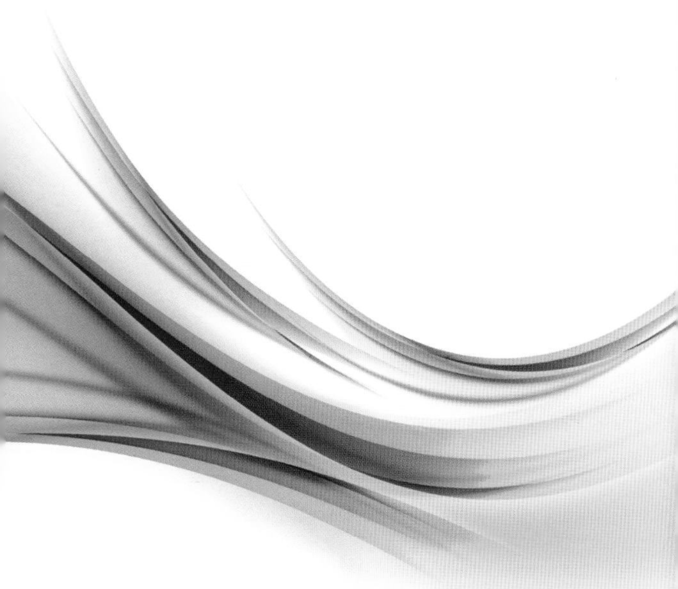

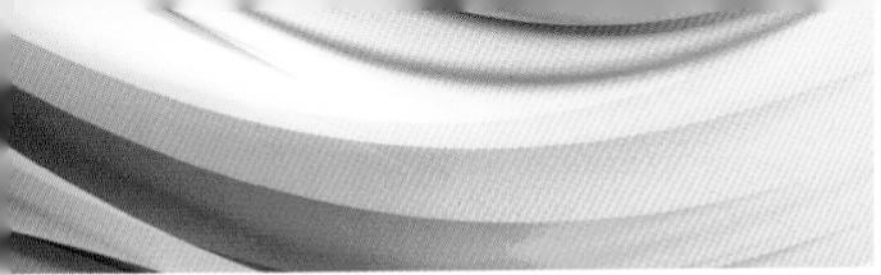

CHAPTER 1

Nutrition Assessment

THE NUTRITION CARE PROCESS

The Nutrition Care Process (NCP), developed by the Academy of Nutrition and Dietetics (the Academy), is a systematic approach to providing high-quality nutrition care, that provides dietetic professionals with a framework for critical thinking, problem-solving, and decision-making to address nutrition-related problems.[1] The NCP was designed to improve the consistency and quality of nutrition care and the predictability of nutrition care outcomes. Dietetic professionals, including registered dietitians (RD) and registered dietitian nutritionists (RDN), use the NCP in diverse venues to provide nutrition services and document the process.

The NCP consists of four steps: nutrition Assessment, nutrition Diagnosis, nutrition Intervention, and nutrition Monitoring and Evaluation. The NCP culminates in documentation of the process, often referred to as being in the ADIME format. A new feature added to this book is a highlight box called "ADIME At-A-Glance," which includes common aspects of each NCP step for a specific condition or disease state.

Nutrition assessment of the patient, client, or resident is the first step in effective nutrition care to identify and diagnose nutrition risks and plan appropriate interventions. It consists of a comprehensive assessment of nutrition status and includes five assessment domains. The following are examples of data collected within each domain, but are not all-inclusive:

1. Anthropometric measurements: Height, weight, body mass index (BMI), weight history, growth pattern indices/percentile ranks, and body measures, including fat, muscle, and bone components and growth
2. Biochemical data, medical tests, and procedures
3. Nutrition-focused physical findings: Findings from a nutrition-focused physical examination (NFPE), interview, or the health record including muscle and subcutaneous fat, oral health, suck/swallow/breathe ability, appetite, and affect
4. Client history: Personal, medical and health (patient/client/family), and social histories
5. Food/Nutrition-related history: Including food and nutrient intake, diet history, medication and complementary/alternative medicine, food and nutrition knowledge, beliefs and behaviors, physical activity and exercise, and food availability

Nutrition diagnosis is the second step in the NCP. After assessment, the patient's nutrition-related problems and needs are determined, which form the nutrition diagnosis. The nutrition diagnosis, in turn, is expressed and documented in a specific format: Problem, etiology, and signs and symptoms (PES). Boxes 1.1 and 1.2 illustrate and provide an example for the PES format.

BOX 1.1 Nutrition Diagnosis: Problem/Etiology/Signs

The problem (P) describes alterations in patient nutritional status:
- A diagnostic label (qualifier) is an adjective that describes the physiologic response (e.g., altered, impaired, risk of)

The etiology (E) refers to cause(s) or contributor(s) to the problem:
- It is linked to the problem by the term "related to" (RT)

The signs/symptoms (S) are clusters of subjective and objective factors that provide evidence that a problem exists:
- They also quantify the problem and describe severity
- Linked to (E) by the term "as evidenced by" (AEB)

BOX 1.2 Writing the Nutrition Diagnosis (ND) Statement

Example for the ND Statement Format

(P)roblem/**(E)**tiology/**(S)**igns/symptoms:

Excessive energy intake **(P)** related to frequent consumption of large portions of high-fat meals **(E)**, as evidenced by:

1. Daily caloric intake exceeding DRI by 500 kcal **(S)**
2. 12 lb weight gain during past 18 months **(S)**

DRI, Daily recommended intake.

The nutrition diagnostic terms are classified according to the following three domains and subclasses:

1. Intake: Caloric energy balance, oral or nutrition support intake, fluid intake, bioactive substances intake, nutrient intake
2. Clinical: Functional, biochemical, weight, malnutrition disorders
3. Behavioral/environmental: Knowledge and beliefs, physical activity and function, food safety and access

Nutrition intervention is the third step in the NCP. The interventions are planned to positively change a nutrition-related behavior, environmental condition, or aspect of health status for the patient/client. The interventions should address the problems identified in the nutrition assessment that have been formulated into the nutrition diagnosis. The intervention is almost always aimed at the etiology of the nutrition diagnosis/problem identified in the PES statement. Less frequently, the nutrition intervention is directed at the signs and symptoms to minimize their impact.[1] The intervention step includes two interrelated components: planning and implementation. Planning involves prioritization of the nutrition diagnoses as to each problem's severity or importance, and the use of evidence-based interventions and practice guidelines to establish patient-focused expected outcomes for each nutrition diagnosis. Implementation of the nutrition intervention is the action phase that includes carrying out and communicating the plan of care to the patient/client, caregivers, and other members of the health care team; continuing data collection; and revising the nutrition intervention strategy, based on the patient/client response. The nutrition intervention terminology is organized into four domains:

1. Food and/or nutrient delivery
2. Nutrition education
3. Nutrition counseling
4. Coordination of nutrition care by a nutrition professional

The final step in the NCP is monitoring and evaluation. This is a critical component of the NCP because it identifies important measures of patient/client outcomes relevant to the nutrition diagnosis and intervention, and describes how best to measure and evaluate these outcomes. During this step, the patient's status is re-examined by gathering new data (monitoring) and assessing to see how it compares with

ADIME 1.1 ADIME At-A-Glance: Nutrition Diagnoses for Malnutrition

- **Severe: Chronic Illness or Condition**
- Chronic Disease/Condition-Related Malnutrition (may have severe protein-calorie malnutrition) RT increased energy expenditure because of catabolic illness AEB estimated energy intake ≤75% over 2 months, severe pectoralis and deltoid muscle loss (shoulder square in appearance), malignancies
- **Severe: Acute Illness or Injury**
- Acute Disease/Condition-Related Malnutrition (may have severe protein-calorie malnutrition) RT alteration in gastrointestinal tract structure AEB weight loss of >5% in 1 month, severe quadriceps wasting (severe depression of muscle on thigh, prominent femur bone), major gastrointestinal surgery
- **Severe: Social or Environmental (Starvation-Related)**
- Starvation-Related Malnutrition (may have severe protein-calorie malnutrition) RT disordered eating pattern AEB intake of ≤50% of estimated energy needs for ≥1 month, severe deltoid muscle loss (prominent acromion protrusion), anorexia nervosa

previous status, expected outcomes, and established standards (evaluation). This fourth step helps to determine whether the patient/client is meeting the nutrition intervention goals or desired outcomes. The domains and terminologies used in monitoring/evaluation are the same as those used in nutrition assessment, except for client history (there is no client history domain in this step because there are no nutrition care outcomes associated with client history).

ANTHROPOMETRIC ASSESSMENT

There are several anthropometric measurements that are useful in the clinical setting. Measurements of body weight, height, and composition can be used by the clinician when evaluating nutritional status.

Estimating Height

An estimation of height is necessary for patients who are confined to bed or a wheelchair, have curvature of the spine or contractures, or are otherwise unable to stand for an actual height measurement.[2]

Demi-span

- This measurement is particularly useful in the clinical setting because it requires no special equipment. It is also helpful to use with patients who have lower limb dysfunction.
- Using the left arm, if possible, measure the distance from the tip of the middle finger to the middle of the sternal notch.
- Make sure the patient's arm is horizontal and in line with the shoulders.
- Height (in cm) is calculated using the following formulas:

Females: Height in cm = (1.35 × demi-span in cm) + 60.1

Males: Height in cm = (1.40 × demi-span in cm) + 57.8

Knee Height

- Knee height is measured using a sliding broad-blade caliper (available commercially at http://www.weighandmeasure.com/).
- Patient should be in the supine position, and the left leg is preferable for measurement.
- With both the knee and ankle at 90-degree angles, place one blade of the caliper under the heel of the foot and the other on the anterior surface of the thigh.
- The shaft of the caliper is held parallel to the long axis of the lower leg, and pressure is applied to compress the tissue.
- Height (in cm) is calculated using the following formulas:

$$\text{Females: Height in cm} = 84.88 - (0.24 \times \text{age in years}) + (1.83 \times \text{knee height in cm})$$

$$\text{Males: Height in cm} = 64.19 - (0.04 \times \text{age in years}) + (2.02 \times \text{knee height in cm})$$

Evaluating Body Weight

Ideal Body Weight

Body weight relative to height is a frequently used measurement to determine risk of morbidity and mortality.[3] Although there is limited published research on their validity, many ideal body weight (IBW) equations and height/weight tables are used to assess an individual's nutrition status by comparing actual body weight with IBW standards in various settings. One common method frequently used in the United States is the Hamwi method, shown below:

Females: IBW = 100 lb for 5 ft + 5 lb for each inch >60 in

Males: IBW = 106 lb for 5 ft + 6 lb for each inch >60 in

For light- or small-framed individuals, the IBW, using this method, can be reduced by 10%, and for heavy- or large-framed individuals, the IBW can be increased by 10%. See the following sections for determining frame size.

TABLE 1.1. Estimating Frame Size Using Wrist Circumference

Female Wrist Measurements

	Height <5′2″	Height 5′2″–5′5″	Height >5′5″
Small	<5.5″	<6.0″	<6.25″
Medium	5.5″–5.75″	6.0″–6.25″	6.25″–6.5″
Large	>5.75″	>6.25″	>6.5″

Male Wrist Measurements

	Height >5′5″
Small	5.5″–6.5″
Medium	6.5″–7.5″
Large	>7.5″

Data from U.S. National Library of Medicine (NLM). Calculating body frame size. Available at: http://www.nlm.nih.gov/medlineplus/ency/imagepages/17182.htm. Accessed December 10, 2015.

Frame Size Adjustment

To adjust for differences in body build (muscularity, bone thickness, and body proportions), it is necessary to determine an individual's frame size when calculating IBW.[4] Frame size can be estimated by two methods. Measuring wrist circumference is easy and straightforward. Measuring elbow breadth is more complex, but tends to provide a more accurate estimate of frame size. Both methods use the measurements in relation to the patient's height.

Wrist Circumference

- Measure the wrist circumference just distal to the styloid process at the wrist crease of the left hand, in inches, using a tape measure. Compare the measurement with the values in Table 1.1.

Elbow Breadth

- Subject should stand, if possible, and extend the arm forward so that it is horizontal and parallel to the ground.
- Turn palm so that it is facing up, and bend elbow so that the forearm is at a 90-degree angle to the ground.
- Measure the distance between the two prominent bones on either side of the elbow (the epicondyles of the humerus). This measurement can be taken with a ruler or tape measure, but using commercially available calipers is preferable.
- Compare the measurement with the values in Table 1.2.

Amputation Adjustment

For patients with amputations, estimation of IBW should be adjusted with the following equation using the factors in Table 1.3.

$$\frac{100 - \%\ \text{amputation}}{100} \times \text{IBW for original height}$$

Spinal Cord Injury Adjustment

For patients with spinal cord injuries, estimation of IBW should be adjusted as follows:

- Paraplegia: Subtract 5% to 10% from IBW
- Quadriplegia: Subtract 10% to 15% from IBW

Interpretation of Body Weight Data

Percentage of Ideal Body Weight

$$\%\ \text{IBW} = \frac{\text{current body weight (CBW)}}{\text{IBW}} \times 100$$

Percentage of Usual Body Weight (UBW)

$$\%\ \text{usual body weight (UBW)} = \frac{\text{CBW}}{\text{UBW}} \times 100$$

Table 1.4 shows how to evaluate % IBW and % UBW data.

Percentage of Weight Change. This calculation is useful in assessing variations from the patient's usual weight, especially

TABLE 1.2. Estimating Frame Size Using Elbow Breadth

Female Elbow Measurements

Medium Frame

If elbow breadth is less than those in the table for a specific height, subject is small framed, and if elbow breadth is greater, subject is large framed.

Height	*Elbow Breadth*
4′10″–4′11″	2 1/4″–2 1/2″
5′0″–5′3″	2 1/4″–2 1/2″
5′4″–5′7″	2 3/8″–2 5/8″
5′8″–5′11″	2 3/8″–2 5/8″
6′0″–6′4″	2 1/2″–2 3/4″

Male Elbow Measurements

Medium Frame

If elbow breadth is less than those in the table for a specific height, subject is small framed, and if elbow breadth is greater, subject is large framed.

Height	*Elbow Breadth*
5′2″–5′3″	2 1/2″–2 7/8″
5′4″–5′7″	2 5/8″–2 7/8″
5′8″–5′11″	2 3/4″–3″
6′0″–6′3″	2 3/4″–3 1/8″
6′4″–6′7″	2 7/8″–3 1/4″

Data from Zeman FJ, Ney DM. *Applications in Medical Nutrition Therapy*. 2nd ed. Upper Saddle River, NJ: Merrill-Prentice Hall; 1996.

in the elderly population where unintentional weight loss is associated with increased morbidity and mortality.[5,6] Once percentage of weight change has been calculated, use Table 1.5 to assess the significance of any weight changes.

$$\%\text{ Weight Change} = \frac{\text{UBW} - \text{CBW}}{\text{UBW}} \times 100$$

TABLE 1.3. Amputation Adjustments for Estimating Ideal Body Weight

Percentage Body Weight Contributed by Body Part	
Hand	0.7%
Forearm and hand (below elbow)	2.3%
Entire arm	5.0%
Foot	1.5%
Lower leg and foot (below knee)	5.9%
Entire leg	16.0%

Data from Osterkamp LK. Current perspective on assessment of human body proportions of relevance to amputees. *J Am Diet Assoc* 1995;95:215–218.

TABLE 1.4. Interpreting % IBW and % UBW

% IBW	% UBW	Nutritional Risk
>120	—	Obesity
110–120	—	Overweight
90–109	—	Not at risk
80–89	85–95	Mild
70–79	75–84	Moderate
<70	<75	Severe

Assessment of Overweight and Obesity

Body Mass Index

BMI, or Quetelet's index, is a direct calculation based on height and weight, regardless of gender, and can be used to assess the severity of obesity. BMI does have limitations, and factors such as age, sex, ethnicity, and muscle mass can

TABLE 1.5. Interpreting Unintentional Weight Changes

Time Frame	Significant Weight Loss	Severe Weight Loss
1 wk	1%–2%	>2%
1 mo	5%	>5%
3 mo	7.5%	>7.5%
6 mo	10%	>10%

Data from Academy of Nutrition and Dietetics. Nutrition Care Manual. Available at: https://www.nutritioncaremanual.org. Accessed December 16, 2015.

influence the relationship between BMI and body fat. In addition, the presence of edema should be considered when interpreting BMI results.[7] See Table 1.6 for classifications of overweight and obesity based on BMI.

$$\text{BMI} = \frac{\text{weight (kg)}}{\text{height (m}^2\text{)}} \quad \text{or} \quad \text{BMI} = \frac{\text{weight (lb)}}{\text{height (in}^2\text{)}} \times 703$$

Waist Circumference and Waist-to-Hip Ratio

The presence of excess fat in the abdomen, out of proportion to total body fat, is an independent predictor of risk factors and morbidity.[7] Two methods for measuring abdominal fat are waist circumference and the waist-to-hip ratio (WHR). Both methods have been used to show increased risk for diabetes, coronary artery disease, and hypertension for those individuals with excess abdominal fat. Some studies suggest that waist circumference is a better predictor of disease risk than WHR, whereas other studies suggest that WHR is the stronger indicator.[7,8] Regardless of which method the clinician uses, measuring abdominal fat can help identify risk level for several chronic diseases (Tables 1.6 and 1.7).

TABLE 1.6. Classification of Overweight and Obesity by BMI, Waist Circumference, and Associated Disease Risk

BMI (kg/m^2)	Weight Status	Obesity Class	Disease Risk[a] Relative to Normal Weight and Waist Circumference	
			Men ≤40" Women ≤35"	**Men >40" Women >35"**
<18.5	Underweight		—	—
18.5–24.9	Normal		—	—
25.0–29.9	Overweight		Increased	High
30.0–34.9	Obesity	I	High	Very high
35.0–39.9	Obesity	II	Very high	Very high
>40.0	Extreme obesity	III	Extremely high	Extremely high

[a]Disease risk for type 2 diabetes, hypertension, and cardiovascular disease.

Data from (i) National Institutes of Health Clinical Guidelines on the identification, evaluation, and treatment of overweight and obesity in adults: The Evidence Report. 1998. Available at: http://www.ncbi.nlm.nih.gov/books/bv.fcgi?rid=obesity. Accessed December 10, 2015, and (ii) Centers for Disease Control and Prevention, Division of Nutrition, Physical Activity, and Obesity. Available at: http://www.cdc.gov/healthyweight/assessing/bmi/adult_bmi/. Accessed December 10, 2015.

TABLE 1.7. Waist-to-Hip Ratio

Male	Female	Health Risk
≤0.95	≤0.80	Low risk
0.96–1.0	0.81–0.85	Moderate risk
≥1.0	≥0.85	High risk

Data from Yusuf S, Hawken S, Ounpuu S, et al. Obesity and the risk of myocardial infarction in 27,000 participants from 52 countries: A case-control study. *Lancet* 2005;366:1640–1650.

ESTIMATING NUTRIENT REQUIREMENTS

Energy Requirements—Noncritical care

Many prediction equations and formulas are available for estimating resting metabolic rate (RMR). The Mifflin–St. Jeor and Harris–Benedict equations are two widely used formulas for estimating energy expenditure in the noncritically ill population. According to the Academy's Evidence Analysis Library (EAL), the Mifflin–St. Jeor equation (MSJE) performed better than the Harris–Benedict equation when predicting RMR in both nonobese and obese, noncritically ill populations.[9] Once RMR has been calculated, the total energy expenditure (TEE) would need to be estimated using a combination of activity and stress factors. Stress factors are used for hospitalized patients in a hypermetabolic state owing to disease, infection, or trauma. The clinician's judgment should be used to determine the appropriate activity and/or stress factor to estimate TEE. See Table 1.8 for activity and stress factors.

Mifflin–St. Jeor Equation

$$\text{Females: REE} = 10W + 6.25H - 5A - 161$$

$$\text{Males: REE} = 10W + 6.25H - 5A + 5$$

where, *REE, resting energy expenditure; W, actual weight in kilograms; H, height in centimeters; A, age in years.*

Harris–Benedict Equation

$$\text{Females: BEE} = 655.1 + 9.6W + 1.9H - 4.7A$$

$$\text{Males: BEE} = 66.5 + 13.8W + 5.0H - 6.8A$$

where, *W, weight in kilograms (use of actual vs. ideal vs. adjusted body weight is determined by the clinician*); H, height in centimeters; A, age in years.*

*The EAL does report that the Harris–Benedict equation was most accurate when used with actual body weight.[10]

TABLE 1.8. Activity and Stress Factors for Determining Total Energy Expenditure

Condition	Factor
Activity Factors	
Confined to bed	1.2
Ambulatory	1.3
Stress Factors	
Burns	
≤20% BSA	1.5
20%–40% BSA	1.8
>40% BSA (use max. of 60% TBSA)	1.8–2.0
Infection	
Mild	1.2
Moderate	1.4
Severe	1.8
Starvation	0.85
Surgery	
Minor	1.1
Major	1.2
Trauma	
Skeletal	1.2
Blunt	1.35
Closed head injury	1.4

TBSA, total body surface area.

Kilocalories per Kilogram

A fast and easy method for estimating energy needs is using kilocalories per kilogram of body weight, with the reference weight as actual or IBW, based on the clinician's judgment (Table 1.9).

Energy Requirements—Critical Care

The Academy's EAL recommends that if indirect calorimetry is not available to determine energy requirements

TABLE 1.9. Energy Requirements Based on Kilocalories per Kilogram of Body Weight

Condition	Energy Requirement (kcal/kg)
Normal	25–30
Obese, critically ill (BMI >30)	11–14 (actual body weight) or 22–25 (ideal body weight)
Stress	
Mild	30–35
Moderate to severe	35–45

Data from (i) Escott-Stump S. *Nutrition and Diagnosis-Related Care*. 8th ed. Philadelphia, PA: Wolters Kluwer; 2015, and (ii) McClave SA, Martindale RG, Vanek VW, et al. Guidelines for the provision and assessment of nutrition support therapy in the adult critically ill patient: Society of Critical Care Medicine and American Society for Parenteral and Enteral Nutrition (A.S.P.E.N.). *JPEN J Parenter Enteral Nutr* 2009;33:277–316.

for critically ill patients, then the Penn State University equations have the best prediction accuracy.[11] For *nonobese*, ventilator-dependent, critically ill patients, and for *obese*, ventilator-dependent, critically ill patients <60 years of age, the EAL recommends using the Penn State equation [PSU(2003b)]. For *obese*, ventilator-dependent, critically ill patients >60 years of age, the Modified Penn State equation [PSU(2010)] has better accuracy.

Penn State Equation [PSU(2003b)]

(Use with nonobese and with obese <60 years of age)

$$\text{RMR} = \text{Mifflin}\ (0.96) + V_E\,(31) + T_{max}\,(167) - 6{,}212$$

Modified Penn State Equation [PSU(2010)]

(Use with obese >60 years of age)

$$\text{RMR} = \text{Mifflin}\ (0.71) + V_E\,(64) + T_{max}\,(85) - 3{,}085$$

where, V_E, *expired minute ventilation; Tmax, maximum body temperature in previous 24 hours in degree Celsius.*

Determining energy requirements for non–ventilator-dependent, critically ill patients is dependent on protocol at each facility and clinician judgment. One method in use is the MSJE modified by a factor of 1.25, although accuracy rates for this equation are only around 50%.[11]

$$\text{RMR} = \text{MSJE} \times 1.25$$

Recommendations by the American Society for Parenteral and Enteral Nutrition (ASPEN) and the Society for Critical Care Medicine (SCCM) for kcal/kg energy requirements for the obese, critically ill patient can be found in Table 1.9.

Protein Requirements

Table 1.10 contains protein recommendations for patients with several general conditions. Disease-specific protein requirements can be found in the respective chapters.

Fluid Requirements

Methods for estimating fluid requirements for the normal person are typically based on kilocalorie intake, body weight, or body surface area (BSA). The caloric intake method uses 1 mL/kcal for adults and 1.5 mL/kg for infants. The BSA method uses 1,500 mL/m^2/day × BSA (see Table 3.7 for calculating BSA).[6] Table 1.11 shows additional methods for estimating fluid requirements based on body weight. Fluid requirements will also depend on the medical condition of the patient, with additional or restricted fluids required in certain situations. The individual disease chapters may list fluid requirements for specific conditions.

BIOCHEMICAL DATA

The purpose of collecting laboratory data for nutrition assessment is to determine status inside the body. Blood and urine samples can be used to directly measure a nutrient

TABLE 1.10. Daily Protein Requirements for Hospitalized Patients

Condition	Protein Requirement (g/kg)
Normal–maintenance	0.8–1.0
Metabolic stress	
Mild	1.2–1.5
Moderate to severe	1.5–2.0
Obese, critically ill	2.0 (when using hypocaloric feeding)
Pressure ulcers	1.2–1.5 (stage 1, 2) 1.5–2.0 (stage 3, 4)
Protein repletion	1.2–2.0
Severe trauma, burns	1.5–2.0

Data from (i) Escott-Stump S. *Nutrition and Diagnosis-Related Care*. 8th ed. Philadelphia, PA: Wolters Kluwer; 2015, (ii) McClave SA, Martindale RG, Vanek VW, et al. Guidelines for the provision and assessment of nutrition support therapy in the adult critically ill patient: Society of Critical Care Medicine and American Society for Parenteral and Enteral Nutrition (A.S.P.E.N.). *JPEN J Parenter Enteral Nutr* 2009;33:277–316, and (iii) National Pressure Ulcer Advisory Panel, European Pressure Ulcer Advisory Panel and Pan Pacific Pressure Injury Alliance. Prevention and Treatment of Pressure Ulcers: Clinical Practice Guideline. In: Haesler E, ed. Osborne Park, WA: Cambridge Media; 2014.

or metabolite that is affected by the nutrient. Each test is associated with a distinctive sensitivity and specificity. Sensitivity indicates the degree to which the assay for a particular constituent is accurate in determining the amount of that constituent in a sample. Specificity refers to how specific the test is in reflecting a particular function or diagnosis, for example, how specific blood urea nitrogen is for assessing renal function.

Basic concepts in the interpretation of laboratory data include the following: No single test is diagnostic on its own; repeated draws are more valid; there can be diurnal variation for some tests; and some constituents can be affected by other superimposed conditions, diseases, and medications.

TABLE 1.11. Estimating Fluid Requirements Based on Body Weight

Method 1 (Adults)	
Body Weight	**Fluid Requirement**
Average adult: 18–54 years	30–35 mL/kg
Older: 55–65 years	30 mL/kg
Elderly: >65 years	25 mL/kg
Method 2 (Commonly Used in Pediatric Populations)	
Body Weight	**Fluid Requirement**
1–10 kg	100 mL/kg
11–20 kg	1,000 mL + 50 mL/kg each kg >10 kg
>20 kg	1,500 mL + 20 mL/kg each kg >20 kg

Data from Academy of Nutrition and Dietetics. Nutrition Care Manual. Available at: https://www.nutritioncaremanual.org. Accessed December 16, 2015.

Protein Status

Protein status, both visceral protein and somatic protein compartments, were historically an important aspect of nutrition assessment in various settings, including acute care. The three major hepatic proteins used to assess visceral protein are albumin, transferrin, and prealbumin (Table 1.12). However, these hepatic proteins also reflect the physiologic response to injury, stress, infection, surgery, and trauma.[6] They are negative acute-phase proteins, in that their levels decrease during the physiologic response to stress when the liver reprioritizes protein synthesis from visceral proteins to acute-phase reactant proteins. Systemic inflammation, a hallmark of the stress response, not only reduces albumin synthesis, but can also increase its degradation and promote transcapillary leakage of albumin.[12] In light of this, markers of protein status, such as albumin and prealbumin, have little value in assessment or monitoring of nutritional status in the acute care setting. Instead, they can be used in conjunction

TABLE 1.12. Visceral Protein Parameters

Protein	Normal Range	Implications and Considerations
Albumin	3.5–5.0 g/dL	Low when visceral protein is depleted; 17–20 d; low in liver disease, malabsorption syndromes, protein-losing nephropathies, ascites, burns, overhydration, inflammation; elevated in dehydration
Fibronectin	220–400 mg/dL	Low when visceral protein is depleted; half-life 15 hr; low in inflammation, injury; affected by coagulation factors
Prealbumin	15–36 mg/dL	Low when visceral protein is depleted; half-life 1.9 d; low in liver disease, burns, inflammation; elevated in nephrotic syndrome, chronic kidney disease, pregnancy, Hodgkin lymphoma
Retinol-binding protein	3–6 mg/dL	Low when visceral protein is depleted; half-life 12 hr; low in chronic pancreatitis or carcinoma, cystic fibrosis, intestinal malabsorption, chronic liver diseases, vitamin A deficiency; elevated in renal failure
Transferrin	188–341 mg/dL	Low when visceral protein is depleted (only if iron status is normal); half-life 8–10 d; low in chronic infection, malignancy; elevated in late pregnancy, use of oral contraceptives, viral hepatitis

Data from Pagana KD. *Mosby's Manual of Diagnostic and Laboratory Tests*. 5th ed. St. Louis, MO: Elsevier: Mosby; 2014.

with positive acute-phase protein lab values, such as C-reactive protein (CRP), to identify patients who might be at nutritional risk because of acute or chronic health conditions that contribute to inflammation. In addition, hypoalbuminemia has been studied extensively among subsets of patients, such as those with burns, pressure ulcers, severe sepsis, cancer, renal disease, and surgical patients, as an important predictor of morbidity and mortality.[13–16] The use of multifactorial prognostic indices may be useful in some situations to predict nutrition risk (see Table 1.13).

Total lymphocyte count (TLC) reflects visceral protein status; although because of its association with immune system function, it will not be accurate in some circumstances (Table 1.14).

Another parameter for assessment of visceral protein status is nitrogen balance, although it more properly reflects total body protein (Table 1.15). Adults are normally in nitrogen balance, in that dietary protein (source of nitrogen) is used for protein synthesis. When protein degradation exceeds synthesis, a person is in negative nitrogen balance, which occurs in malnutrition. Children and pregnant women are in positive nitrogen balance, because protein synthesis exceeds degradation during phases of growth.

The somatic protein compartment is assessed using both anthropometric and biochemical measurements, the latter through the use of creatinine excretion and nitrogen balance. Creatinine is a catabolic product of creatine phosphate, a compound needed in muscular contraction. It is excreted at a constant daily rate proportional to muscle mass. Kidney disorders and high intake of meat products can raise levels. Table 1.16 provides the formula for calculating creatinine height index and standards for comparison to determine protein depletion severity.

Biochemical assessment also includes review of hematologic parameters, as they may be indicators of nutritionally related anemia (Table 1.17). Several of these parameters can also be expected to be affected by compromised visceral protein status.

TABLE 1.13. Formulas for Assessment of Nutrition Risk

Risk Assessment	Formula	Interpretation
Nutrition Risk Index	(1.519 × albumin) + (41.7 × % IBW)	>100, no risk 97.5–100, mild risk 83.5–97.5, moderate risk <83.5, severe risk
Prognostic Nutrition Index	158 – 16.6 (albumin) – 0.78 (triceps skin fold in mm) – 0.2 (transferrin) – 5.8 (delayed skin hypersensitivity)	<40, normal ≥40, compromised
Prognostic Inflammatory and Nutritional Index	$\frac{\text{C-reactive protein} \times \text{alpha 1-acid-glycoprotein}}{\text{prealbumin} \times \text{albumin}}$	≤1, no risk 1–10, low risk 11–20, moderate risk 21–30, severe risk

TABLE 1.14. Total Lymphocyte Count and Visceral Protein Status

Formula: TLC = % of lymphocytes × No. of WBCs (10^3)	
Interpretation (Values in cells/mL^3)	
Normal:	>1,500
Mild degree of depletion:	1,200–1,500
Moderate degree of depletion:	800–1,199
Severe degree of depletion:	<800
Affected by:	
Injury, viral infection, radiation therapy, surgery, chemotherapy, and other immunosuppressive medications.	

Note: TLC may not be reliable indicator of malnutrition in the elderly.
WBCs, white blood cells.
Data from (i) Academy of Nutrition and Dietetics. Nutrition Care Manual. Available at: https://www.nutritioncaremanual.org. Accessed December 16, 2015, and (ii) Pagana KD. *Mosby's Manual of Diagnostic and Laboratory Tests*. 5th ed. St. Louis, MO: Elsevier: Mosby; 2014.

TABLE 1.15. The Use of Nitrogen Balance in Assessment of Total Body Protein

1. Monitor dietary intake of protein (PRO) for 24 hr
2. Convert dietary protein intake to nitrogen intake:

$$\text{Nitrogen} = \frac{\text{PRO intake}}{6.25 \text{ g nitrogen}}$$

3. Collect 24-hr urine; obtain urinary urea nitrogen (UUN)
4. Nitrogen Balance = nitrogen intake – (UUN + 3[a])
5. Interpretation: Adults are normally in nitrogen balance (0); pregnant women and children (growth states) are in positive balance; negative balance may suggest malnutrition.

[a]Insensible losses.

TABLE 1.16. Calculation and Interpretation of Creatinine Height Index

24-Hour Urine Collection; Meat-Free Diet (Ideally); Compare Creatinine with Standard for Height/Gender

$$\%\ \text{CHI} = \frac{24°\text{urinary creatinine} \times 100}{\text{expected 24-hr urinary excretion (mg)}}$$

Interpret: 60%–80%, mild depletion
40%–59%, moderate depletion
<40%, severe depletion

Affected by: Renal dysfunction, advanced age, stress, trauma, sepsis, strenuous exercise, use of corticosteroids

24-Hour Urinary Creatinine Excretion in Adults

Males: 23 mg/kg/IBW		Females: 18 mg/kg/IBW	
Height (cm)	Creatinine (mg)	Height (cm)	Creatinine (mg)
157.5	1,288	147.3	830
160.0	1,325	149.9	851
162.6	1,359	152.4	875
165.1	1,386	154.9	900
167.6	1,426	157.5	925
170.2	1,467	160.0	949
172.7	1,513	162.6	977
175.3	1,555	165.1	1,006
177.8	1,596	167.6	1,044
180.3	1,642	170.2	1,076
182.9	1,691	172.7	1,109
185.4	1,739	175.3	1,141
188.0	1,785	177.8	1,174
190.5	1,831	180.3	1,206
193.0	1,891	182.9	1,240

CHI, creatine height index.

Data from Blackburn GL, Bistrain BR, Maini BS, et al. Nutritional and metabolic assessment of the hospitalized patient. *JPEN J Parenter Enteral Nutr* 1977;1:11–12.

TABLE 1.17. Hematologic Parameters Related to Anemia

Constituent	Normal Range	Implications and Considerations
Erythrocyte protoporphyrin	<5 μg/dL RBCs	High in later stages of iron-deficiency anemia
Ferritin	Males: 18.0–350 ng/mL Females: 15–49 years: 12.0–156 ng/mL >49 years: 18.0–204 ng/mL	Low in early deficiency state in the presence of depleted iron stores
Folate, RBC content	95 ng/mL	Low in later stages of folate-deficiency anemia
Folate, serum	1.9 ng/mL	Low as folate-deficiency progresses
Hematocrit	Males: 41%–50% Females: 35%–46%	Low in anemia; represents percentage of RBCs in total blood volume
Hemoglobin	Males: 14.0–17.2 g/dL Females: 12.0–15.6 g/dL	Low in anemia; represents total amount of hemoglobin in RBCs
Mean corpuscular hemoglobin concentration	32–36 g/dL	Low in iron-deficiency anemia (hypochromic); normal in B_{12} and folate deficiency (normochromic); represents hemoglobin (pigmentation) contained in an average RBC
RBC count	Male: 4.4–5.8 × 10^6 μL Female: 3.9–5.2 × 10^6 μL	Low in anemia; the number of RBCs in sample

TABLE 1.17. Hematologic Parameters Related to Anemia (*continued*)

Constituent	Normal Range	Implications and Considerations
Transferrin	188–341 mg/dL	High in iron-deficiency anemia as transport of iron increases
Vitamin B_{12}	200–800 pg/mL	Low in B_{12} deficiency

RBC, red blood cell.
Data from Pagana KD. *Mosby's Manual of Diagnostic and Laboratory Tests*. 5th ed. St. Louis, MO: Elsevier: Mosby; 2014.

NUTRITION-FOCUSED PHYSICAL EXAMINATION

Physical assessment is a vital part of the nutrition assessment of a patient. The goal is to identify signs and symptoms that may be associated with specific nutrient deficiencies and compromised nutritional status or malnutrition.

In 2010, an etiology-based approach to the diagnosis of adult malnutrition in the clinical setting was developed by an international committee.[17] Adult malnutrition is now described in the context of acute illness or injury, chronic diseases or conditions, and starvation-related malnutrition. Six characteristics were identified as vital in the detection and diagnosis of malnutrition: insufficient energy intake, weight loss, loss of subcutaneous body fat, loss of muscle mass, fluid accumulation that may mask weight loss, and diminished functional status. As no single parameter is definitive for adult malnutrition, two or more of the six characteristics are recommended for diagnosis (Table 1.18).

The NFPE is conducted to help identify malnutrition by determining fat loss, muscle loss, and presence of edema (Table 1.19), as well as to identify possible nutrient deficiencies (Table 1.20).

TABLE 1.18. Determining Adult Malnutrition

Context of Malnutrition	Chronic Illness		Acute Illness or Injury		Social/Environmental Circumstances	
Degree of Malnutrition	Malnutrition of Moderate Degree	Severe Protein-Calorie Malnutrition	Malnutrition of Moderate Degree	Severe Protein-Calorie Malnutrition	Malnutrition of Moderate Degree	Severe Protein-Calorie Malnutrition
Energy intake: Compare recent intake with estimated energy needs and report inadequate intake as a percentage of estimated needs over time.	<75% of estimated energy requirement for ≥1 mo	≤75% of estimated energy requirement for ≥1 mo	<75% of estimated energy requirement for >7 d	≤50% of estimated energy requirement for ≥5 d	<75% of estimated energy requirement for ≥3 mo	≤50% of estimated energy requirement for ≥1 mo
Weight loss: Evaluate weight in light of other clinical findings, including hydration. Report weight change over time as a percentage of weight	5% in 1 mo 7.5% in 3 mo 10% in 6 mo 20% in 12 mo	>5% in 1 mo >7.5% in 3 mo >10% in 6 mo >20% in 12 mo	1%–2% in 1 wk 5% in 1 mo 7.5% in 3 mo	>2% in 1 wk >5% in 1 mo >7.5% in 3 mo	5% in 1 mo 7.5% in 3 mo 10% in 6 mo 20% in 12 mo	>5% in 1 mo >7.5% in 3 mo >10% in 6 mo >20% in 12 mo

Body fat: Loss of subcutaneous fat (orbital, triceps, fat overlying ribs).	Mild depletion	Severe depletion	Mild depletion	Moderate depletion	Mild depletion	Severe depletion
Muscle mass: Loss of muscle (temples, clavicles, shoulders, scapula, thigh, calf).	Mild depletion	Severe depletion	Mild depletion	Moderate depletion	Mild depletion	Severe depletion
Fluid accumulation: General or local fluid accumulation (extremities, ascites, or vulvar/scrotal edema).	Mild	Severe	Mild	Moderate to severe	Mild	Severe
Functional status: Based on standards supplied by manufacturer of dynamometer	Not applicable	Measurably reduced	Not applicable	Not recommended in intensive care setting	Not applicable	Measurably reduced

TABLE 1.19. Nutrition-Focused Physical Examination: Malnutrition Assessment

Fat Area	Normal	Mild to Moderate	Severe
Orbital region—surrounding the eye (fluid retention may mask loss)	Slightly bulged fat pads	Slightly darker circles; somewhat hallow look	Dark circles; hallow look; depression; loose skin
Upper arm region—triceps/biceps	Large space between fingers when pinching	Some depth pinch but not ample; fingers almost touch	Very little space between folds, fingers touch
Thoracic and lumbar region—ribs, lower back, midaxillary line	Chest is full; ribs do not show; slight to no protrusion of the iliac crest	Ribs apparent; depressions between them less pronounced; iliac crest somewhat prominent	Depression between the ribs very apparent; iliac crest very prominent
Muscle Area	**Normal**	**Mild to Moderate**	**Severe**
Temple region—temporalis muscle	Can see/feel well-defined muscle	Slight depression	Hollow; scooping depression
Clavicle and acromion bone region—deltoid muscle	Rounded curves at arm/shoulder/neck	Acromion process may slightly protrude	Shoulder to arm joint looks square; bones prominent; acromion protrusion very prominent
Clavicle bone region—pectoralis major, deltoid,	Not visible in male; visible but not prominent in female	Visible in male; some protrusion in female	Protruding, prominent bone

Scapular bone region—trapezius, supraspinatus, infraspinatus muscles	Bones not prominent; no significant depressions	Mild depression or bone may show slightly	Prominent, visible bones; depressions between ribs/scapula or shoulder/spine
Dorsal hand—interosseous muscle	Muscle bulges could be flat in some well-nourished people	Slightly depressed	Depressed area between thumb–forefinger
Patellar region—quadricep muscle	Muscles protrude; bones not prominent	Knee cap less prominent; more rounded	Bones prominent; little sign of muscle around knee
Anterior thigh region—quadriceps muscles	Well rounded; no depressions	Mild depression on inner thigh	Depression/line on thigh; obviously thin
Posterior calf region—gastrocnemius muscle	Well-developed bulb of muscle	Not well developed	Thin; minimal to no muscle definition
Edema	Normal	Mild to Moderate	Severe
Edema—rule out other causes of edema; patient at dry weight	No sign of fluid accumulation	Mild to moderate pitting; slight swelling of the extremity; indentation subsides quickly (0–30s)	Deep to very deep pitting; depression lasts a short to moderate time (31–60s); extremity looks swollen (3–4+)

Adapted with permission from TouchPoint Support Services. Atlanta, GA. Available at: http://www.iamtouchpoint.com/pages/home.aspx.

TABLE 1.20. Nutrition-Focused Physical Examination: Nutrient Deficiency Assessment

	Observed Conditions		
Body System	Healthy	Abnormal	Implications
Hair	Normal distribution, shiny	Thin, dull, dry, brittle, corkscrew hairs	Chemotherapy, protein or biotin deficit, vitamin C deficiency
Eyes	Bright, clear, pink conjunctiva	Sunken, dull, pale, dry conjunctiva, photophobia, xerosis	Deficiency of: Vitamin A, zinc, riboflavin
Lips	Moist, good color	Swollen, dry, red, cracked	Deficiency of riboflavin, pyridoxine, niacin
Gums	Pink, firm	Sore, spongy, red, swollen, bleed easily	Vitamin C deficiency
Tongue	Pink, presence of papillae	Purple, white or gray coating, smooth, slick	Deficiency of riboflavin, pyridoxine, folic acid, niacin, vitamin B_{12}, iron
Teeth	Clean, intact, all present	Dentures, missing teeth, loss of tooth enamel	Calcium deficiency, poor diet
Neck	No swelling	Presence of nodule(s), goiter	Excess or deficiency of iodine

Skin	Smooth, slightly moist, good color	Pale, dry, scaly, bruises easily, pressure ulcers, dermatitis	Deficiency of iron, vitamins A or C, zinc, essential fatty acid, protein; excess of niacin
Legs	Well-developed, firm musculature, no joint or bone pain	Calf tenderness, flaccid muscles, pain, edema, rickets, bone or joint pain	Deficiency of protein; vitamins A, C, or D; calcium
Abdomen	No swelling or pain	Mildly edematous, diarrhea, ascites	Deficiency of protein, niacin, zinc
Hands/nails	Smooth	Brittle nails, atrophied fine muscles, spoon-shaped nails	Deficiency of protein, iron
Musculoskeletal, adipose	Normal bone, muscle, and fat development	Calf tenderness, loss of subcutaneous fat, emaciated appearance, pain, decreased grip strength, hollow cheeks, fractures, osteoporosis	Deficiency of protein, thiamin, vitamin C; energy or fluid deficit
Neurologic	Normal reflexes	CVA, limited reflexes, disorientation, paralysis, convulsions, dementia	Deficiency of thiamin, niacin, vitamins B_6 or B_{12}, folic acid, iodine, phosphorus, calcium, magnesium

CVA, cerebrovascular accident.

Data from Escott-Stump S. *Nutrition and Diagnosis-Related Care*. 8th ed. Philadelphia, PA: Wolters Kluwer; 2015.

The Subjective Global Assessment (SGA) is another nutrition assessment tool that has been found to be highly predictive of nutrition-associated complications.[18] The SGA uses patient assessment data such as weight, intake, functional status, disease state, symptoms, metabolic stress, and physical examination to assess and monitor risk for malnutrition and to evaluate effects of interventions. An online, Scored Patient-Generated SGA is available for health professionals to utilize at http://pt-global.org.

PATIENT HISTORY

A comprehensive nutrition assessment includes many aspects of the patient's history. The main types of history include health or medical, medications, personal, and food and nutrition. Sources for the historical information include the medical record, the patient, and significant others.

The health or medical history identifies factors that affect nutrient needs or nutrition education needs or that place the client at risk for poor nutrition status. One important component is the nutritional relevance of the current diagnosis (Table 1.21). The diagnosis may present a specific level of risk based on the potential to adversely affect nutritional status. In addition to the disease's potential to alter nutritional status, the degree of risk posed to an individual patient depends on several factors, including its duration and severity, the presence of other physiologic stressors, and the individual (genetics, age, and nutritional status). Some diseases are nutritionally relevant because of the likelihood of the need for nutrition intervention.

The medication history identifies substances that can affect nutrient needs or alter nutritional status. This includes prescribed medications, over-the-counter (OTC) medications, and dietary supplements (see Appendix B). Personal history includes several aspects of psychosocial and lifestyle patterns that may affect nutrient needs, influence food choices, or limit therapy options. The food and nutrition history

TABLE 1.21. Nutritionally Relevant Conditions

AIDS-HIV	Dehydration	Multiple sclerosis
Alcohol and/or drug abuse	Diabetes	Nephrotic syndrome
Cachexia	Dysphagia	Neutropenia
Cancer	Eating disorders	Obesity
Celiac disease	Gastrointestinal bleeding	Pancreatitis
Cerebrovascular accident	Hepatic encephalopathy	Parkinson disease
Chronic obstructive pulmonary disease	Hepatitis	Peritonitis
	Hypertension	Pressure ulcers
Cirrhosis	Inflammatory bowel disease	Renal failure
Coronary heart disease (MI)	Malabsorption	Sepsis
Crohn disease	Malnutrition	Tuberculosis

MI, myocardial infarction.
Data from Academy of Nutrition and Dietetics, Evidence Analysis Library. *Energy Expenditure: Evidence Analysis: Estimating RMR with Prediction Equations*. 2006. Available at: http://www.eatrightpro.org/resources/research/evidence-based-resources/evidence-analysis-library. Accessed December 10, 2015.

identifies food consumption patterns, specific nutrient intake and imbalances, reasons for potential nutrition problems, and dietary factors important to shaping the nutrition care plan. Table 1.22 lists general information for all categories of history in addition to specific information to collect from the patient or the medical record.

Food and Nutrition History

A comprehensive food and nutrition history (diet history) is generally not possible with most patients in the acute care setting, although components of the history are vital

TABLE 1.22. Patient History Categories

History Category	Specific Information
Health/Medical	
Current health status and diagnoses	Date of first diagnosis Previous education on diagnosis
Previous medical history and health status	Specific family members affected by nutritionally relevant disease and onset age
Family history	Recent diagnostic procedures requiring NPO status
Surgical history	Difficulty chewing (state of dentition) or swallowing Chronic gastrointestinal problems (diarrhea, constipation, nausea, vomiting)
Medications	
Prescription medications	Use of multiple medications
OTC meds	Duration of medication use
Dietary supplements (nutrient, herbal, essential nutrients)	Frequency of use (chronic or as needed) Changes in sense of smell or taste related to medications
Illegal drugs	Previous education on potential interactions
Personal	
Age	Income
Gender	Use of or eligibility for government programs
Cultural/ethnic identity	Communication barriers
Occupation/economic status	Cognitive function
Role in family	Smoking
Educational level	Ability to perform daily functions

TABLE 1.22. Patient History Categories (*continued*)

History Category	Specific Information
Motivational level	Person responsible for grocery shopping, meal preparation Access to transportation Recent loss of spouse
Food and Nutrition/Diet	
Food intake	Food intolerances or allergies
Eating habits and patterns	Appetite (current and prior to admission) Weight history (recent weight loss in particular) Physical handicaps affecting food preparation or intake Typical daily intake (types and amounts of foods and beverages consumed) Meal pattern Religious dietary restrictions
Lifestyle patterns	Ethnic dietary habits Alcohol consumption Frequency of dining out; types Exercise, physical activity (type and frequency) Attitude regarding diet and health Previous diet instruction (location, year, topic) Interest in diet instruction or outpatient counseling Stage of change/readiness to learn

OTC, over the counter.

TABLE 1.23. Typical Daily Intake Form

Meal Timing	Food Item	Amount	Where Eaten
	Sample Form		

in nutrition assessment. In other practice settings, it is both possible and desirable to collect detailed information of this type. The goal of a food and nutrition history is to identify nutrient intake and imbalances, the reasons for potential food and nutrition problems, and all dietary factors important in generating the nutrition diagnosis and subsequent intervention. The following types of data are needed: Food intake, eating habits and patterns, and lifestyle patterns related to nutrition and health. If it is likely the patient will require bedside instruction, and depending on the diagnosis, more detailed information about the patient's food intake may need to be collected.

Of the various methods for obtaining a patient's food intake, the most practical in the acute or extended care settings are the typical daily intake (TDI) (Table 1.23) and simplified food frequency (FF) (Table 1.24). In the TDI, the patient is asked what he or she typically eats on a daily basis. In contrast to a 24-hour food recall, in which the patient recounts his or her intake beginning with the last meal eaten, the TDI begins with the first meal of the day. To avoid a judgmental approach, it is best not to label meals as breakfast, lunch, and dinner, but rather based on time of day. For example, you could ask, "What is the first thing you would eat or drink when you get up in the morning?"

A simplified FF is not as detailed as a comprehensive FF questionnaire, but is advantageous for two reasons. The first advantage is that the simplified FF is a quick method for

TABLE 1.24. Food Frequency Form

Food Item/Group	Amount/Day	Amount/Week
Milk or other dairy products (yogurt, cheese)		
Meat, poultry, eggs		
Fish		
Nuts, legumes, and legume products		
Fruits		
Vegetables		
Starches (breads, cereals, grains)		
Fats, added (oils, margarine, salad dressing)		
Snack foods (chips, pretzels, crackers)		
Desserts/sweets		
Dining out		
Fast food		
Restaurant dining		
Beverages		
Alcohol		
Coffee, tea		
Carbonated beverages		
Fruit juices		

determining whether the patient avoids any major category of food, and the second is that it will provide a crosscheck of the TDI. After collecting the food intake information, it is compared with an appropriate standard, such as the Dietary Guidelines for Americans or the Dietary Reference Intakes. A simplified evaluation form of general aspects of diet can also be used (Table 1.25).

TABLE 1.25. Evaluation of Dietary Intake

Group	Servings/Day	Recommended	Adequate/Excess
Dairy			
Protein			
Fruit			
Vegetable			
Starch			
Fat/sweets			
	Overall Diet Adequacy: ___yes ___no		

Specific Nutrients:

Deficit of: ___kcals ___PRO ___fiber ___Vit A ___Vit C ___Fe ___Ca ___Other

Excess of: ___kcals ___Fat ___SFA ___Chol ___Sugar ___Alcohol ___Na

Other: ____________

Summary: ______________________________________

____

PRO, protein; Fe, iron; Ca, calcium; SFA, saturated fatty acid; Chol, cholesterol; NA, Sodium.

References

1. Academy of Nutrition and Dietetics. Nutrition Terminology Reference Manual (eNCPT): Dietetics Language for Nutrition Care. Available at: http://ncpt.webauthor.com. Accessed November 12, 2015.
2. Estimating height in bedridden patients. Available at: http://www.rxkinetics.com/height_estimate.html. Accessed December 9, 2015.
3. Shah B, Sucher K, Hollenbeck CB. Comparison of ideal body weight equations and published height-weight tables with body mass index tables for healthy adults in the United States. *Nutr Clin Pract* 2006;21:312–319.
4. U.S. National Library of Medicine (NLM). Calculating body frame size. Available at: http://www.nlm.nih.gov/medlineplus/ency/imagepages/17182.htm. Accessed December 10, 2015.

5. Gaddey HL, Holder K. Unintentional weight loss in older adults. *Am Fam Physician* 2014;89(9):718–722.
6. Academy of Nutrition and Dietetics. Nutrition Care Manual. Available at: https://www.nutritioncaremanual.org. Accessed December 16, 2015.
7. National Institutes of Health Clinical Guidelines on the identification, evaluation, and treatment of overweight and obesity in adults: The Evidence Report. 1998. Available at: http://www.ncbi.nlm.nih.gov/books/bv.fcgi?rid=obesity. Accessed December 10, 2015.
8. Singh R, Prakash M, Dubey R, et al. Body composition parameters as correlates of coronary artery disease. *Indian J Med Res* 2013;138(6):1016–1019.
9. Academy of Nutrition and Dietetics, Evidence Analysis Library. *Energy Expenditure: Evidence Analysis: Estimating RMR with Prediction Equations*. 2006. Available at: http://www.eatrightpro.org/resources/research/evidence-based-resources/evidence-analysis-library. Accessed December 10, 2015.
10. Academy of Nutrition and Dietetics, Evidence Analysis Library. *Energy Expenditure: Evidence Analysis: Harris-Benedict*. 2005. Available at: http://www.eatrightpro.org/resources/research/evidence-based-resources/evidence-analysis-library. Accessed December 10, 2015.
11. Academy of Nutrition and Dietetics, Evidence Analysis Library. *Critical Illness: Critical Illness Guidelines: Determination of Resting Metabolic Rate*. 2012. Available at: http://www.eatrightpro.org/resources/research/evidence-based-resources/evidence-analysis-library. Accessed December 11, 2015.
12. Huckleberry Y. Nutritional support and the surgical patient. *Am J Health Syst Pharm* 2004;61(7):671–682. Available at: http://www.medscape.com/viewarticle/474066_6. Accessed December 16, 2015.
13. Aguayo-Becea OA, Torres-Garibay C, Macia-Amerzxua MD, et al. Serum albumin level as a risk factor for mortality in bur patient. *Clinics (Sao Paulo)* 2013;6(7):940–945.
14. Lin MY, Liu WY, Tolan AM, et al. Preoperative serum albumin but not prealbumin is an excellent predictor of postoperative complications and mortality in patients with gastrointestinal cancer. *Am Surg* 2011;77(10):1286–1289.
15. Peralta R. *Hypoalbuminemia*. Available at: http://emedicine.medscape.com/article/166724-overview#a6. Accessed December 15, 2015.

16. Eljaiek R, Dubois MJ. Hypoalbuminemia in the first 24 hours of admission with organ dysfunction in burned patients. *Burns* 2012;39(1):113–118.
17. White JV, Guenter P, Jensen G, et al. Consensus statement of the Academy of Nutrition and Dietetics/American Society for Parenteral and Enteral Nutrition: Characteristics recommended for the identification and documentation of adult malnutrition (undernutrition). *J Acad Nutr Diet* 2012;112(5):275–283,730–738.
18. Jeejeebhoy K. Subjective global assessment. Available at: http://subjectiveglobalassessment.com/. Accessed December 16, 2015.

Notes

Notes

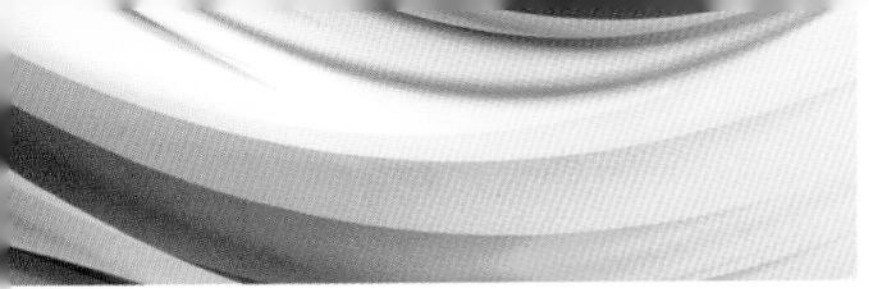

CHAPTER 2

Pregnancy

Lynn Kuligowski, RD

Pregnancy represents a vulnerable life stage relative to a woman's nutritional status. In addition, both the dietary intake and the nutritional status of a woman before and during pregnancy greatly influence fetal development and, in turn, pregnancy outcome. In 2006, the Centers for Disease Control and Prevention (CDC) issued special recommendations to improve preconception care and health (Box 2.1).[1–3] Research has also shown the profound impact of maternal nutritional status and intake on the infant's risk in adulthood for several chronic diseases such as hypertension and diabetes, largely via birth weight.[4] Several of the complications of pregnancy can also adversely affect nutritional status. For these reasons, nutritional assessment is imperative to help ensure optimal pregnancy outcome.

One of the most important aspects of pregnancy is body weight. Both prepregnancy weight and weight gain during gestation significantly influence pregnancy outcome.[5] A woman with either excess or low body weight before pregnancy has a higher risk for poor outcome. In addition, weight gain during pregnancy, specifically total amount and rate, is correlated with infant birth weight, which in turn is associated with infant mortality.[6]

BOX 2.1 Special Recommendations for Women Before Pregnancy

1. Have a reproductive life plan.
2. See your doctor. Discuss any known medical conditions and STIs.
3. Be active. Exercise according to physician recommendations.
4. Maintain a healthy weight. If BMI $\geq$26 kg/m^2, consider a structured weight loss program. If BMI $\leq$19.8 kg/m^2, consider counseling to achieve weight gain.
5. Stop smoking, and/or limit exposure to smoking.
6. Consume 400 µg of folic acid daily (from fortified foods or a dietary supplement) and foods rich in folate.
7. Take a multivitamin supplement if unable to meet RDAs from food sources.
8. Avoid toxic substances and environmental contaminants.
9. Avoid alcohol. There is no safe level of consumption at any time during pregnancy.
10. Stop using street drugs.
11. Review immunization status and update, if necessary.
12. Learn your family health history.
13. Get help for violence.
14. Address mental health issues.

RDAs, recommended dietary allowances.

Data from (i) Centers for Disease Control and Prevention. Recommendations to improve preconception health and health care—United States: A report of the CDC/ATSDR Preconception Care Work Group and the Select Panel on Preconception Care. *MMWR Recomm Rep* 2006;55(RR-6):1–23. Available at: http://www.cdc.gov/mmwr/PDF/rr/rr5506.pdf. Accessed October 30, 2015, (ii) Centers for Disease Control and Prevention. Planning for Pregnancy. Available at: http://www.cdc.gov/preconception/planning.html. Updated January 9, 2015. Accessed October 30, 2015, and (iii) Moos MK, Dunlop AL, Jack BW, et al. Healthier women, healthier reproductive outcomes: Recommendations for the routine care of all women of reproductive age. *Am J Obstet Gynecol* 2008;199(6):S280–S289. doi:10.1016/j.ajog.2008.08.060.

GUIDELINES FOR PREGNANCY WEIGHT GAIN

The Institute of Medicine (IOM) issued pregnancy weight gain recommendations based on current body weight for both total weight and rate of weight gain, which were reviewed again in 2009 (Table 2.1).[6] The Committee to Reexamine IOM Pregnancy Weight Guidelines made recommendations for weight gain during pregnancy for all women, regardless of age or racial/ethnic background. These differ from the previous guidelines in that they are based on the World Health Organization (WHO) body mass index (BMI) categories and not the categories of the Metropolitan Life Insurance tables. In addition, they provide a more specific weight gain range for obese women.

Provisional recommendations are also provided for twin pregnancies, encouraging women with a normal prepregnancy (BMI 18.5 to 24.9) to gain 37 to 54 lb, overweight women (BMI 25.0 to 29.9) to gain 31 to 50 lb, and obese women (BMI ≥30) to gain 25 to 42 lb. It was determined that insufficient data exist to provide weight gain recommendations for other multifetal pregnancies (Table 2.2).[6] As these pregnancies typically result in a higher rate of low birth weight, it is necessary to ensure adequate weight gain.

TABLE 2.1. Guidelines for Pregnancy Weight Gain

Category	BMI (WHO)	Weight Gain (lb)	Rate of Weight Gain for 2nd and 3rd Trimesters
Underweight	<18.5	28–40	1–1.3 lb/wk
Normal weight	18.5–24.9	25–35	0.8–1 lb/wk
Overweight	25.0–29.9	15–25	0.5–0.7 lb/wk
Obese (all classes)	≥30.0	11–20	0.4–0.6 lb/wk

Data from Institute of Medicine and National Research Council Committee to Reexamine IOM Pregnancy Weight Guidelines. *Weight Gain During Pregnancy: Reexamining the Guidelines*. Washington, DC: The National Academies Press; 2009.

TABLE 2.2. Weight Gain Recommendations for Multifetal Pregnancy

Twin Gestation:	
Normal BMI (18.5–24.9)	37–54 lb
Overweight BMI (25.0–29.9)	31–50 lb
Obese BMI (≥30.0)	25–42 lb
Triplet Gestation:	
Any BMI	Insufficient data to determine

Data from Institute of Medicine and National Research Council Committee to Reexamine IOM Pregnancy Weight Guidelines. *Weight Gain During Pregnancy: Reexamining the Guidelines*. Washington, DC: The National Academies Press; 2009.

NUTRIENT RECOMMENDATIONS FOR PREGNANCY

Requirements for most essential nutrients increase during pregnancy over nonpregnant status (Table 2.3).[7–9] Meeting energy needs during pregnancy is crucial for adequate maternal weight gain to prevent low birth weight (Table 2.4). Although the dietary reference intakes (DRIs) consider only single-fetus pregnancy, data from research have generated an energy recommendation for multifetal pregnancy of an additional 500 to 600 kcal to the single-fetus pregnancy level, based on prepregnancy weight.[10]

Specific nutrients become "nutrients of concern," as described by the U.S. Department of Agriculture, because of their role in gestation and/or low intake by the American population (Table 2.5).[11] Pregnant women are routinely prescribed a vitamin and mineral supplement, but a healthful daily eating pattern is important. The MyPlate Daily Food Plan can serve as the basis for such a pattern (Table 2.6).[12]

TABLE 2.3. Percentage of Increase Over Nonpregnant Women for Recommended Nutrient Intakes

	Female, 14–18 yr	Pregnant, 14–18 yr	% Increase	Female, 19–30 yr	Pregnant, 19–30 yr	% Increase	Female, 31–50 yr	Pregnant, 31–50 yr	% Increase
Macronutrient									
Carbohydrates	130 g	175 g	35%	130 g	175 g	35%	130	175	35%
Protein[a]	0.85 g/kg	1.1 g/kg	30%	0.8 g/kg	1.1 g/kg	38%	0.8 g/kg	1.1 g/kg	38%
Fiber	26 g	28 g	8%	25 g	28 g	12%	25 g	28 g	12%
Vitamin									
Vitamin A	700 µg	750 µg	7%	700 µg	770 µg	10%	700 µg	770 µg	10%
Vitamin D	600 IU	600 IU	0%	600 IU	600 IU	0%	600 IU	600 IU	0%
Vitamin C	65 mg	80 mg	24%	75 mg	85 mg	13%	75 mg	85 mg	13%
Vitamin E	15 mg	15 mg	0%	15 mg	15 mg	0%	15 mg	15 mg	0%
Vitamin K	75 µg	75 µg	0%	90 µg	90 µg	0%	90 µg	90 µg	0%
Thiamin B_1	1.0 mg	1.4 mg	40%	1.1 mg	1.4 mg	28%	1.1 mg	1.4 mg	28%
Riboflavin	1.0 mg	1.4 mg	40%	1.1 mg	1.4 mg	28%	1.1 mg	1.4 mg	28%
Niacin	14 mg	18 mg	29%	14 mg	18 mg	29%	14 mg	18 mg	29%
Vitamin B_6	1.2 mg	1.9 mg	59%	1.3 mg	1.9 mg	46%	1.3 mg	1.9 mg	46%
Vitamin B_{12}	2.4 µg	2.6 µg	8%	2.4 µg	2.6 µg	8%	2.4 µg	2.6 µg	8%

(*continued*)

TABLE 2.3. Percentage of Increase Over Nonpregnant Women for Recommended Nutrient Intakes (*continued*)

	Female, 14–18 yr	Pregnant, 14–18 yr	% Increase	Female, 19–30 yr	Pregnant, 19–30 yr	% Increase	Female, 31–50 yr	Pregnant, 31–50 yr	% Increase
Folate	400 μg	600 μ/d	50%	400 μg	600 μg	50%	400 μg	600 μg	50%
Pantothenic acid	5 mg	6 mg	20%	5 mg	6 mg	20%	5 mg	6 mg	20%
Biotin	25 μg	30 μg	20%	30 μg	30 μg	0%	30 μg	30 μg	0%
Choline	400 mg	450 mg	12.5%	425 mg	450 mg	6%	425 mg	450 mg	6%
Mineral									
Calcium	1,300 mg	1,300 mg	0%	1,000 mg	1,000 mg	0%	1,000 mg	1,000 mg	0%
Fluoride	3 mg	3 mg	0%	3 mg	3 mg	0%	3 mg	3 mg	0%
Iodine	150 μg	220 μg	47%	150 μg	220 μg	47%	150 μg	220 μg	47%
Iron	15 mg	27 mg	80%	18 mg	27 mg	50%	18 mg	27 mg	50%
Magnesium	360 mg	400 mg	11%	310 mg	350 mg	13%	320 mg	360 mg	13%
Phosphorus	1,250 mg	1,250 mg	0%	700 mg	700 mg	0%	700 mg	700 mg	0%
Selenium	55 μg	60 μg	9%	55 μg	60 μg	9%	55 μg	60 μg	9%
Zinc	9 mg	12 mg	34%	8 mg	11 mg	38%	8 mg	11 mg	38%

[a]For the 2nd and 3rd trimester.

Data from (i) Institute of Medicine. *Dietary Reference Intakes: The Essential Guide to Nutrient Requirements*. Washington, DC: National Academies Press; 2009, and (ii) Institute of Medicine. Committee to Review Dietary Reference Intakes for Vitamin D and Calcium. In: Ross AC, Taylor CL,

TABLE 2.4. Energy Needs in Pregnancy

Trimester	Additional Energy Needs (kcal/d) Estimated Energy Requirement (kcal/d)
1st trimester	EER = Nonpregnant EER + 0
2nd trimester	EER = Nonpregnant EER + 340
3rd trimester	EER = Nonpregnant EER + 452

EER, estimated energy requirement.

Data from (i) Institute of Medicine. *Dietary Reference Intakes: The Essential Guide to Nutrient Requirements*. Washington, DC: National Academies Press; 2009, and (ii) Academy of Nutrition and Dietetics. Nutrition Care Manual. Available at: https://www.nutritioncaremanual.org. Accessed November 16, 2015.

TABLE 2.5. Recommendations for Nutrients of Concern in Pregnancy

Nutrient	Age (yr)	Amount
Calcium	14–18	1,300 mg
	19 and older	1,000 mg
Folate	All ages	600 µg (daily folate equivalents)
Iron	All ages	27 mg
Protein	All ages	1.1 (g/kg/d)[a]

[a]In the 2nd and 3rd trimesters.

Data from Institute of Medicine. *Dietary Reference Intakes: The Essential Guide to Nutrient Requirements*. Washington, DC: National Academies Press; 2009.

TABLE 2.6. The MyPlate Daily Food Plan for Moms[a,b]

Food Group	Servings	Serving Size/Types
Whole grain breads, cereal, rice, and pasta	6 oz[a] 8 oz[b]	1 slice of bread 3–4 crackers ½ English muffin or bagel ½ cup cooked cereal 1 cup ready-to-eat cereal ½ cup cooked pasta, rice, or other grain

(continued)

TABLE 2.6. The MyPlate Daily Food Plan for Moms[a,b] (*continued*)

Food Group	Servings	Serving Size/Types
Fruits	2 cups[a,b]	1 medium item (apple, orange, banana) 1 cup raw/cooked fruit or 100% juice ½ cup canned or dried fruit
Vegetables	2.5 cups[a] 3 cups[b]	1 cup raw/cooked vegetables 1 cup 100% vegetable juice 2 cups raw leafy salad greens
Protein foods: lean meat, poultry, fish, dry beans, eggs, and nuts	5.5 oz[a] 6.5 oz[b]	1 oz cooked, lean meat, poultry, or seafood 1 egg ¼ cup cooked, dry beans, or peas ½ oz nuts 1 tbsp peanut butter
Milk and dairy products	3 cups[a,b]	1 cup skim or low-fat milk 1 cup fortified soy milk (soy beverage) 8 oz yogurt 1½ oz natural cheese (e.g., Cheddar) 2 oz processed cheese (e.g., American)
Fats and sweets	6 tsp[a] 7 tsp[b]	1 tsp vegetable oil 1½ tsp mayonnaise 2 tsp tub margarine 2 tsp French dressing
Alcohol	Avoid	Avoid all alcoholic beverages

[a]Based on a 2,000 kcal diet (1st trimester).

[b]Based on a 2,400 kcal diet (2nd and 3rd trimesters).

Data from USDA Food and Nutrition Service. Tips for Pregnant Moms [fact sheet]. FNS-457. 2013. Available at: http://www.gchd.us/clinic_services/wic/docs/PregnancyFactSheettipspg.pdf. Accessed October 15, 2015.

NUTRITION ASSESSMENT

An early nutrition assessment is crucial in pregnancy, given the relationship between nutritional status of the mother and pregnancy outcome. In addition to the standard nutrition assessment categories, it is important to consider key risk factors, which may be present prior to pregnancy or arise during prenatal care (Box 2.2).[10,13]

BOX 2.2 Nutrition Assessment Risk Factors in Pregnancy

Age: ≥35 years or ≤16 years
Prepregnancy weight: >120% desirable BMI for age or <85% of desirable BMI
Chronic disease (e.g., diabetes, cardiovascular disease, gastrointestinal diseases)
Multiple pregnancy (twins, triplets, etc.)
Use of alcohol, illegal drugs
Smoking
High parity; close birth spacing
Previous low-birth-weight pregnancy
Pica (eating/craving unusual food or nonfood items)
Poorly managed vegetarian/vegan diet
History of food avoidance (may be owing to allergy/intolerance, cultural/religious beliefs, self-imposed dietary restrictions)
Eating disorders (anorexia/bulimia), or poor eating habits
Following a weight reduction diet, or imposed dietary restrictions
History of bariatric surgery
Poor eating habits
Late initiation of prenatal care
Weight loss during pregnancy
Hyperemesis with weight loss
Risk of anemia
Risk of preeclampsia/eclampsia
Socioeconomic difficulties (low income, lack of family or social support, homeless, inability to prepare meals)
History of adverse gynecologic or obstetrical conditions

(continued)

BOX 2.2 Nutrition Assessment Risk Factors in Pregnancy (*continued*)

History of poor birth outcome (low birth weight, prematurity, congenital anomalies, death of infant or stillborn >20 weeks, SGA, preterm labor, or miscarriage)

Data from (i) Academy of Nutrition and Dietetics. Nutrition Care Manual. Available at: https://www.nutritioncaremanual.org. Accessed November 16, 2015, and (ii) Escott-Stump S. *Nutrition and Diagnosis-Related Care.* 8th ed. Philadelphia, PA: Wolters Kluwer; 2015.

Anthropometric Measurement

As an assessment category, anthropometric measure is perhaps the most important because of the relationship between prenatal weight gain and pregnancy outcome. Using the IOM weight gain guidelines, based on prepregnancy weight and multifetal pregnancy, allows the establishment of weight gain goals. Recording prenatal weight gain on a growth grid to monitor weight gain is important in assuring both adequate total weight gain and appropriate rate of gain.[6]

Variations in weight gain goals (amount or rate) require further scrutiny to determine whether the cause is pathophysiologic or related to inadequate dietary intake. Fluid retention may cause a sudden surge in weight after the 20th gestational week, and this may indicate development of preeclampsia.

Biochemical Data: Laboratory Data

Because of the nearly 50% increase in blood volume during pregnancy, there is a dilution of solids in the blood of pregnant women, which causes changes in specific laboratory constituents (Table 2.7).[10,14]

Patient History

The history component of nutrition assessment in pregnancy is vital in identifying problems and risk factors related to dietary intake and lifestyle, many of which will greatly

TABLE 2.7. Laboratory Values in Pregnancy

Constituent (Serum[a])	Normal Level/Range (Common Units)	
Albumin	1st trimester: 3.1–5.1 g/dL	
	2nd trimester: 2.6–4.5 g/dL	
	3rd trimester: 2.3–4.2 g/dL	
Calcium (total)	1st trimester: 8.8–10.6 mg/dL	
	2nd trimester: 8.2–9.0 mg/dL	
	3rd trimester: 8.2–9.7 mg/dL	
Creatinine (s/p)	1st trimester: 0.4–0.7 mg/dL	
	2nd trimester: 0.4–0.8 mg/dL	
	3rd trimester: 0.4–0.9 mg/dL	
Glucose (OGTT, 100-g test load to diagnose GDM) (s/p)	Time (hr)	mg/dL
–GDM diagnosed:	0	>105
2 abnormal values	1	190
	2	165
	3	145
Hematocrit (whole blood)	1st trimester: 31%–41%	
	2nd trimester: 30%–39%	
	3rd trimester: 28%–40%	
Hemoglobin (whole blood)	1st trimester:11.6–13.9 g/dL	
	2nd trimester: 9.7–14.8 g/dL	
	3rd trimester: 9.5–15 g/dL	
White blood cell count	1st trimester: 5.7–13.6 × $10^3/mm^3$	
	2nd trimester: 5.6–14.8 × $10^3/mm^3$	
	3rd trimester: 5.6–16.9 × $10^3/mm^3$	
Lipids: cholesterol	1st trimester: 141–210 mg/dL	
	2nd trimester: 176–299 mg/dL	
	3rd trimester: 219–349 mg/dL	

(*continued*)

TABLE 2.7. Laboratory Values in Pregnancy (*continued*)

Constituent (Serum[a])	Normal Level/Range (Common Units)
Lipids:	
Triglyceride	1st trimester: 40–159 mg/dL
	2nd trimester: 75–382 mg/dL
	3rd trimester: 131–453 mg/dL
Osmolality	1st trimester: 275–280 mmol/kg
	2nd trimester: 276–289 mmol/kg
	3rd trimester: 278–280 mmol/kg
Thyroid Hormones:	
Thyroxine total, T_4	1st trimester: 6.5–10.1 μg/dL
	2nd trimester: 7.5–10.3 μg/dL
	3rd trimester: 6.3–9.7 μg/dL
TSH	1st trimester: 0.1–2.5 mIU/L
	2nd trimester: 0.2–3.0 mIU/L
	3rd trimester: 0.3–3.0 mIU/L
Thyroxin-binding globulin (TBG)	1st trimester: 10–40 mg/L
	2nd trimester: 23–46 mg/L
	3rd trimester: 19–49 mg/L
Urea nitrogen	1st trimester: 7–12 mg/dL
	2nd trimester: 3–13 mg/dL
	3rd trimester: 3–11 mg/dL
Uric acid	1st trimester: 2.0–4.2 mg/dL
	2nd trimester: 2.4–4.9 mg/dL
	3rd trimester: 3.1–6.3 mg/dL

[a]Serum values, unless denoted as (p), plasma, or s/p, serum or plasma, or as noted.

TSH, thyroid-stimulating hormone.

Data from Perinatology.com. Focus Information Technology, Inc. Normal reference ranges and laboratory values in pregnancy. 2010–2015. Available at: http:/perinatology.com/Reference/Reference%20Ranges/Reference%20for%20Serum.htm. Accessed November 12, 2015.

influence pregnancy outcome. The following relevant historical components provide detailed descriptions of such factors.

Food and Nutrition History

The importance of nutritional intake during pregnancy, in particular for specific nutrients, necessitates a thorough food and nutrition history as part of nutrition assessment. Potential nutrients of concern, because of their importance or increased need in pregnancy, include calcium, vitamin D, iron, zinc, magnesium, folate, vitamin B_6, and energy and protein. Box 2.3 provides dietary intake details and lifestyle factors, which are a critical component of a complete food and nutrition history.[10,13] Pregnant women are routinely prescribed a prenatal vitamin and mineral supplement containing key nutrients (Table 2.8).[15]

BOX 2.3 Food and Nutrition History

I. Socioeconomic, Lifestyle, and Health Beliefs/Attitudes

1. Perceived nutrition/dietary problems
2. Follows a special diet (e.g., vegan, food allergy/intolerance)
3. Economics: adequate resources/availability of food. Adequate housing and transportation.
4. Ethnic/cultural background
5. Home life/meal patterns
6. Appropriate physical activity

II. Physiologic Problems

1. Nausea, vomiting, diarrhea
2. Constipation
3. Gastroesophageal reflux
4. Recent weight change

III. Nutritional Adequacy: Food Groups/Nutrients

1. Appetite
2. Multiple gestation
3. Dairy products (calcium, vitamins D and B_{12})
4. Fruits and vegetables (folate, vitamin C, fiber, magnesium)
5. Whole grains (B_6, folic acid, fiber)
6. Protein foods (iron, zinc, B_{12}, B_6, iodine)

(continued)

Pregnancy

BOX 2.3 Food and Nutrition History (*continued*)

IV. Medical Problems

1. Chronic disease
2. Medications
3. Oral/dental health

V. Contaminants/Other Substances

1. Fish (mercury/contaminants: check local health department for advisories)
2. Pica
3. Excessive caffeine (>2 cups coffee/day)
4. Alcohol
5. Smoking
6. Foodborne pathogens (*Listeria monocytogenes, Toxoplasma gondii*)

Data from (i) Academy of Nutrition and Dietetics. Nutrition Care Manual. Available at: https://www.nutritioncaremanual.org. Accessed November 16, 2015, and (ii) Escott-Stump S. *Nutrition and Diagnosis-Related Care.* 8th ed. Philadelphia, PA: Wolters Kluwer; 2015.

TABLE 2.8. Nutrients in a Prenatal Supplement

Vitamins	Amount	% DV[a]
A	4,000 IU	156
B_1	1.8 mg	129
B_2	3 mg	215
B_6	10 mg	527
B_{12}	12 µg	460
Folic acid	1 mg	170
Niacin	20 mg	111
C	120 mg	141
D	400 IU	150
E	22 mg	150

TABLE 2.8. Nutrients in a Prenatal Supplement (*continued*)

Minerals	Amount	
Calcium	200 mg	20
Iron	27 mg	100
Zinc	25 mg	227

[a]Daily values for pregnant and lactating women.

Data from (i) Institute of Medicine. *Dietary Reference Intakes: The Essential Guide to Nutrient Requirements*. Washington, DC: National Academies Press; 2009, and (ii) Drugs.com [Inernet] Prenatal Plus information from Drugs.com; c 2000–2015 [Revised June 2014; Cited November 12, 2015]. Available at: http://www.drugs.com/pro/prenatal-plus.htm. Accessed November 12, 2015.

Medication and Supplement History

Many common medications, both prescription and over-the-counter, and dietary supplements can exert adverse effects during pregnancy. In some cases, timing of the medication determines the potential for an adverse effect. However, many women (up to 70%) must take medications for a chronic disease or condition, and the physician weighs the risks and benefits in those instances.[16] In 2014, the Food and Drug Administration (FDA) changed its format for labeling prescription drugs for use in pregnancy. Previously, medications were categorized by letter (A, B, C, D, or X) to indicate their safety for use in pregnancy.

However, the FDA determined that these categories were often misunderstood and misused. Therefore, to provide a more consistent format for presenting risk and benefit information, a final rule was enacted in 2014. It requires that product labels provide essential information such as a risk summary of use during pregnancy and lactation, supporting data for the summary, and information to assist health care providers with prescribing and patient counseling. In addition, it requires labeling to include information about pregnancy testing, contraception, and infertility to assist health care providers with prescribing and counseling for males and females with reproductive potential.[17]

Because there is very little research on how they may affect pregnancy, dietary supplements, including herbs, botanicals, and herbal teas, should be avoided. As a registration process with the FDA is lacking, the agency only takes action if a supplement is found to be unsafe after marketing.[18] Box 2.4 provides a listing, although not comprehensive, of common medications and supplements, which should be avoided during pregnancy.[19]

BOX 2.4 Medications and Dietary Supplements to Avoid During Pregnancy

Prescription Drugs	
ACE inhibitors	Captopril (Capoten)
Acne medications	Isotretinoin (Accutane, Amnesteem, Claravis, and Sotret)
Anticonvulsants	Carbamazepine (Carbatrol, Epitol, Equetro, Tegretol), valproic acid (Depacon, Depakene, Depakote, Stavzor, Valproic)
MAO inhibitors	Isocarboxazid (phenelzine)
Tranquilizers	Librium, Miltown, Valium
Opioids	Morphine, codeine, hydrocodone (Vicodin), oxycodone (OxyContin, Percocet), tramadol (ConZip, Ryzolt, Ultram)
Antidepressants	Fluoxetine (Prozac), paroxetine (Paxil)
Others	Thalidomide (Thalomid), warfarin (Coumadin, Jantoven), medical marijuana
Drugs that interfere with folic acid	Phenobarbital, phenytoin (Dilantin), primidone (Mysoline), sulfasalazine (Sulfazine, Azulfidine

BOX 2.4 Medications and Dietary Supplements to Avoid During Pregnancy (*continued*)

Over-the-Counter Drugs	
Pain relievers (NSAIDs)	Ibuprofen[a] (Motrin, Advil, Nuprin), naproxen[b], aspirin[c]
Cold preparations	Guaifenesin[a], pseudoephedrine[b], phenylephrine[c]
Dietary Supplements	
Herbs and other substances	Black cohosh, blue cohosh, chaste berry, echinacea, ephedra, feverfew, goldenseal, juniper berry, mugwort, pennyroyal oil, rue, St. John's wort

[a]3rd trimester.
[b]1st trimester.
ACE, angiotensin-simulating enzyme; MAO, monoamine oxidase; NSAIDs, nonsteroidal anti-inflammatory drugs.
Data from (i) March of Dimes [Internet]. Prescription drugs, over-the-counter drugs, supplements and herbal products; c 2015 [Revised July 2015; Cited November 28, 2015]. Available at: http://www.marchofdimes.org/pregnancy/prescription-drugs-over-the-counter-drugs-supplements-and-herbal-products.aspx. Accessed November 12, 2015, (ii) Servey J, Chang J. Over-the counter medications in pregnancy. *Am Fam Physician* 2014;90(8):548–555, and (iii) March of Dimes [Internet]. Mood-altering drug use during pregnancy—the risks of medical marijuana and prescription opioids; c 2015. Available at: http://www.marchofdimes.org/mood-altering-drug-use-during-pregnancy-the-risks-of-medical-marijuana-and-prescription-opioids.aspx. Accessed November 12, 2015.

PROBLEMS DURING PREGNANCY

The most common problems during pregnancy include preexisting diabetes, gestational diabetes, hyperemesis gravidarum (HG), morning sickness, and pregnancy-induced hypertension. Such problems, either preexisting or arising during pregnancy, pose varying degrees of risk to maternal and fetal health. In addition, other factors such as a woman's preconception health and nutritional status also influence the risk of low birth weight, preterm birth, and intrauterine growth restriction (IUGR).[20] This emphasizes the importance of nutritional assessment with regard to specific conditions to help ensure a positive pregnancy outcome.

Nausea and Vomiting of Pregnancy

Nausea and vomiting of pregnancy (NVP), also known as morning sickness, occurs in approximately 44% to 89% of all pregnancies and is not confined to only morning hours.[21] It generally begins between 4 and 6 weeks' gestation, with the symptomatic acme at weeks 8 to 12, and resolution for most pregnancies between weeks 16 and 20. A small number of women, 2.5% to 10%, experience continued symptoms beyond 20 weeks gestation.[22] A severe form of NVP—hyperemesis gravidarum—effects up to 1.2% of pregnant women and sometimes requires hospitalization. As HG can have significant impact on energy and nutrient intake, parenteral nutrition may become necessary. Strategies to combat NVP are varied, and sometimes contradictory, so a highly individualized approach is necessary (Box 2.5).[21–23]

BOX 2.5 Strategies for Nausea and Vomiting of Pregnancy

Eat small, more frequent meals and snacks with added protein.
Avoid an empty stomach.
Drink fluids between meals instead of with meals.
Consume adequate liquids throughout the day (2 L/day).
Avoid stimuli such as strong odors from food/perfume and visual stimuli.
Eat a higher amount of protein (vs. carbohydrates and fats), although higher amounts of carbohydrate may be helpful for some women.
Avoid high-fat and fried foods, as this may delay gastric emptying.
Eat dry food or carbohydrate before rising from bed in the morning.
Try sour foods as this is helpful for some women.

BOX 2.5 Strategies for Nausea and Vomiting of Pregnancy (*continued*)

Avoid highly spiced foods if this exacerbates nausea.
Take prenatal vitamins for 3 months before conception.
Treatment with ginger has been shown to be beneficial in reducing nausea (250 mg 2 to 4 times/day).
First-line pharmacotherapy is pyridoxine (B_6) plus doxylamine (Diclegis) (2 to 4 tabs/day).

Data from (i) Niebyl JR, Briggs GG. The pharmacological management of nausea and vomiting of pregnancy. *J Fam Pract* 2014;63(2 Suppl):S31–S37, (ii) Tyler S, Nagtalon-Ramos J. Managing nausea and vomiting of pregnancy. *Women's Healthcare* 2015;3(2):7–13, and (iii) American College of Obstetrics and Gynecology. ACOG Practice Bulletin 153: Nausea and vomiting of pregnancy. *Obstet Gynecol* 2015;126(3):687–688. doi:10.1097/AOG.0000000000001048.

ADIME 2.1 ADIME At-A-Glance: Nausea and Vomiting of Pregnancy

Assessment

- Prepregnancy BMI and weight, weight loss
- Frequency/severity of nausea and vomiting
- Use of herbal supplements for nausea, adherence to prescribed prenatal vitamin
- Dietary intake, meal pattern (eating one large meal per day in the evening when foods are better tolerated)

Nutrition Diagnosis

- Inadequate oral food and beverage intake related to nausea and vomiting of pregnancy, AEB weight loss of 2 lb in 9 weeks
- Inadequate vitamin/mineral intake related to nausea and vomiting of pregnancy, AEB inability to consume prescribed nutrient supplement
- Increased nutrient needs related to pregnancy, AEB diet history of low intake and weight loss
- Harmful nutrition practices related to taking over-the-counter (OTC) herbal supplement, AEB diet history of unsafe dietary supplements

(*continued*)

ADIME 2.1 ADIME At-A-Glance: Nausea and Vomiting of Pregnancy (*continued*)

Intervention

- Nutrition counseling for small, frequent meals with adequate protein and avoidance of high-fat foods
- Nutrition counseling for safe alternatives to OTC herbal supplement (i.e., ginger, B_6, or prescribed medication)
- Nutrition counseling for adequate fluid intake between meals vs. with meals
- Suggest temporary alternatives to prenatal vitamins such as a chewable/liquid children's vitamin

Monitoring and Evaluation

- Body weight
- PO intake (food, fluid)
- Vitamin/mineral supplement tolerance/usage
- Status of nausea and vomiting
- Usage of non-FDA-approved herbal supplements

Diabetes Mellitus

Diabetes affects up to 4.6% to 9.2% of all pregnancies in the United States.[24] Women may enter pregnancy with preexisting diabetes (type 1 or type 2), or develop gestational diabetes during pregnancy. All forms of diabetes during pregnancy increase the risk for adverse outcomes for the mother and infant. These risks include congenital anomalies, macrosomia, (birth weight of 9 lb or more), shoulder dystocia, postpartum hypoglycemia, neonatal hyperinsulinemia, and cesarean section.[25] However, management of blood glucose levels via daily self-monitoring of blood glucose (SMBG), physical activity, nutrition therapy, and/or medications significantly reduces these risks and provides improved birth outcomes.[26]

Gestational Diabetes

The American Diabetes Association (ADA) defines gestational diabetes as "Diabetes diagnosed in the 2nd or 3rd trimester of pregnancy that is not clearly overt diabetes," and it is one of the most common complications of pregnancy. The ADA has recommended two options for gestational diabetes mellitus (GDM) diagnostic criteria: A "one-step" strategy using a 2-hour, 75-g oral glucose tolerance test (OGTT), which is the consensus of the International Association of Diabetes and Pregnancy Study Groups (IADPSG), or a "two-step" approach consisting of a 1-hour 50-g (nonfasting) screening with a subsequent 3-hour 100-g OGTT for those with a positive screen, which is the consensus of the National Institutes of Health (NIH) (Table 2.9).[27] Many women who develop GDM are overweight/obese, or have additional risk factors (Box 2.6),[28] and benefit from following the IOM weight gain and energy intake guidelines for their prepregnancy weight category.[6,8]

TABLE 2.9. Detection and Diagnosis of Gestational Diabetes

One-Step Strategy (IADPSG Consensus)

- Perform a 75-g OGTT, with plasma glucose measurement at fasting and at 1 and 2 hr, at 24–28 wk of gestation in women not previously diagnosed with overt diabetes.
- The OGTT should be performed in the morning after an overnight fast of at least 8 h.
- The diagnosis of GDM is made when any of the following plasma glucose values are exceeded:
  - Fasting: >92 mg/dL (5.1 mmol/L)
  - 1 h: >180 mg/dL (10.0 mmol/L)
  - 2 h: >153 mg/dL (8.5 mmol/L)

Two-Step Strategy (NIH Consensus)

- Step 1: Perform a 50-g glucose load test (GLT) (nonfasting), with plasma glucose measurement at 1 hr, at 24–28 wk of gestation in women not previously diagnosed with overt diabetes. If the plasma glucose level measured 1 hr after the load is >140 mg/dL[a] (7.8 mmol/L), proceed to 100-g OGTT.
- Step 2: The 100-g OGTT should be performed when the patient is fasting.

(continued)

TABLE 2.9. Detection and Diagnosis of Gestational Diabetes (*continued*)

- The diagnosis of GDM is made when at least two of the following four plasma glucose levels (measured fasting, 1, 2, 3 hr after the OGTT) are met or exceeded:

	Carpenter/Coustan	NDDG
Fasting	95 mg/L (5.3 mmol/L)	105 mg/dL (5.8 mmol/L)
1 hr	180 mg/dL (10.0 mmol/L)	190 mg/dL (10.6 mmol/L)
2 hr	155 mg/dL (8.6 mmol/L)	165 mg/dL (9.2 mmol/L)
3 hr	140 mg/dL (7.8 mmol/L)	145 mg/dL (8.0 mmol/L)

[a]The American College of Obstetricians and Gynecologists (ACOG) recommends a lower threshold of 135 mg/dL (7.5 mmol/L) in high-risk ethnic minorities with higher prevalence of GDM; some experts also recommend 130 mg/dL (7.2 mmol/L).

NDDG, National Diabetes Data Group.

Data from American Diabetes Association. Standards of medical care in diabetes—2014. *Diabetes Care* 2014;37(Suppl 1):S14–S80.

Although adequate energy intake is crucial for appropriate fetal weight gain, a modest reduction (to 24 kcal/kg of present pregnancy weight for overweight women) is associated with improved glycemic control. Aerobic exercise (i.e., 30 minutes of brisk walking most days of the week) may also be helpful in delaying the need for medication and improving glycemic control.[26] However, energy restriction must be approached cautiously, with some evidence that 1,800 kcal/day should be the minimum because of the risk of ketonuria and ketonemia. In an effort to standardize nutrition therapy for GDM, the Academy of Nutrition and Dietetics developed evidence-based nutrition practice guidelines.[29] Three key components include SMBG with

BOX 2.6 Questionnaire for Gestational Diabetes Risk[a]

Question	Yes	No
1. Are you overweight or very overweight?		
2. Are you related to anyone who has diabetes now or had diabetes in his or her lifetime?		
3. Are you Hispanic/Latina, African American, American Indian, Alaska Native, Asian American, or Pacific Islander?		
4. Are you older than 25?		
5. In a previous pregnancy, did you have any of the following? • Gestational diabetes • Stillbirth or miscarriage • Large baby (weighing more than 9 lb)		
6. Do you have polycystic ovary syndrome (PCOS) or another health condition linked to problems with insulin?		
7. Have you ever had problems with insulin or blood sugar, such as insulin resistance, glucose intolerance, or "prediabetes"?		
8. Do you have high blood pressure, high cholesterol, and/or heart disease?		

[a]High risk, Yes to two or more questions; average risk, Yes to only one question; low risk: No to all questions.
Data from National Institutes of Health Publication No. 12-4818. June 2012. Available at: https://www.nichd.nih.gov/publications/pubs/Documents/gestational_diabetes_2012.pdf. Accessed November 16, 2015.

medical nutrition therapy (MNT), diet modifications including adjustment of carbohydrate intake, and physical activity. In addition, they developed guidelines for nutrition monitoring and evaluation (Box 2.7).

BOX 2.7 Recommended MNT Guidelines for GDM

Screening/Referral

1. Screen for GDM risk at first prenatal visit.
2. Most women with low risk screened using OGTT between 24 and 28 wk gestation.
3. For women with average to high risk, screen for type 2 diabetes at first prenatal visit. Monitor nutritional intake, weight gain, and physical activity. Risk increases with obesity, excessive weight gain prior to pregnancy, and increased intake of saturated fat.
4. Initiate MNT within 1 week of GDM diagnosis. Provide minimum of three nutrition visits.

Nutrition Assessment

1. Food intake (i.e., dietary patterns, food preferences, nausea/vomiting)
2. Physical activity (consistency, frequency)
3. Medications (special medical concerns or conditions)
4. Prepregnancy BMI as a basis for weight gain recommendations

Nutrition Intervention

1. Encourage adequate calories for weight gain in underweight/normal weight women (use DRIs).
2. Encourage slow weight gain and mild calorie restriction in obese/overweight women (24 kcal/kg/day in overweight and 12 kcal/kg/day in obese).
3. Recommend carbohydrate intake of at least 175 g/day and <45% of energy.
4. Consume adequate amounts of protein and fat based on DRIs.
5. Prevent nutritional deficiencies by recommending a multivitamin/mineral supplement for women whose intake does not meet the DRIs.

BOX 2.7 Recommended MNT Guidelines for GDM (*continued*)

6. Perform physical activity 3 or more days/week for at least 30 minutes unless contraindicated.
7. Perform daily self-blood glucose monitoring (SBGM): fasting and 1 to 2 hours after meals.
8. Use only FDA-approved nonnutritive sweeteners in moderation.
9. Encourage breastfeeding.
10. Avoid consuming alcohol, even in cooking.
11. Recommend initiation of pharmacologic therapy (insulin) if MNT has been unsuccessful.
12. Recommend ketone testing for women with weight loss or inadequate carbohydrate/calorie intake.

Nutrition Monitoring and Evaluation

At each prenatal visit, monitor blood glucose levels, change in weight, food/nutrient intake, physical activity, and pharmacologic therapy (if necessary).

Outcomes Management

After delivery, recommend weight loss via dietary modifications and physical activity if woman is overweight/obese or gained more weight than recommended during pregnancy.

MNT, medical nutrition therapy.

Data from Academy of Nutrition and Dietetics. GDM: Executive summary of recommendations (2008). Available at: https://www.andeal.org/topic.cfm?menu=5288&cat=3731. Accessed November 16, 2015.

Specific dietary measures are outlined in Box 2.8, and if this fails to control blood glucose levels, exogenous insulin will be necessary as is the case in up to 15% of women with GDM.[29] Oral hypoglycemic agents currently used off label in pregnancy (glyburide and metformin) have not been approved by the FDA and may not be safe during pregnancy. Studies of the drug's ability to provide glycemic control and their potential risk for pregnancy complications have yielded mixed results.[30]

BOX 2.8 Specific Dietary Measures for GDM

Reduce energy intake:
- 30 kcal/kg present pregnancy weight for normal weight
- 24 kcal/kg present pregnancy weight for overweight
- 12 kcal/kg for morbidly obese

Restrict carbohydrate intake to 33%–40% of total energy (min. 175 g):
- 10% to 35% of calories from protein
- 20% to 35% of calories from fat (<10% from saturated fat)

Reduce carbohydrate intake in morning meals to 15–30 g.

Space carbohydrate evenly throughout the day (other than morning meals).

Eat several small meals and snacks versus large meals without snacks.

Data from Toiba R. Gestational diabetes. *Today's Dietitian* 2013;15(8):48.

Preexisting Diabetes

Pregnancy requires heightened vigilance with regard to glycemic control, and so women who enter pregnancy with diabetes may need to increase the frequency of SMBG and adjust insulin dose. In addition, insulin requirements (IRs) generally increase up to the first 9 weeks possibly because of peaking levels of chorionic gonadotropin, progesterone, and thyroid hormones. IRs then drop during weeks 9 to 16 likely because of decreasing levels of progesterone, thyroid hormones, an increase of C-peptide, and possibly morning sickness. The need for insulin increases again between weeks 16 and 37 principally because of gestational hormones and tumor necrosis factor.[31] A woman with preexisting type 2 diabetes, who previously managed glycemic control without insulin, may require insulin. Those using oral hypoglycemic agents to control diabetes before pregnancy will also require insulin, because of a lack of consensus on their use and potential complications.

ADIME 2.2 ADIME At-A-Glance: Gestational Diabetes

Assessment

- Prepregnancy BMI and weight, current weight
- OGTT results
- Previous history of GDM or large for gestational age deliveries
- Access to transportation, social support
- Dietary intake, physical activity

Nutrition Diagnosis

- Excessive oral food/beverage intake related to nutrition knowledge deficit and inactivity, AEB prepregnancy BMI of 30 and weight gain of 20 lb at 28 weeks' gestation
- Excessive carbohydrate intake related to knowledge deficit and lack of social support, AEB 1 hour nonfasting OGTT result of 150 mg/dL
- Limited access to food related to lack of transportation and social support, AEB consumption of high-calorie convenience/fast foods
- Physical inactivity related to lack of safe environment, AEB reported sedentary lifestyle

Intervention

- Provide nutrition counseling for IOM weight gain recommendations.
- Provide nutrition counseling for carbohydrate-controlled diet (<45% of energy, at least 175 g/day and 12 kcal/kg/day).
- Ensure consumption of multivitamin/mineral supplement to prevent nutritional deficiencies.
- Counsel regarding indoor exercise for 30 minutes 3 or more times/week with physician approval.
- Refer to WIC and Maternal Infant Health Programs for assistance with food availability and transportation.
- Refer to Certified Diabetes Educator for self-blood glucose monitoring instruction.

Monitoring and Evaluation

- Body weight
- PO intake
- SBGM diaries (BGL—fasting and postprandial)
- Exercise logs
- Verification of enrollment in social support programs
- Attendance at prenatal appointments

Preeclampsia (Pregnancy-Induced Hypertension)

Preeclampsia is a form of hypertension that arises during pregnancy, typically in the 3rd trimester, and complicates approximately 2% to 8% of pregnancies.[32] The term is derived from the potential culminating event of eclampsia, or convulsions, which represents an obstetric emergency. Preeclampsia poses significant risks for the mother and infant. In addition to a spike in blood pressure (140/90 mm Hg on two separate occasions ≥4 hours apart), a woman with preeclampsia will also exhibit proteinuria (≥0.3 g in a 24-hour urine collection) usually after the 20th week of gestation.

The condition is thought to result from impaired placental perfusion and subsequent oxidative stress in the presence of systemic inflammation and other maternal risk factors.[33] Early identification of preeclampsia and careful management are essential to prevent adverse outcomes for mother and fetus. There are several risk factors for preeclampsia to consider early in pregnancy, several of which are moderated by parity status and preexisting conditions (Box 2.9).[32]

In the past, sodium restrictions were standard practice, but the current recommendation by the WHO is that healthy dietary practices should be promoted and the avoidance of excessive dietary salt intake is considered a healthy dietary practice.[34] Therefore, the Dietary Approaches to Stop Hypertension, or DASH diet, may be useful (Table 2.10).[35] In populations where calcium intake is low or inadequate, supplementation of 1.5 to 2.0 g/day is recommended for the prevention of preeclampsia, especially for those at high risk. The WHO found insufficient evidence to recommend supplementation of vitamins C, D, and E.[34]

Medical management of preeclampsia involves the use of low-dose aspirin (prior to 12 weeks gestation until 36 weeks) to reduce the risk of developing preeclampsia in high-risk women. Oral antihypertensive medications such as labetalol or methyldopa are commonly used to treat pregnancy hypertension. Delivery of the fetus is the only known cure for preeclampsia, although women with chronic hypertension should continue with their recommended treatment postnatally.[33]

BOX 2.9 Risk Factors for Preeclampsia

High Risk	Moderate Risk
Early-onset hypertensive disease during a previous pregnancy	First pregnancy (nulliparity)
Chronic kidney disease	Age 40 years or older
Autoimmune disease such as lupus erythematosis or antiphospholipid syndrome	Pregnancy interval of more than 10 years
Type 1 or type 2 diabetes	BMI of ≥35 kg/m^2 at first visit
Chronic hypertension	Family history of preeclampsia
Preexisting medical conditions	Multiple pregnancy
	Pregnancy achieved via donor eggs, donor insemination/embryo

Data from English FA, Kenny LC, McCarthy FP. Risk factors and effective management of preeclampsia. *Integr Blood Press Control* 2015;8:7–12.

TABLE 2.10. The DASH Diet in Pregnancy (Based on a 2,000 Calorie Diet)

Nutrient	Dietary Amount
Carbohydrate	45%–55% total energy
Protein	15%–20% total energy
Fat	25%–30% total energy
Sodium	2–3 g
Food Item	**Servings/d**
Fruits	4–5
Vegetables	4–5
Grains (whole grains recommended)	6–8

(*continued*)

TABLE 2.10. The DASH Diet in Pregnancy (Based on a 2,000 Calorie Diet) (*continued*)

Nutrient	Dietary Amount
Dairy (low or nonfat)	3 or more
Lean meats/poultry/fish	6 or less
Nuts, seeds, and legumes	4–5 per wk
Fats and oils	2–3
Sweets and added sugars	5 or less per wk

DASH, Dietary Approaches to Stop Hypertension.

Data from National Heart, Lung, and Blood Institute. In Brief: Your guide to lowering your blood pressure with DASH (Publication No. 06-5834). 2006. Revised August 2015. Available at: https://www.nhlbi.nih.gov/files/docs/public/heart/dash_brief.pdf. Accessed November 18, 2015.

References

1. Centers for Disease Control and Prevention. Recommendations to improve preconception health and health care—United States: A report of the CDC/ATSDR Preconception Care Work Group and the Select Panel on Preconception Care. *MMWR Recomm Rep* 2006;55(RR-6):1–23. Available at: http://www.cdc.gov/mmwr/PDF/rr/rr5506.pdf. Accessed October 30, 2015.
2. Centers for Disease Control and Prevention. Planning for pregnancy. Available at: http://www.cdc.gov/preconception/planning.html. Updated January 9, 2015. Accessed October 30, 2015.
3. Moos MK, Dunlop AL, Jack BW, et al. Healthier women, healthier reproductive outcomes: Recommendations for the routine care of all women of reproductive age. *Am J Obstet Gynecol* 2008;199(6):S280–S289. doi:10.1016/j.ajog.2008.08.060.
4. Mu M, Wang S-F, Sheng J. Birth weight and subsequent blood pressure: A meta-analysis. *Arch Cardiovasc Dis* 2012;105(2):99–113. doi:10.1016/j.acvd.2011.10.006.
5. Shin D, Song WO. Prepregnancy body mass index is an independent risk factor for gestational diabetes, preterm labor, and small- and large-for-gestational-age infants. *J Matern Fetal Neonatal Med* 2014;28(14):1679–1686. doi:10.3109/14767058.2014.964675.

6. Institute of Medicine and National Research Council Committee to Reexamine IOM Pregnancy Weight Guidelines. *Weight Gain During Pregnancy: Reexamining the Guidelines*. Washington, DC: The National Academies Press; 2009.
7. Institute of Medicine. *Dietary Reference Intakes: The Essential Guide to Nutrient Requirements*. Washington, DC: National Academies Press; 2009.
8. Butte NF, Wong WW, Treuth MS, et al. Energy requirements during pregnancy based on total energy expenditure and energy deposition. *Am J Clin Nutr* 2004;79(6):1078–1087.
9. Institute of Medicine. Committee to Review Dietary Reference Intakes for Vitamin D and Calcium. In: Ross AC, Taylor CL, Yaktine AL, et al, eds. *Dietary Reference Intakes for Calcium and Vitamin D*. Washington, DC: National Academies Press; 2011. doi:10.17226/13050.
10. Academy of Nutrition and Dietetics. Nutrition Care Manual. Available at: https://www.nutritioncaremanual.org. Accessed November 16, 2015.
11. U.S. Department of Agriculture and U.S. Department of Health and Human Services. *Dietary Guidelines for Americans, 2010*. 7th ed. Washington, DC: U.S. Government Printing Office; 2010.
12. USDA Food and Nutrition Service. Tips for Pregnant Moms [fact sheet]. FNS-457. 2013. Available at: http://www.gchd.us/clinic_services/wic/docs/PregnancyFactSheettipspg.pdf. Accessed October 15, 2015.
13. Escott-Stump S. *Nutrition and Diagnosis-Related Care*. 8th ed. Philadelphia, PA: Wolters Kluwer; 2015.
14. Perinatology.com. Focus Information Technology, Inc. Normal reference ranges and laboratory values in pregnancy. 2010–2015. Available at: http:/perinatology.com/Reference/Reference%20Ranges/Reference%20for%20Serum.htm. Accessed November 12, 2015.
15. Drugs.com [Internet] Prenatal Plus information from Drugs.com; c 2000–2015 [Revised June 2014; Cited November 12, 2015]. Available at: http://www.drugs.com/pro/prenatal-plus.htm. Accessed November 12, 2015.
16. March of Dimes [Internet]. Prescription drugs, over-the-counter drugs, supplements and herbal products; c 2015 [Revised July 2015; Cited November 28, 2015]. Available at: http://www.marchofdimes.org/pregnancy/prescription-drugs-over-the-counter-drugs-supplements-and-herbal-products.aspx. Accessed November 12, 2015.

17. 79 FR 72063-72103 (December 4, 2014).
18. Servey J, Chang J. Over-the counter medications in pregnancy. *Am Fam Physician* 2014;90(8):548–555.
19. March of Dimes [Internet]. Mood-altering drug use during pregnancy—the risks of medical marijuana and prescription opioids; c 2015. Available at: http://www.marchofdimes.org/mood-altering-drug-use-during-pregnancy-the-risks-of-medical-marijuana-and-prescription-opioids.aspx. Accessed November 12, 2015.
20. Abu-Saad K, Fraser D. Maternal nutrition and birth outcomes. *Epidemiol Rev.* 2010;32:5–25. doi:10.1093/epirev/mxq001.
21. Niebyl JR, Briggs GG. The pharmacological management of nausea and vomiting of pregnancy. *J Fam Pract* 2014;63(2 Suppl):S31–S37.
22. Tyler S, Nagtalon-Ramos J. Managing nausea and vomiting of pregnancy. *Women's Healthcare* 2015;3(2):7–13.
23. American College of Obstetrics and Gynecology. ACOG Practice Bulletin 153: Nausea and vomiting of pregnancy. *Obstet Gynecol* 2015;126(3):687–688. doi:10.1097/AOG.0000000000001048.
24. DeSisto CL, Kim SY, Sharma AJ. Prevalence estimates of gestational diabetes mellitus in the United States, Pregnancy Risk Assessment Monitoring System (PRAMS), 2007–2010. *Prev Chronic Dis* 2014;11:130415.
25. Gupta Y, Kalra B, Baruah MP, et al. Updated guidelines on screening for gestational diabetes. *Int J Womens Health* 2015;7:539–550.
26. Toiba R. Gestational diabetes. *Today's Dietitian* 2013;15(8):48.
27. American Diabetes Association. Standards of medical care in diabetes—2014. *Diabetes Care* 2014;37(Suppl 1):S14–S80.
28. National Institutes of Health Publication No. 12-4818. June 2012. Available at: https://www.nichd.nih.gov/publications/pubs/Documents/gestational_diabetes_2012.pdf. Accessed November 16, 2015.
29. Academy of Nutrition and Dietetics. GDM: Executive summary of recommendations (2008). Available at: https://www.andeal.org/topic.cfm?menu=5288&cat=3731. Accessed November 16, 2015.
30. Castorino K, Jovanovic L. Pregnancy and diabetes management: Advances and controversies. *Clin Chem* 2011;57(2):221–230.
31. García-Patterson A, Gich I, Amini SB, et al. Insulin requirements throughout pregnancy in women with type 1 diabetes mellitus: Three changes of direction. *Diabetologia* 2010;53:446–451.

32. English FA, Kenny LC, McCarthy FP. Risk factors and effective management of preeclampsia. *Integr Blood Press Control* 2015;8:7–12.
33. National Institute for Health and Care Excellence. Hypertension in pregnancy: Diagnosis and management. NICE Guidelines [CG107]. 2010. Available at: http://www.nice.org.uk/guidance/cg107/chapter/1-recommendations. Accessed November 18, 2015.
34. World Health Organization (WHO). WHO recommendations for prevention and treatment of pre-eclampsia and eclampsia. Geneva, Switzerland: WHO; 2011, 38 p. Available at: https://www.guideline.gov/content.aspx?id=39384#Section420. Accessed November 18, 2015.
35. National Heart, Lung, and Blood Institute. In Brief: Your guide to lowering your blood pressure with DASH (Publication No. 06-5834). 2006. Revised August 2015. Available at: https://www.nhlbi.nih.gov/files/docs/public/heart/dash_brief.pdf. Accessed November 18, 2015.

Notes

NOTES

NOTES

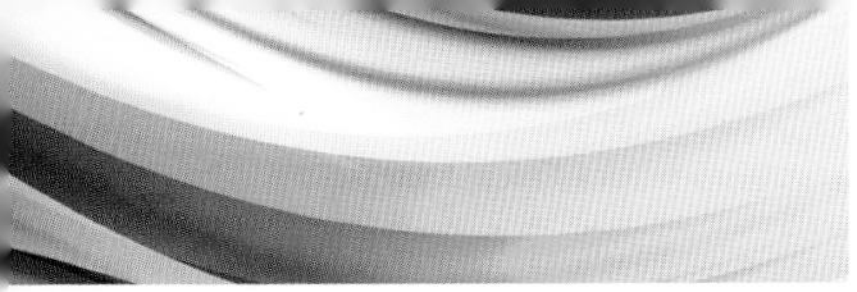

CHAPTER 3

Assessing Pediatric Patients

Ellen McCloy, MS, RDN

Nutrition assessment of the pediatric patient is unique in many ways. Nutrition screening is most useful in identifying high-risk infants, children, and adolescents in all settings of health care. Box 3.1 lists some "red flags" that warrant nutrition intervention in inpatient units, in outpatient clinics, or in the community setting. Box 3.2 lists some common classifications used when assessing infants.

BOX 3.1 Indicators of Need for Nutrition Assessment

Infants/NICU	Toddler/Child/Adolescent
≤37 weeks gestational age	Weight for length <10th percentile or BMI <10th percentile
Very low birth weight	Weight for length >95th percentile or BMI >95th percentile
Insufficient weight gain	Significant weight loss or gain
Nonstandard formula	Enteral or parenteral feeding
Formula concentrated to nonstandard dilution	Special diet
Food allergies/intolerances	Food allergies/intolerances

(continued)

BOX 3.1 Indicators of Need for Nutrition Assessment (*continued*)

Infants/NICU	Toddler/Child/Adolescent
Poor/inappropriate intake	Eating disorder
Malnutrition or at risk for malnutrition owing to diagnosis, comorbidities, social or economic status, etc.	Malnutrition or at risk for malnutrition owing to diagnosis, comorbidities, social or economic status, etc.
Inborn errors of metabolism	Omitting foods for religious reasoning
	Adolescent pregnancy

BOX 3.2 Infant Classification and Associated Terms

Classification	Parameters
Chronological or birth age	Time since birth (days, weeks, months)
Gestational age	Estimated time since conception or postconceptional age
Corrected age	Age adjusted for prematurity
Preterm infant	<37 weeks gestation
Full-term infant	37 to 42 weeks gestation
Postterm infant	>42 weeks gestation
Low birth weight	<2,500 g
Very low birth weight	<1,500 g
Extremely low birth weight	<1,000 g
Small for gestational age	Weight <10th percentile
Appropriate for gestational age	Weight ≥10th percentile and ≤90th percentile
Large for gestational age	Weight >90th percentile

Data from (i) Nevin-Folino N, ed. *Pediatric Manual of Clinical Dietetics*. 2nd ed. Chicago, IL: American Dietetic Association; 2003, and (ii) Davis A. *Pediatrics: Contemporary Nutrition Support Practice*. Philadelphia, PA: Saunders; 1998:356.

ANTHROPOMETRIC ASSESSMENT

Measurement of growth is essential for assessing the health and nutritional status of the pediatric patient. Serial measurements are best measures of growth and are more conclusive than isolated measurements. Below are the recommended anthropometric measurements to use based on age:

- **0 to 24 months**
  - Body weight
  - Recumbent length
  - Head circumference
  - Weight for length
- **2 to 18 years**
  - Body weight
  - Height
  - Waist circumference
  - Body mass index (BMI)

Weight

Weight should be obtained using consistency in technique and scales. Infants should be nude and without diaper. Children and adolescent patients should wear minimal clothing. Weight should be obtained to nearest 0.1 kg.

Length

Length is measured crown to heel. Recumbent length should be measured by use of a length board in infants aged birth to 24 months. Two people may be needed for this process. Standing height or stature, using a perpendicular stadiometer, should be measured in children aged 24 months and older who are able to stand. Measurement should be taken to nearest 0.5 cm. Knee/heel measurement may be used for older patients who are unable to stand (Table 3.1).

Head Circumference

Head circumference is measured at the largest frontal–occipital plate. Head circumference is a useful tool until about 3 years of age when head growth slows dramatically. Measurement should be taken to nearest 0.5 cm.

TABLE 3.1. Knee/Heel Measurement Equations

Stevenson method	Height = (2.69 × knee height) + 24.2 *Based on data obtained from children under 12 years of age with cerebral palsy*
Chumlea method	Male: Height = 64.19 – (0.04 × age) + (2.02 × knee height) Female: Height = 84.88 – (0.24 × age) + (1.83 × knee height) *Equations derived from recumbent knee height in the elderly*

Data from Bunting KD, Mills J, Ramsey E, et al. *Texas Children's Hospital Pediatric Nutrition Reference Guide*. 10th ed. Houston, TX: Texas Children's Hospital; 2013.

Body Mass Index 5 kg/m^2

The BMI for children and adolescents is unique, and it is not appropriate to use the adult BMI categories to interpret the value. BMI-for-age must be interpreted using the growth charts to compare age- and sex-specific percentile (see "Relevant Web Sites Relating to Growth Charts").

Waist Circumference

Waist circumference is measured midway between the top of the iliac crest and the lowermost portion of the rib cage. A nonstretchable measuring tape should be used. This measurement is most accurate if the patient has not recently consumed a large meal and is demonstrating normal expiration (not "sucking in").

Mid-Upper Arm Circumference

Mid-upper arm circumference (MUAC) is a valuable tool in the assessment of pediatric patients since, unlike other indicators, it can be used as an independent anthropometric assessment tool because normal values change little during early years. Measurements can be compared with the standards developed by the World Health Organization (WHO), or serial measurements can be used to monitor changes using the patient as his or her own control. The WHO standards can be found at http://www.who.int/childgrowth/standards/ac_for_age/en/.

Nutrition-Focused Physical Examination

Similar to the adult patient population, pediatric practitioners should conduct a nutrition-focused physical exam in addition to using data from the physical examination assessments conducted by other health care practitioners. See Tables 1.19 and 1.20 in Chapter 1 for nutrition-focused physical exam information.

EVALUATION OF GROWTH

Measurements should be plotted on growth charts and trends monitored. In 2010, the Centers for Disease Control and Prevention (CDC) adopted the WHO growth charts for children less than 24 months. The WHO growth charts are based on an international sample of healthy children living under optimal health conditions to support growth (single births, breast-fed, nonsmoking environment, etc.). Therefore, the WHO growth charts should be considered standard curves (or prescriptive) rather than reference (or descriptive) as were the CDC 2000 curves. The appropriate chart for age and gender should be used. In addition to standard growth charts, there are specialty growth charts for some select conditions. Tables 3.2 and 3.3 list interpretations of percentiles on the growth charts.

If using a standard growth chart for a preterm infant, postnatal age (age of infant calculated, in weeks, from the date of birth) needs to be corrected for gestational age (age of infant calculated, in weeks, from the date of conception,

TABLE 3.2. Interpretation of Height-for-Age and Weight-for-Age Plotted on Standard CDC Growth Charts

Percentile	Interpretation[a]
50th	Average for age
10th–90th	Healthy for most pediatric patients
3rd–10th or 90th–97th	Further investigation needed
<3rd or >97th	Unhealthy until proven otherwise

[a]If the patient plots higher or lower than expected potential, or if there are large changes in measurements, pathologic or nutritional factors should be considered. Further assessment may include consideration of parental height, growth velocity, bone age, pubertal status, and development.

TABLE 3.3. Interpretation of BMI-for-Age Plotted on Standard CDC Growth Charts

Percentile	Interpretation
<5th	Underweight
≥5th and <85th	Normal weight
≥85th and <95th	At risk of overweight
≥95th	Overweight

Data from BMI—Body Mass Index: About BMI for Children and Teens. Available at: http://www.cdc.gov/nccdphp/dnpa/bmi/childrens_BMI/about_childrens_BMI.htm. Accessed December 16, 2006.

determined by ultrasound examination) until at least 24 months of age.[1] Box 3.3 gives an example of calculating gestation-adjusted age.

As the mode of feeding (breast-fed vs. formula-fed) influences trends, it is important to note that formula-fed infants will plot differently on the WHO charts. Whereas breast-fed infants have a higher growth velocity in the first 3 months of life, more formula-fed infants may be identified

BOX 3.3 Gestation-Adjusted Age for Preterm Infants

Adjustment for Prematurity = 40 weeks (full term) – gestational age at birth (in weeks)

Gestation-Adjusted Age = postnatal age – adjustment for prematurity

Example: Michael was born March 1, 2006. His gestational age at birth was determined to be 30 weeks based on ultrasound examination. At the time of his admission into the hospital on May 24, 2006, his postnatal age was 12 weeks. Based on the previous equations, what is his gestation-adjusted age?

Adjustment for Prematurity = 40 weeks – 30 weeks = 10 weeks

Gestation-Adjusted Age = 12 weeks – 10 weeks = 2 weeks

If this were plotted on a standard WHO growth chart, anthropometric measurements would be plotted for a 2-week-old infant.

as low weight-for-age during this time. After this time, there is a slower rise in weight, and so fewer 6- to 23-month-old children may be identified as low weight. Differences in length for age are small, and so significant clinical differences are not expected.[2]

Relevant Web Sites Relating to Growth Charts

- Standard WHO growth charts for infants and children under the age of 2 and CDC growth charts (including BMI-for-age) can be accessed at http://www.cdc.gov/growthcharts.
- The WHO multicultural growth charts for ages 0 to 5 years can be accessed at http://www.who.int/childgrowth/standards/en/.
- Premature infant growth charts can be found in the following publication: Fenton TR, Kim JH. A systematic review and meta-analysis to revise the Fenton growth chart for

preterm infants. *BMC Pediatr* 2013;13:59. Available at: http://www.ncbi.nlm.nih.gov/pmc/articles/PMC3637477/

- Growth chart for children with cerebral palsy can be accessed at http://www.kennedykrieger.org/kki_misc.jsp?pid=2694.
- Growth chart for children with Down syndrome can be found in the following publication: Zemel BS, Pipan M, Stallings VA, Hall W, Schadt K, Freedman DS, Thorpe P. Growth Charts for Children with Down Syndrome in the United States. *Pediatrics* 2015;136:5. Available at: http://pediatrics.aappublications.org/content/136/5/e1204

ASSESSMENT OF WEIGHT CHANGES

Newborn weight loss is expected after birth secondary to body composition shifts and total body water decrease. Normal weight loss is 7% to 10% of birth weight in term infants. A preterm infant may lose ≤15% of birth weight. An infant born at extremely low birth weight may lose ≤20% of birth weight. Birth weight should be regained by the second week of life.[3] Weight typically doubles by 5 to 6 months of age and triples by 12 months. Weight is typically affected during acute periods of undernutrition and will be examined later in this chapter.

Usual Body Weight

Usual body weight (UBW) is useful in assessing weight status:

$$\% \text{ UBW} = (\text{actual weight}/\text{usual weight}) \times 100$$

$$\% \text{ Weight change} = [(\text{actual} - \text{usual weight})/\text{usual weight}] \times 100$$

Significant weight loss:

- >2% in 1 week
- >5% in 1 month
- >7.5% in 3 months
- >10% in 6 months

GROWTH VELOCITY

Height or weight velocity measures the change in measurement over time. Alterations in normal growth velocity indicate need for further investigation.

$$\text{Velocity} = \frac{\text{height (cm) or weight (g) at Time 2} - \text{height (cm) or weight (g) at Time 1}}{\text{Time 2 (month or day)} - \text{Time 1 (month or day)}}$$

Example: At her 4-month well-baby visit, Stephanie weighed 5.8 kg and was 60 cm long. At her 6-month well-baby visit, she weighed 6.5 kg and was 64 cm long. Based on the equation, what is Stephanie's height and weight growth velocity? ***Note:*** It is best to use actual days old for the weight velocity calculation, but if this data are not readily available, it is acceptable to estimate how old the child is, in days, by using 30 days/month.

Weight velocity in grams per day =

$$\frac{6{,}500\text{ g} - 5{,}800\text{ g}}{180\text{ days old (6 months)} - 120\text{ days old (4 months)}}$$

$$= \frac{700\text{ g}}{60\text{ days old}}$$

$$= 11.67\text{ g/day}$$

Height velocity in centimeters per week

$$= \frac{63.5\text{ cm} - 60\text{ cm}}{24\text{ weeks} - 16\text{ weeks}}$$

$$= \frac{3.5\text{ cm}}{8\text{ weeks}}$$

$$= 0.44\text{ cm/week}$$

According to Table 3.4, both weight and height growth velocity are within the ideal range of average growth between 3 and 6 months of age (Table 3.5 lists normal growth velocity values for children aged 2 to 10 years).

TABLE 3.4. Average Normal Growth Velocity for Children Aged 0–24 mo

Age	Weight (g/d)	Length (cm/wk)
Preemie <2 kg	15–20 g/kg/d	0.8–1.1
Preemie >2 kg	20–30	0.8–1.1
<4 mo	23–34	0.8–0.93
4–8 mo	10–16	0.37–0.47
8–12 mo	6–11	0.28–0.37
12–16 mo	5–9	0.24–0.33
16–20 mo	4–9	0.21–0.29
20–24 mo	4–9	0.19–0.26

Data from (i) Bunting KD, Mills J, Ramsey E, et al. *Texas Children's Hospital Pediatric Nutrition Reference Guide*. 10th ed. Houston, TX: Texas Children's Hospital; 2013, and (ii) Ekvall S, Bandini L, Ekvall V. *Pediatric Nutrition in Chronic Disease and Developmental Disorders*. Oxford, UK: Oxford University Press; 2005:140.

TABLE 3.5. Average Normal Growth Velocity for Children Aged 2–10 yr

Age (yr)	Weight (g/d)	Length (cm/mo)
2–3	4–10	0.7–1.1
4–6	5–8	0.5–0.8
7–10	5–12	0.4–0.6

Data from Fomon SJ, Haschke F, Ziegler EE, et al. Body composition of reference children from birth to age 10 years. *Am J Clin Nutr* 1982;35:1169–1175.

ESTIMATING NUTRIENT NEEDS

Fluid Needs

Fluid needs may be estimated using the formula in Table 3.6, or by using body surface area:[4]

$$\text{Fluid needs} = 1{,}500 \text{ mL fluid/m}^2\text{/day}$$

Example: John weighs 15 kg. Using the equation in Table 3.7, what is his body surface area in m^2?

$$\text{Body surface area (m}^2) = (15 \text{ kg} \times 0.03) + 0.2 = 0.45 + 0.2 = 0.65 \text{ m}^2$$

Based on the calculated body surface area, what are John's fluid requirements?

$$\text{Fluid needs} = 1{,}500 \text{ mL} \times 0.65 \text{ m}^2 = 975 \text{ mL/day}$$

Energy and Protein Needs

In the pediatric population, as in the adult, a variety of methods are used to estimate energy and protein needs. Tables 3.8 and 3.9 provide commonly used methods. These methods are based on values determined for the pediatric population who display normal body composition, metabolism, and activity level.

TABLE 3.6. Baseline Fluid Requirements

Weight (kg)	Fluid Needs
1–10	100 mL/kg
11–20	1,000 mL + 50 mL/kg for each kg >10 kg
>20	1,500 mL + 20 mL/kg for each kg >20 kg

Data from Engorn B, Flerlage J. *Harriet Lane Handbook*. 20th ed. Philadelphia, PA: Saunders; 2014.

TABLE 3.7. Calculating Body Surface Area (m^2)

Weight (kg)	Body Surface Area (m^2)
<5	kg × 0.05 + 0.05
5–10	kg × 0.04 + 0.1
10–20	kg × 0.03 + 0.2
20–40	kg × 0.02 + 0.4
>40	kg × 0.01 + 0.8

The use of basal energy metabolism is useful in estimating the energy needs of compromised infants and children.

kcal/day = Basal Metabolic Rate × Activity Factor × Stress Factor

TABLE 3.8. Estimated Energy and Protein Requirements

Category	Age	Reference Weight (kg)	DRI kcal/kg	Pro g/kg
Infants (mo)	0–2	N/A	—	1.52
	2–3	6	102	1.52
	7–12	9	80	1.2
	13–35	12	82	1.08
Boys (yr)	3	12	85	1.08
	4–5	20	70	0.95
	6–7	20	64	0.95
	8	20	59	0.95
Girls (yr)	3	12	82	1.08
	4–5	20	65	0.95
	6–7	20	61	0.95
	8	20	59	0.95
Boys (yr)	9–11	36	49	0.94
	12–13	36	44	0.94
Girls (yr)	14–16	61	39	0.85
	17–18	61	37	0.85
	>18	70	36	0.8
	9–11	37	42	0.92
	12–13	37	40	0.92
	14–16	54	33	0.85
	17–18	54	31	0.85
	>18	57	34	0.8

Data from (i) Bunting KD, Mills J, Ramsey E, et al. *Texas Children's Hospital Pediatric Nutrition Reference Guide*. 10th ed. Houston, TX: Texas Children's Hospital; 2013, and (ii) Otten J, Pitz H, Meyers L. *Dietary Reference Intakes: The Essential Guide to Nutrition Requirements*. Washington, DC: National Academy Press; 2006.

TABLE 3.9. Dietary Reference Intakes of Estimated Energy Requirement (EER)

Sex and Age	Calculation of Estimated Energy Requirements	Physical Activity (PA) Coefficient Based on Physical Activity Level (PAL)
All infants and toddlers		
0–3 mo	(89 × wt [kg] – 100) + 175	N/A
4–6 mo	(89 × wt [kg] – 100) + 56	N/A
7–12 mo	(89 × wt [kg] – 100) + 22	N/A
13–35 mo	(89 × wt [kg] – 100) + 20	N/A
Boys 3–8 years	EER = 88.5 – 61.9 × age [y] + PA × (26.7 × wt [kg] + 903 × ht [m]) + 20	PA = 1.0 if PAL is estimated to be ≥1 <1.4 (sedentary) PA = 1.13 if PAL is estimated to be ≥1.4 <1.6 (low active)
Boys 9–18 years	EER = 88.5 – 61.9 × age [y] + PA × (26.7 × wt [kg] + 903 × ht [m]) + 25	PA = 1.26 if PAL is estimated to be ≥1.6 <1.9 (active) PA = 1.42 if PAL is estimated to be ≥1.9 <2.5 (very active)
Girls 3–8 years	EER = 135.3 – 30.8 × age [y] + PA × (10 × wt [kg] + 934 × ht [m]) + 20	PA = 1.0 if PAL is estimated to be ≥1 <1.4 (sedentary)
Girls 9–18 years	EER = 135.3 – 30.8 × age [y] + PA × (10 × wt [kg] + 934 × ht [m]) + 25	PA = 1.16 if PAL is estimated to be ≥1.4 <1.6 (low active)

(continued)

TABLE 3.9. Dietary Reference Intakes of Estimated Energy Requirement (EER) (*continued*)

Sex and Age	Calculation of Estimated Energy Requirements	Physical Activity (PA) Coefficient Based on Physical Activity Level (PAL)
		PA = 1.31 if PAL is estimated to be ≥1.6 <1.9 (active) PA = 1.56 if PAL is estimated to be ≥1.9 <2.5 (very active)

Data from Otten J, Pitz H, Meyers L. *Dietary Reference Intakes: The Essential Guide to Nutrition Requirements*. Washington, DC: National Academy Press; 2006.

See Tables 3.10 to 3.12 for equations to estimate basal metabolic rate (BMR), as well as common activity and stress factors.

Estimating Energy Needs for Catch-up Growth

For patients who are malnourished or for those whose growth is compromised, the nutritional goal is to accelerate growth. This increase in normal weight and height velocity is referred to as "catch-up growth." Catch-up growth is optimal to facilitate normalized weight and height. Total energy needs for catch-up growth may be as high as 150% of expected needs.

General Method of Estimating Energy Needs for Catch-up Growth[2]:

$$\text{kcal/kg/day}^{*} = \frac{\text{IBW in kg (50th percentile wt/ht)} \times \text{kcal/kg/day (DRI for age)}}{\text{Actual weight (kg)}}$$

where, IBW, ideal body weight; DRI, dietary reference intake.

*Note that protein needs for catch-up growth are calculated using the same formula by substituting DRI of kcal (kcal/kg/day) with DRI of protein (g/kg/day).

TABLE 3.10. Schofield Method to Estimate BMR

Age (yr)	Male	Female
0–3	(0.167 × wt) + (15.174 × ht) – 617.6	(16.252 × wt) + (10.23 × ht) – 413.5
3–10	(19.59 × wt) + (1.303 × ht) + 414.9	(16.969 × wt) + (1.618 × ht) + 371.2
10–18	(16.25 × wt) + (1.372 × ht) + 515.5	(8.365 × wt) + (4.65 × ht) + 200
>18	(15.057 × wt) – (1.004 × ht) + 705.8	(13.623 × wt) + (2.83 × ht) + 98.2

Data from Bunting KD, Mills J, Ramsey E, et al. *Texas Children's Hospital Pediatric Nutrition Reference Guide*. 10th ed. Houston, TX: Texas Children's Hospital; 2013.

TABLE 3.11. Activity Factors

Condition	Factor
Ambulatory	1.2–1.3
Confined to bed	1.1
Paralyzed	1.0

TABLE 3.12. Stress Factors

Condition	Factor
Burn	1.5–2.5
Growth failure	1.5–2.0
Infection	1.2–1.6
Starvation	0.70
Surgery	1.2–1.5
Trauma	1.1–1.8

Data from Page C, Hardin T, Melnik G. *Nutritional Assessment and Support*. Baltimore, MD: Williams & Wilkins; 1994.

Example: Andrea is 5 years and 6 months old. She weighs 13 kg (<5th percentile) and is 106 cm tall (between the 10th and 25th percentiles). Using the standard CDC growth chart, what is Andrea's ideal body weight for her height?

$$\begin{aligned}\text{IBW in kg} &= \text{50th percentile BMI} \times \text{height (in meters)}^2 \\ &= 15.2 \times 1.06^2 \\ &= 17.1 \text{ kg}\end{aligned}$$

Using the general equation for catch-up growth, how many kilocalories per kilogram per day does Andrea require?

kcal/kg/day =

$$\frac{17.1 \text{ kg (IBW for height)} \times 65 \text{ (DRI for girls age } 4-5)}{13 \text{ kg (actual weight)}}$$

$$= 86 \text{ kcal/kg/day}$$

How many total kilocalories per day does Andrea require?

$$86 \text{ kcal/kg} \times 13 \text{ kg} = 1{,}471 \text{ kcal/day for catch-up growth}$$

MacLean Method for Estimating Energy Needs for Catch-up Growth

kcal/kg/day =

$$\frac{120 \text{ kcal /kg } \text{ IBW in kg (50th \%tile weight for height)}}{\text{actual weight (kg)}}$$

Example: Andrea is 5 years and 6 months old. She weighs 13 kg (<5th percentile) and is 106 cm tall (between the 10th and 25th percentiles). Using the standard CDC growth chart, what is Andrea's ideal body weight for her height?

IBW in kg = weight at the 50th percentile BMI = 17.1 kg

Using the MacLean equation for catch-up growth, how many kilocalories per kilogram per day does Andrea require?

$$\text{kcal/kg/day} = \frac{120 \text{ kcal/kg} \ \ 17.2 \text{ kg (IBW for height)}}{13 \text{ kg (actual weight)}}$$

$$= 157 \text{ kcal/kg/day}$$

How many total kilocalories per day does Andrea require?

$$157 \text{ kcal/kg} \times 13 \text{ kg} = 2{,}041 \text{ kcal/day for catch-up growth}$$

Children with Developmental Disabilities

Table 3.13 lists methods for estimating energy needs of children with developmental disabilities.

TABLE 3.13. Estimating Energy Needs for Children with Developmental Disabilities

Diagnosis	Calorie Needs
Cerebral Palsy (Age 5–11 Years Old)	
Mild to moderate activity	13.9 kcal/cm ht
Severe physical restrictions	11.1 kcal/cm ht
Athetoid cerebral palsy	Up to 6,000 kcal/d
Down Syndrome (Age 5–12 Years Old)	
Males	16.1 kcal/cm ht
Females	14.3 kcal/cm ht
Myelomeningocele (Spina Bifida)	
Weight maintenance requirements	9–11 kcal/cm ht
Weight loss requirements	7 kcal/cm
>1 year old	~50% DRI/RDA for age
Prader–Willi Syndrome	
Weight maintenance requirements	10–11 kcal/cm ht
Weight loss requirements	8.5 kcal/cm ht

DRI, dietary reference intake.

Data from (i) Ekvall S, Bandini L, Ekvall V. *Pediatric Nutrition in Chronic Disease and Developmental Disorders*. Oxford, UK: Oxford University Press; 2005:140, and (ii) Davis A. *Pediatrics: Contemporary Nutrition Support Practice*. Philadelphia, PA: Saunders; 1998:356.

Vitamins and Minerals

A few key micronutrients require special attention in the assessment of the pediatric population.

- Iron: The combination of rapid growth and relatively low iron intake places children at risk for iron-deficiency anemia. Adolescent females and those who partake in high levels of activity are also at risk. This can be prevented with appropriate feeding choices. If iron deficiency is suspected, it should be confirmed with laboratory testing. The following are laboratory values to consider: hemoglobin, hematocrit, mean corpuscular volume, ferritin, serum iron, and total iron-binding capacity.
- Vitamin D: Exclusively breast-fed infants should receive a vitamin D supplement of 400 international units (IU) per day in the first few days of life. Supplementation for compromised children and adolescents who do not get regular exposure to sunlight may also be indicated, and needs may be above the recommended dietary allowance (RDA) of 600 IU.[9]
- Zinc: Some studies show that infants and children are at risk for zinc deficiency because of altered absorption of the nutrient. It is important to assess dietary intake of sources of zinc. These sources are meat, eggs, legumes, and whole grains.
- Fluoride: Fluoride is necessary for reduction of dental decay. If using bottled water, it may or may not contain fluoride; therefore, individual products need to be investigated. Recommendation of a supplement depends on the assessment of a child's total daily fluoride intake based on fluid sources. From 0 to 6 months of age, no supplementation is required. After 6 months of age, supplementation amount should be based on the child's total fluoride exposure.[9]
- Calcium: Adequate calcium intake in all children and adolescents is required for optimum growth, prevention of future skeletal abnormalities, and bone weakness. Dairy and nondairy sources of calcium need to be evaluated. For those whose intake is deficient, education regarding sources of calcium should be complete. Supplementation may be considered if deemed necessary by clinical judgment.

A comprehensive list of standard DRIs for vitamins and elements can be found at https://ods.od.nih.gov/Health_Information/Dietary_Reference_Intakes.aspx

Supplementation

Routine vitamin and mineral supplementation is unnecessary for the normal, healthy child older than 1 year. The following is a list of individuals who are at risk. Supplementation should be considered for these patients (see Table 3.14).

- Infants with malabsorption and liver or pancreatic disease
- Children and adolescents from deprived families or children who experience neglect or abuse
- Children and adolescents with anorexia or inadequate appetites
- Children with chronic disease
- Children following dietary regimens for weight loss
- Pregnant teenagers
- Children or adolescents who omit any one food group from their diet

Fiber

Table 3.15 lists fiber recommendations for children and adolescents.

TABLE 3.14. Common Vitamin/Mineral Supplements[a]

Supplement	Age Group (yr)	Daily Dose
Poly-Vi-Sol (with or without iron)	0–3	1 mL
Tri-Vi-Sol (with or without iron)	0–3	1 mL
Nano VM	1–3	2 packets
Nano VM	4–8	2 packets
Nano VM T/F	9–18	41 mL
Centrum kids (complete)	2–3	½ tablet
	≥4	1 tablet

(*continued*)

TABLE 3.14. Common Vitamin/Mineral Supplements[a] (continued)

Supplement	Age Group (yr)	Daily Dose
Flintstones (complete)	2–3	½ tablet
	≥4	1 tablet
Vitamax Pediatric Liquid	<1	1 mL
	1–3	2 mL
Vitamax Chewable	4–11	1 tablet
	>11	2 tablets

[a]Check hospital formulary for available supplements. Please note that mineral and vitamin contents vary among products. Refer to manufacturer for complete listing of contents. Many generic MVIs are available and chosen by consumers; these are typically equal to national brand unless found otherwise.

Data from (i) Nevin-Folino N, ed. *Pediatric Manual of Clinical Dietetics*. 2nd ed. Chicago, IL: American Dietetic Association; 2003, and (ii) Bunting KD, Mills J, Ramsey E, et al. *Texas Children's Hospital Pediatric Nutrition Reference Guide*. 10th ed. Houston, TX: Texas Children's Hospital; 2013.

TABLE 3.15. Fiber Requirements in Children Through Adolescents

Age (yr)	Fiber/d (g)
1–3	19
4–8	25
Girls 9–13	26
Boys 9–13	31
Girls 14–18	26
Boys 14–18	38

Data from Bunting KD, Mills J, Ramsey E, et al. *Texas Children's Hospital Pediatric Nutrition Reference Guide*. 10th ed. Houston, TX: Texas Children's Hospital; 2013.

GUIDELINES FOR COMPLETING DIETARY ASSESSMENT

In addition to any information available in the medical record, a thorough dietary history should be gathered by means of interviewing any and all caregivers and/or patients when appropriate. The accuracy of information will be highly variable and is dependent on the skill of the interviewer as well as on the data collection method. Some important areas of focus include but are not limited to the following:

- Maternal, prenatal, and postnatal history (exposure of toxic agents, medications, infections, maternal nutrition, length of pregnancy, etc.)
- Birth weight and weight history
- Feeding history (duration of breast-feeding, type of formula, age at introduction to solid foods)
- Typical eating habits, food preferences, amounts (use visual models as needed), frequency of consumption
- Chewing and swallowing function
- Past or present gastrointestinal problems (gastroesophageal reflux disease [GERD], history of feeding disorders, nausea, vomiting, diarrhea, constipation)
- Number of caregivers and households involved in child's care
- Food and/or formula preparation, including location, methods, and sanitation habits
- Sleep habits
- Food allergies/intolerances
- Necessary feeding aids, or special utensils or nipples
- Access to and use of community resources

NORMAL FEEDING GUIDELINES

Tables 3.16 and 3.17 list feeding guidelines for infants, toddlers, and adolescents.

BREAST-FEEDING

The American Academy of Pediatrics supports breast-feeding as the preferred method of feeding for all infants, including premature newborns (Box 3.4). Breast-feeding is recommended for the first year of life or as long as desired or feasible. Exclusive breast-feeding will provide adequate nutrition until approximately 6 months of age. This is the point at which complementary foods should be offered.[9]

TABLE 3.16. Feeding Guidelines for Infants 0–12 Months Old

	Breast Milk and/or Fortified Infant Formula	Cereal, Bread, Grains, and Starches	Fruits and Vegetables	Meats and Other Protein-Rich Foods
Birth–4 mo	8–12 feedings 2–6 oz/feeding (18–32 oz/d)	None	None	None
4–6 mo	4–6 feedings 4–6 oz/feeding (27–45 oz/d)	None	None	None
6–8 mo	3–5 feedings 6–8 oz/feeding (24–32 oz/d)	2–3 servings of iron-fortified infant cereal, soft cooked breads and starches (serving = 1–2 Tbsp)	Introduce plain, cooked, mashed, or strained infant vegetables and fruits. Avoid meat-containing dinners. 2–4 oz 100% fruit juice in cup.	Begin to offer plain, cooked, pureed meats. Avoid combination dinners.

8–10 mo	3–4 feedings 7–8 oz/feeding (24–32 oz/d)	2–3 servings of iron-fortified infant cereal, soft cooked breads and starches (serving = 1–2 Tbsp)	2–3 servings of soft, cut-up, and mashed vegetables and fruits (serving = 1–2 Tbsp). 3–4 oz 100% fruit juices in cup.	Offer plain, well-cooked, soft, finely cut, or pureed meats, cheeses, and casseroles
10–12 mo	24–32 oz/d	4 servings of iron-fortified infant cereal, soft cooked breads and starches (serving = 1–2 Tbsp)	4 servings of soft, cut-up, and mashed vegetables and fruits (serving = 1–2 Tbsp). 3–4 oz 100% fruit juices in cup.	1–2 oz of soft, finely cut, or chopped meat or other protein foods

Data from (i) Bunting KD, Mills J, Ramsey E, et al. *Texas Children's Hospital Pediatric Nutrition Reference Guide*. 10th ed. Houston, TX: Texas Children's Hospital; 2013, and (ii) Becker PJ, Carney LN, Corkins MR, et al. Consensus statement of the Academy of Nutrition and Dietetics/American Society for Parenteral and Enteral Nutrition: Indicators recommended for the identification and documentation of pediatric malnutrition (undernutrition). *J Acad Nutr Diet* 2014;114:1988–2000.

TABLE 3.17. Feeding Guidelines for Toddlers to Adolescents

	Milk and Milk Products	Cereal, Bread, Grains, and Starches	Fruits and Vegetables	Meats and Other Protein-Rich Foods	Fats and Oils	Sweets, Jellies, Jams, Soft Drinks
12–23 mo	2 cups/d (whole milk or milk products)	2 oz/d (1 oz equivalent = 1 slice whole grain bread, ½ cup cooked cereal, rice or pasta, 1 cup dry cereal)	1¾ cup/d (1 cup raw or cooked fruit or vegetable or 1 cup fruit or vegetable juice or ½ cup dried fruit, 2 cups raw leafy greens)	1.5 oz/d (1 oz beef, poultry, or fish; ¼ cup cooked beans; 1 egg; 1 Tbsp peanut butter; ½ oz nuts)	Do not restrict	Provide small amount if desired
2–3 years[a]	2–2.5 cups/d (1 cup milk, 1.5 oz natural cheese, 2 oz processed cheese, 1/3 cup shredded cheese)	3 oz/d (1 oz equivalent = 1 slice whole grain bread, ½ cup cooked cereal, rice or pasta, 1 cup dry cereal)	2 cups/d (1 cup raw or cooked fruit or vegetable or 1 cup fruit or vegetable juice or ½ cup dried fruit, 2 cups raw leafy greens)	2 oz/d (1 oz beef, poultry, or fish; ¼ cup cooked beans; 1 egg; 1 Tbsp peanut butter; ½ oz nuts)	3 teaspoons/d (1 teaspoon oil, margarine, butter, or mayonnaise; 1 Tbsp salad dressing; sour cream or light mayonnaise)	165–170 discretionary calories

4–8 years	2.5–3 cups/d (1 cup milk, 1.5 oz natural cheese, 2 oz processed cheese, 1/3 cup shredded cheese)	4–5 oz/d (1 oz equivalent = 1 slice whole grain bread, ½ cup cooked cereal, rice or pasta, 1 cup dry cereal)	2½— 3 cups/d (1 cup raw or cooked fruit or vegetable or 1 cup fruit or vegetable juice or ½ cup dried fruit, 2 cups raw leafy greens)	3–4 oz/d (1 oz beef, poultry, or fish; ¼ cup cooked beans; 1 egg; 1 Tbsp peanut butter; ½ oz nuts)	4 teaspoons/d (1 teaspoon oil, margarine, butter, or mayonnaise; 1 Tbsp salad dressing; sour cream or light mayonnaise)	170–195 discretionary calories
9–13 years	3 cups/d (1 cup milk, 1.5 oz natural cheese, 2 oz processed cheese, 1/3 cup shredded cheese)	5–6 oz/d (1 oz equivalent = 1 slice whole grain bread, ½ cup cooked cereal, rice or pasta, 1 cup dry cereal)	3½—4 cups/d (1 cup raw or cooked fruit or vegetable or 1 cup fruit or vegetable juice or ½ cup dried fruit, 2 cups raw leafy greens)	5 oz/d (1 oz beef, poultry, or fish; ¼ cup cooked beans; 1 egg; 1 Tbsp peanut butter; ½ oz nuts)	5 teaspoons/d (1 teaspoon oil, margarine, butter, or mayonnaise; 1 Tbsp salad dressing; sour cream or light mayonnaise)	Limit amount, use sparingly (130–140 discretionary calories)

(*continued*)

TABLE 3.17. Feeding Guidelines for Toddlers to Adolescents (*continued*)

	Milk and Milk Products	Cereal, Bread, Grains, and Starches	Fruits and Vegetables	Meats and Other Protein-Rich Foods	Fats and Oils	Sweets, Jellies, Jams, Soft Drinks
14–18 years	3 cups/d (1 cup milk, 1.5 oz natural cheese, 2 oz processed cheese, 1/3 cup shredded cheese)	6–7 oz/d (1 oz equivalent = 1 slice whole grain bread, ½ cup cooked cereal, rice or pasta, 1 cup dry cereal)	3½—5 cups/d (1 cup raw or cooked fruit or vegetable or 1 cup fruit or vegetable juice or ½ cup dried fruit, 2 cups raw leafy greens)	5–6 oz/d (1 oz beef, poultry, or fish; ¼ cup cooked beans; 1 egg; 1 Tbsp peanut butter; ½ oz nuts)	5–6 teaspoons/d (1 teaspoon oil, margarine, butter, or mayonnaise; 1 Tbsp salad dressing; sour cream or light mayonnaise)	Limit amount, use sparingly (265–650 discretionary calories)

[a]Some foods are considered choking hazards to the developing toddler and should be avoided until the child is >3 years old. Such foods are peanut butter, hot dogs, grapes, hard pieces of fruit and vegetables, and tough or chewy meats.

Data from Bunting KD, Mills J, Ramsey E, et al. *Texas Children's Hospital Pediatric Nutrition Reference Guide*. 10th ed. Houston, TX: Texas Children's Hospital; 2013.

BOX 3.4 Breast-feeding Benefits and Contraindications

Benefits of Breast-feeding

Breast milk contains the most complete nutrition composition in terms of fat, carbohydrate, and protein.
There is optimal growth associated with breast-feeding.
Protein quality differs from that of cow's milk, making human milk better tolerated.
Calcium and phosphorus are more bioavailable than those found in milk formulas.
Many factors in human milk enhance maturity of the digestive tract.
Breast-feeding has been proven to reduce the risk of infection.
Decreased risk of over feeding
Breast-feeding has been shown to enhance cognitive and motor skill development.
Reduced costs by eliminating formula
Reduced risk of premenopausal breast cancer in the infant's mother
Increased mother/infant bonding
Aids in postpartum weight loss and uterine involution

Contraindications of Breast-feeding[a]

Infants with galactosemia
Infants with other inborn errors of metabolism, unless as directed by physician
Mothers infected with HIV
Mothers with herpetic lesion of the breast or other abscesses
Mothers receiving chemotherapy
Mothers with substance abuse
Mothers with untreated syphilis

[a]Refer to pharmaceutical reference when determining safety of maternal medications in relation to breast-feeding.

ASSESSMENT OF ADEQUACY OF FEEDINGS

- Monitor infant's growth and weight losses and gains.
- Monitor stooling and urine output.
- By the third day of life, breast-fed infants should produce
  - approximately 6 wet diapers/day.[3]

- approximately 3 stools/day. Stool consistency should progress from meconium to greenish-yellow to yellow and seedy.[3]
- Recommended feeding schedule:
  - At least 8 to 12 feedings/24 hour. Typically, every 1½ to 3 hour during first few weeks of life. Feed 10 to 20 minutes per breast during each feeding.[3]

Human milk contains approximately 20 kcal/oz. If it is determined that the infant is not obtaining adequate kilocalories from the breast milk, the milk may be fortified to a higher caloric density using human milk fortifier or standard formula powder (Table 3.18).

INFANT FORMULAS

Commercial infant formulas provide adequate kilocalories, protein, fat, vitamins, and minerals to those infants who are not breast-fed. Infant formulas are available in ready-to-feed, concentrated, or powdered forms. Most infants thrive on a standard cow's milk-based formula. However, if intolerance or allergy occurs, alternative formulas are available. Table 3.19 lists common types of infant formulas, and Table 3.20 shows standard formula preparation.

TABLE 3.18. Increasing Caloric Density of Human Breast Milk (by Adding Powdered Formula to 100 mL of Expressed Breast Milk)

Desired Caloric Concentration (kcal/oz)	Similac Advance Powder (g)	Enfamil Infant Powder (g)	Similac NeoSure Advance Powder (g)	Enfamil EnfaCare Powder (g)
22	1.3	1.3	1.3	1.4
24	2.5	2.6	2.6	2.7
27	4.4	4.5	4.6	4.7
30	6.3	6.4	6.5	6.8

TABLE 3.19. Common Types of Infant Formulas[a]

Type of Formulas	Indications	Examples[b]
Cow's milk-based	The standard type of formula traditionally used. The distribution of nutrients is similar to that of breast milk. Most are iron fortified. Contains 19–20 kcal/oz (dependent on brand)	• Enfamil Infant • Good Start Gentle • Good Start Supreme DHA and ARA • Good Start Essentials • Similac Advance (all may be available in lactose-free or other versions)
Soy-based	Standard formula derived from soy protein rather than from bovine milk protein. Used in patients with milk protein allergy. It should be noted that many infants who have milk protein allergy may also present with soy protein allergy. Contains 19–20 kcal/oz (dependent on brand).	• Enfamil ProSobee • Gerber Good Start Soy • Similac Soy Isomil
Formulas for low birth weight babies	Increased caloric density and/or mineral concentration for premature infants.	• Enfamil EnfaCare (22 kcal/oz) • Enfamil Premature (20 kcal/oz or 24 kcal/oz) • Similac Expert Care NeoSure (22 kcal/oz) • Similac Special Care Advance (20 or 24 kcal/oz)

(*continued*)

TABLE 3.19. Common Types of Infant Formulas[a] *(continued)*

Type of Formulas	Indications	Examples[b]
Protein hydrolysate	Formulas containing hydrolyzed proteins that are easier to digest. Indicated for use in infants who are not tolerating standard milk or soy formulas. Many contain additional medium-chain triglyceride (MCT) oil for infants with compromised gastrointestinal function. 20 kcal/oz.	• Similac Alimentum • Nutramigen • Pregestimil • Gerber Extensive HA
Free amino acids	Indicated for infants with extreme allergies to intact proteins. 20 kcal/oz.	• Neocate • EleCare
Follow-up formulas	Iron-fortified formulas for toddlers who may be in need of higher iron or more nutrient-dense fluid source than whole milk.	• Enfagrow Toddler Transitions • Enfamil Toddler Next Step • Good Start Graduates Gentle • Similac Go & Grow Stage 3

[a]Please note that the above list is not complete and does not contain all infant formulas available. Refer to product labels or manufacturers' references for nutrient values and ingredients.

[b]The manufacturers have copyrighted the terms "Lipil" and "Advance" to indicate the inclusion of docosahexaenoic (DHA) and arachidonic acid (ARA) polyunsaturated fatty acids.

TABLE 3.20. Standard Formula Preparation 19–20 kcal/oz (Calories Vary by Brand, Preparation Does Not Vary by Brand)

Concentrate	Powder	Ready to Feed
13 fl oz concentrate (1 can) + 13 fl oz water = 26 oz total formula	1 scoop powder + 2 fl oz water = 2 fl oz formula	Do not add water

TABLE 3.21. Increasing Formula Calories Based on Patient Goals

Goal	Adjustment to Formula
Increase overall nutrient density (most common)	Concentrate and/or add carbohydrate or fat modular
Increase caloric density only	Add carbohydrate and/or fat modular
Increase protein density only	Add modular protein supplement

If nutrition assessment indicates the need for a higher calorie formula, the formula recipe can be modified to concentrate more kilocalories into the same amount of total formula. When concentrating formulas, symptoms of intolerance may occur because of increased osmolality and renal solute load. Table 3.21 shows methods of increasing kilocalories of formulas. The patient's goals need to be considered before making any changes to a formula. When formulas are concentrated to >20 kcal/oz, all nutrients are concentrated unless a modular supplement is added.

PEDIATRIC FORMULAS

There are many formulas designed to meet the needs of children >1 year (Table 3.22). Many products can be used as both enteral feeding and oral supplementation when required.

TABLE 3.22. Common Pediatric Formulas[a] by Brand

Formula	Route	Amount Required to Meet DRIs	Caloric Strength (kcal/oz)	Comments
Compleat Pediatric	Enteral	1,400 mL for 1–13-year-olds	30	Lactose free, gluten free, blenderized tube feeding
EleCare Junior	Oral or enteral	NL	30	Elemental formula, lactose free, gluten free, soy free, milk protein free, fructose free, galactose free
Neocate Junior	Oral or enteral	NL	30	Elemental formula for children with multiple protein allergies, lactose free, gluten free
Nutren Junior (with or without fiber)	Oral or enteral	1,000 mL for 1–8-year-olds 1,500 mL for 9–13-year-olds	30	Lactose free, gluten free, kosher, low residue
PediaSure (with or without fiber)	Oral and enteral	1,000 mL for 1–8-year-olds 1,500 mL for 9–13-year-olds	30	Lactose free, gluten free, kosher

Peptamen Junior	Oral and enteral	1,000 mL for 1–8-year-olds 1,500 mL for 9–3-year-olds	30	Elemental formula designed for children with severe GI tract disturbances
Vivonex pediatric	Oral or enteral	1,000 mL for 1–8-year-olds 1,500 mL for 9–13-year-olds	24	Elemental, lactose-free, gluten-free, low-residue formula

GI, gastrointestinal; NL, not listed by manufacturer.

[a]The above list is not complete and does not contain all pediatric formulas available. Refer to product labels or manufacturers' references for most current nutrient values and ingredients. In some cases, it is appropriate to utilize an adult formula for nutrition supplementation. Refer to the guidelines for use provided by the manufacturers of those products.

It should be noted that it is preferable to increase energy intake with common nutrient-dense foods rather than by formula supplementation (e.g., fortifying the child's meals with peanut butter, avocado, oils, whole milk, heavy cream, and addition of evaporated milk to casseroles and soups). This method encourages healthful feeding practices, lowers cost, and improves taste.

BIOCHEMICAL EVALUATION OF NUTRITIONAL STATUS IN THE PEDIATRIC PATIENT

See Table 3.23.

TABLE 3.23. Normal Laboratory Values[a]

Measure	Range
Albumin (serum), g/dL	
Infants	2.9–5.5
Other children	3.7–5.5
Calcium	
Serum total calcium, mg/dL	
Preterm infants	6–10
Term infants	7–12
Other children	8–10.5
Serum ionized calcium, mg/dL	4.48–4.92
Folate (serum)	>6–7 ng/mL
Hemoglobin (blood), g/dL	
Newborns	≥14.0
12–35-month-old children	≥11.0
3.0–4.9-year-old children	≥11.0
5.0–7.9-year-old children	≥11.5
8.0–11.9-year-old children	≥11.9
12.0–15.0-year-old boys	≥12.5
12.0–15.0-year-old girls	≥11.8
>15-year-old boys	≥13.0
>15-year-old girls	≥12.0

TABLE 3.23. Normal Laboratory Values[a] (*continued*)

Measure	Range
Iron (serum), mg/dL	
Neonates	>30
Infants	>40
Children < 4 years	>50
Other children	>60
Phosphorus (serum), mg/dL	
Newborns	4.0–8.0
1 year	3.8–6.2
2- to 5-year-old child	3.5–6.8
Other children	2.9–5.6
Prealbumin (serum), mg/dL	
Premature infants	4–14
Term infants	4–20
6–12-month-old children	8–24
1–6-year-old children	17–30
Other children	17–42
Blood urea nitrogen, mg/dL	7–22
Transferrin, mg/dL	170–440
Vitamin A (plasma retinol), µg/dL	
Infants	13–50
Other children	20–72
Vitamin D	
25-Hydroxyvitamin-D, ng/mL (preferred)	20–30
1,25-OH-D3, ng/mL	15–60
Vitamin E	
Plasma alpha-tocopherol, mg/dL	
Preterm infants	0.5–3.5
Other children	0.7–10
Red blood cell hemolysis test, %	10

(*continued*)

TABLE 3.23. Normal Laboratory Values[a] (*continued*)

Measure	Range
Vitamin K	
Prothrombin time, sec	11–15
PIVKA-II, ng/mL	≤3
Thiamin	
Red blood cell transketolase stimulation, %	<15
Vitamin B_{12}, pg/mL	200–900
Absorption test	Excretion of more than 7.5% of ingested labeled vitamin B_{12}
Vitamin C (plasma), mg/dL	0.2–2.0
Magnesium (serum), mEq/L	1.5–2.0
Zinc (serum), mcg/dL	60–120

PIVKA, Proteins induced by vitamin K absence.

[a]Results of a single lab test should be interpreted with caution and normal values may vary among laboratories.

Data from (i) Fenton TR, Kim JH. A systematic review and metaanalysis to revise the Fenton growth chart for preterm infants. *BMC Pediatr* 2013;13:59, (ii) Barlow SE; Expert Committee. Expert Committee recommendations regarding the prevention, assessment and treatment of child and adolescent overweight and obesity: Summary report. *Pediatrics* 2007;120(Suppl 4):S164–S192, and (iii) Baker RD, Greer FR; The Committee on Nutrition. Clinical report—diagnosis and prevention of iron deficiency and iron deficient anemia in infants and young children (0–3 years of age). *Pediatrics* 2010;126:1040–1050.

COMMON NUTRITIONAL DISTURBANCES

Anemia

Iron deficiency is the most prevalent single nutrient deficiency in children in the United States. As discussed previously, true iron-deficiency anemia needs to be determined to properly treat the condition. An iron-rich diet may be indicated for infants, children, and adolescents at risk for iron-deficiency anemia.

Constipation

Nutrition intervention is warranted for patients who experience pain associated with the passage of stool, the hard nature of stool, or the failure to pass at least three stools per week. Painful stools, despite frequency, may also be considered constipation. Major causes include inadequate fluid and fiber, abnormal muscle tone, motor skill impairments, medications, or debilitating disorders. Therapy for children 1 year and older includes modifications in fiber, fluid, and activity level.

Gastroesophageal Reflux

Gastroesophageal reflux (GER) is a common occurrence in infants. It is typically resolved by 18 months of age and rarely requires corrective surgery. Medical nutrition therapy for GER is usually used in combination with drug therapy. Recommendations should be individualized based on the child's age and developmental status. Commercially prepared thickened formulas are available, and feeds thickened with infant cereal remain common along with positioning techniques and avoidance of known irritants.

Failure to Thrive

Failure to thrive is an outdated term used to describe a child's growth that is significantly lower than normal for the child's age and gender.[9] It has now been recognized that malnutrition is the proximate cause of organic (presence of an underlying medical cause) or inorganic (psychological, social, or economic cause) in nature. The goals of medical nutrition therapy are centered on the assessment of and therapy for malnutrition.

Lead Poisoning

Rates of lead poisoning in children are highest in older cities and among low-income communities. Medical nutrition therapy for lead poisoning consists of a high-iron, high-fiber, and fat-modified diet. A multivitamin may also be recommended. Iron deficiency increases the absorption and storage of lead in the body. Fiber speeds the transport of food through the body and thus decreases the length of stay of lead in the gut, whereby decreasing its absorption. High-fat foods should be limited in the diet because they enhance the absorption and storage of lead in the body.

Malnutrition

Pediatric malnutrition is typically examined in the context of its chronicity, severity, and etiology. Acute versus chronic malnutrition is determined by the National Center for Health Statistics (NCHS) definition of a chronic disease as one that lasts 3 months or longer. Stunting (decreased height velocity) is the characteristic sign of chronic malnutrition, whereas weight is usually affected during acute periods of malnutrition. Use of z-scores (standard deviation comparisons) of growth measurements have replaced previously used criteria such as the Gomez Classification, Waterlow criteria, or McClaren criteria to define severity. Various online tools are available to easily determine z-scores (see Tables 3.24 to 3.26).

TABLE 3.24. Resources for Determining Z-Scores for Anthropometrics

CDC Growth Charts	WHO Growth Charts
STAT GrowthCharts (compatible with iPod Touch, iPhone, iPad [Apple Inc])	STAT GrowthCharts WHO (compatible with iPod Touch, iPhone, iPad [Apple Inc])
Epi Info NutStat (available for download): http://www.cdc.gov/growthcharts/computer_programs.htm	WHO z-score charts: http://www.who.int/childgrowth/standards/chart_catalogue/en/index.htm
CDC website: z-score data files available as tables: http://www.cdc.gov/growthcharts/zscore.htm	WHO Multicentre Growth Study website: http://www.who.int/childgrowth/software/en/
	All four macros (SAS, S-plus, SSPS, and STATA) calculate the indicators of the attained growth standards

TABLE 3.24. Resources for Determining Z-Scores for Anthropometrics (*continued*)

CDC Growth Charts	WHO Growth Charts
PediTools Home: www.peditools.org Clinical tools for pediatric providers; growth charts, calculators, etc.; mobile compatible	PediTools Home: www.peditools.org Clinical tools for pediatric providers; growth charts, calculators, etc.; mobile compatible

Data from Fenton TR, Kim JH. A systematic review and metaanalysis to revise the Fenton growth chart for preterm infants. *BMC Pediatr* 2013;13:59.

TABLE 3.25. Pediatric Malnutrition Criteria (Single Data Point)

Primary Indicators	Mild Malnutrition	Moderate Malnutrition	Severe Malnutrition
Weight for height z-score	−1 to −1.9 z-score	−2 to −2.9 z-score	−3 or greater z-score
BMI-for-age z-score	−1 to −1.9 z-score	−2 to −2.9 z-score	−3 or greater z-score
Length/height z-score	No data	No data	−3 z-score
Mid-upper arm circumference	Greater than or equal to −1 to −1.9 z-score	Greater than or equal to −2 to −2.9 z-score	Greater than or equal to −3 z-score

Data from Fenton TR, Kim JH. A systematic review and metaanalysis to revise the Fenton growth chart for preterm infants. *BMC Pediatr* 2013;13:59.

TABLE 3.26. Pediatric Malnutrition Criteria (Two or More Data Points)

Primary Indicators	Mild Malnutrition	Moderate Malnutrition	Severe Malnutrition
Weight gain velocity (<2 years)	<75% of the norm for expected weight gain	<50% of the norm for expected weight gain	<25% of the norm for expected weight gain
Weight loss (2–20 years)	5% usual body weight	7.5% usual body weight	10% usual body weight
Deceleration in weight for length/height z-score	Decline of 1 z-score	Decline of 2 z-score	Decline of 3 z-score
Inadequate nutrient intake	51%–75% estimated energy/ protein need	26%–50% estimated energy/ protein need	25% estimated energy/ protein need

Data from Fenton TR, Kim JH. A systematic review and metaanalysis to revise the Fenton growth chart for preterm infants. *BMC Pediatr* 2013;13:59.

Obesity

Weight management intervention should be completed in children whose BMI is greater than the 85th percentile for age with comorbidities and/or complications, and also in those whose BMI is above the 95th percentile for age. Basic framework for intervention should include nutrition education, exercise plan, and behavior modifications (see Table 3.27).

TABLE 3.27. Expert Panel Intervention Stages According to Age and BMI-for-Age Percentile

Counseling Stage	Age (yr)	BMI-for-Age Percentile	Presence of Health Risk	Goal of Intervention
Stage 1	<18	<94th	No	Weight maintenance until BMI-for-age is <85th percentile or a slower rate of weight gain
Stages 1–2	2–18	85th–94th	Yes	Weight maintenance until BMI-for-age is <85th percentile or a slower rate of weight gain
Stages 1–2	6–18	95th–98th	Yes	Either weight maintenance until BMI-for-age is <85th percentile or gradual weight loss of 1 lb/mo
Stages 1–3	2–5	95th–98th	Yes	Weight maintenance until BMI-for-age is <85th percentile or a slower rate of weight gain; weight loss should be <1 lb/mo
Stages 1–3	2–5	≥99th	Yes	Gradual weight loss of ≤1 lb/mo
Stages 1–3	6–11	>99th	Yes	Weight loss of 2 lb/mo
Stages 1–4	12–18	>95th	Yes	Weight loss of ≤2 lb/wk until BMI-for-age is <85th percentile

Data from (i) Mehta NM, Corkins MR, Malon A, et al. Defining pediatric malnutrition: A paradigm shift towards etiology-related definitions. *JPEN J Parenter Enteral Nutr* 2013;37:460–481, and (ii) Barlow SE; Expert Committee. Expert Committee recommendations regarding the prevention, assessment and treatment of child and adolescent overweight and obesity: Summary report. *Pediatrics* 2007;120(Suppl 4):S164–S192.

ADIME 3.1 ADIME At-A-Glance: Pediatric Malnutrition

Assessment

- Breast- or bottle-fed, feeding regimen, appetite
- Labs (electrolytes, BUN, creatinine, glucose, albumin)
- Physical findings: GI symptoms, diarrhea, constipation, NFPE findings (loss of muscle mass/fat stores, edema)
- Anthropometrics (weight, length, BMI, head circumference, WHO growth chart percentiles, z-scores)
- Food availability

Nutrition Diagnosis

- Malnutrition (acute, mild) RT improper feeding regimen AEB weight for length z-score −1.85

Intervention

- 3 oz formula per feeding (concentrate formula to 24 kcal/oz) every 4 hours, including through the night, with goal intake of 18 oz/24 hours

Monitoring and Evaluation

- Weekly weights; goal ≥35 g/day
- Confirm enrollment in WIC Program

References

1. Center for Disease Control and Prevention Growth Charts 2000. Available at: http://www.cdc.gov/nccdphp/dnpao/growthcharts/who/index.htm. Accessed December 10, 2006.
2. American Academy of Pediatrics Committee on Nutrition. *Pediatric Nutrition Handbook*. 7th ed. Washington, DC: American Academy of Pediatrics; 2013: 44, 48, 619, 635, 663, 684, 1173.
3. Nevin-Folino N, ed. *Pediatric Manual of Clinical Dietetics*. 2nd ed. Chicago, IL: American Dietetic Association; 2003.
4. Engorn B, Flerlage J. *Harriet Lane Handbook*. 20th ed. Philadelphia, PA: Saunders; 2014.

NOTES

NOTES

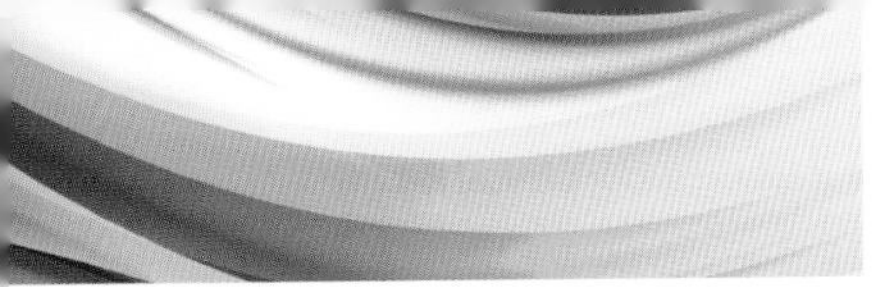

CHAPTER

4

Older Adults

Vikki Lasota, RDN

Aging produces numerous physical and physiologic changes, which in turn alter nutritional requirements and affect nutritional status (Box 4.1). The presence of chronic disease, and/or use of multiple medications, polypharmacy, can enhance potential disparities between nutrient needs and dietary intake, leading to malnutrition. Indeed, research suggests that malnutrition is a common condition among the elderly, with a prevalence of 12% to 50% of those hospitalized and 23% to 60% of elderly in extended care facilities.[1,2] A key predictor of malnutrition in older adults is loss of appetite. Often referred to as anorexia of aging, food intake and appetite typically decline in older adults compared with younger adults, as a result of physiologic, psychological, social, and cultural factors.[3]

NUTRITION ASSESSMENT

Screening for Nutrition Risks in the Elderly

Nutrition assessment in elderly patients consists of the typical nutrition assessment parameters (refer to Chapter 1), with particular emphasis on risk factors in this population. The Nutrition Screening Initiative was a collaborative effort of several lead agencies whose goal was to identify and treat

BOX 4.1 Physiologic Changes in Aging and Nutrition Implications

Body System or Function	Changes in Aging	Nutrition Implications
Body composition	Increase in body fat, especially intra-abdominal; decrease in muscle (sarcopenia); bone loss (including tooth)	Increased risk for obesity, cardiovascular disease, diabetes
Cardiovascular function	Reduced blood vessel elasticity, higher peripheral resistance, and blood flow to heart	Higher risk for hypertension and other cardiovascular disease
Gastrointestinal function	Reduction in secretions, especially acid, achlorhydria or hypochlorhydria (a consequence of atrophic gastritis [AG], which occurs in 33% of elderly)	Impairment of digestion and absorption (iron, B_{12}, zinc, folate, biotin, calcium); AG causes inflammation and reduction in intrinsic factor, which can cause B_{12} deficiency; AG can also cause B_6 deficiency, dysphagia, constipation
Immunocompetence	Reduced function, especially T-cell component	In combination with poor nutritional status, higher susceptibility to infection
Oral health	Reduction in saliva, leading to dry mouth (xerostomia); tooth loss	Problem chewing and swallowing

BOX 4.1 Physiologic Changes in Aging and Nutrition Implications (*continued*)

Body System or Function	Changes in Aging	Nutrition Implications
Neurologic function	Reduction in neurotransmitter synthesis; less efficient nerve conduction; central nervous system (CNS) changes cause problems in balance/coordination; depression; dementia	Depression can cause loss of appetite and food intake, leading to malnutrition
Nutrient metabolism	Lower synthesis of cholecalciferol in skin and renal activation; increased retention of vitamin A owing to reduced clearance	Vitamin D deficiency; vitamin A retention could be toxic if high-dose supplement used
Renal function	Reduction in number of nephrons (therefore, lower glomerular filtration rate (GFR) and total renal function)	Fluid balance aberrations; acid–base balance problems; metabolism of nutrient medications may be altered
Sensory losses	Decreased sensitivity in taste (dysgeusia), smell (hyposmia), sight, hearing, tactile	Dysgeusia and hyposmia cause loss of appetite and intake, and also increase risk for foodborne illness

nutritional problems in the elderly.[4] Simple screening tools from both that project and others focusing on all aspects of elderly health, including psychosocial and environmental factors, were developed (Determine and Meals-on-Wheels),[4,5] and continue to be used by health care providers working with the elderly (Boxes 4.2 and 4.3).

BOX 4.2 Determine Your Nutrition Health Checklist

D	Presence of chronic disease or condition
E	Eating poorly; too little or poor quality of diet
T	Tooth loss or mouth pain
E	Economic hardship
R	Reduced social contact
M	Multiple medicines
I	Involuntary weight loss or gain
N	Needing assistance in self-care
E	Elder years; older than age 80

BOX 4.3 Meals-on-Wheels: Assess Malnutrition Risks

M	Medications
E	Emotional problems
A	Anorexia nervosa and other eating behavior problems
L	Late-life paranoia
S	Swallowing problems
O	Oral problems
N	No money
W	Wandering and other dementia behaviors
H	Hyperthyroidism, hyperparathyroidism
E	Entry problems (malabsorption)
E	Eating problems (both physical and cognitive)
L	Low-salt, Low-saturated-fat/cholesterol diets
S	Shopping (lack of food availability, access to foods)

ADIME 4.1 ADIME-At-A-Glance

Assessment

- BMI <23, UWL, decrease in appetite and food intake, dehydration
- Change in ADLs/IADLs, cognitive decline, depression
- Neurologic disease, swallowing difficulty, infection, pressure ulcers
- Multiple medications, recent hospitalization

Nutrition Diagnosis

- Inadequate oral intake RT decreased appetite, AEB recent UWL of 5% × 2 weeks, and PO intake of <50%
- Inadequate fluid intake RT Alzheimer disease, AEB dry skin and mucosal tissues, UWL of 5% × 6 days, and high blood urea nitrogen
- Swallowing difficulty RT recent CVA, AEB coughing when drinking thin liquids
- Unintended weight loss RT Alzheimer disease, AEB UWL of 10% × 5 weeks
- Self-feeding difficulty RT multiple sclerosis, AEB dropping of utensils, and decreased PO intake of <75%
- Impaired ability to prepare foods/meals RT recent hip fracture, AEB reduced mobility

Intervention

- Provision of commercial beverage product
- Increased fluid diet
- Liquid consistency—nectar-thick liquids
- Insert enteral feeding tube
- Feeding assistance
- Referral to Home-Delivered Meals Program

Monitoring and Evaluation

- Body weight
- PO intake (food, fluid)

CVA, cerebrovascular accident.

Anthropometric Measurements

In adults over the age of 65, the risk of mortality is increased in those with a body mass index (BMI) of less than 23.[6] In addition, regardless of usual body weight, one of the most significant anthropometric risk factors in the elderly is involuntary or unintentional weight loss (IWL, UWL). For this reason, the use of ideal body weight is not necessarily appropriate, although it continues to be widely used. A more important parameter is usual body weight and percentage of body weight lost, as described in Chapter 1.

Patient History

Patient history is a significant area of assessment in the elderly, as a change in various functional abilities is correlated with morbidity and mortality. The typical daily functions are described as activities of daily living (ADLs) and instrumental activities of daily living (IADLs) (Box 4.4). Health care practitioners should ask questions regarding any change in the patient's ADLs and IADLs of both the patient and the significant others. In addition, patient history risk factors include cognitive decline, depression, neurologic disease, dehydration, presence of infection and/or pressure ulcers, and recent hospitalization.

Estimation of Energy and Protein Needs

The use of energy expenditure equations, as described in Chapter 1, to determine energy needs is varied and depends on factors such as body weight and disease or condition.

BOX 4.4 Activities of Daily Living and Instrumental Activities of Daily Living

ADLs	IADLs
Bathing	Doing light housework
Dressing	Preparing meals
Eating	Using the telephone
Maintaining continence	Managing money
Mobility indoors and outdoors	Shopping
Moving into and out of bed and chairs	Traveling
Toileting	Taking medications

Based on a validation study, the Academy of Nutrition and Dietetics Evidence Analysis Library concluded that in critical illness, "the Penn State (modified) equation should be used for patients 60 years or older with BMI of 30 kg/m^2 or higher."[7,8] For nonobese critically ill patients of all ages, the original Penn State equation appears to be most accurate.[9] For the relatively healthy elderly individual, the practitioner can use any of the energy expenditure equations in Chapter 1, particularly those which take into account age.

There is growing consensus that the elderly, those not affected by chronic kidney disease, may require higher protein intake to maintain "metabolic, physical, and functional status".[10] The current recommended dietary allowance (RDA) for protein for adults over the age of 18 is 0.8 g/kg of body weight and 46 and 56 g per day for females and males, respectively. The suggested optimal level is 1.0 to 1.5 g/kg, 58 to 86 g/day for females, and 70 to 105 g/day for males.

Essential Nutrient Recommendations

The physiologic changes associated with aging affect requirement for several essential nutrients. In general, the requirement for many nutrients decreases, concomitant with the decrease in energy needs. However, some nutrients are needed in higher amounts. Additionally, various psychosocial and socioeconomic changes that often attend aging may also alter dietary intake (Box 4.5).[11]

The age category for older adults is divided into two separate categories in the dietary reference intakes (DRIs) (Tables 4.1 to 4.3).[12] The adult age groups are 51 to 70 years and 70 and above, although the nutrient levels are the same for both adult categories for essential nutrients. One exception is the tolerable upper intake level (UL) for phosphorus, which decreases from 4,000 to 3,000 mg for both males and females at the higher age group, and this is not a recommended level but rather an upper limit to avoid toxicity. Two nutrients of particular concern in the elderly are B_{12} and vitamin D.

BOX 4.5 Psychosocial and Socioeconomic Problems Affecting Dietary Intake with Aging

Problem	Approach
Limited income	1. Buy low-cost food, such as dried beans/peas, rice, and pasta
	2. Use coupons for money off on foods used, and check store weekly circular to buy foods on sale
	3. Buy store-brand foods
	4. Check with local place of worship for free or low-cost meals
	5. Participate in local senior nutrition programs[a], offered at senior congregate feeding sites or home-delivered meals
	6. Check for eligibility for the Food Stamp Program[a]
	7. Contact local food banks or emergency food program[a]
Inability to grocery shop	1. Ask a friend or relative to grocery shop
	2. Contact local grocery store to bring groceries to your home
	3. Contact food delivery companies
	4. Check with local place of worship or senior center for volunteers who will shop
	5. Hire a home health worker (listed under "Home Health Services" in phone book)

Inability to prepare food	1. Use a microwave oven to cook frozen meals and foods 2. Buy easily prepared nutritious foods (fresh fruits, whole grain breads, peanut butter, tuna in foil pouch) 3. Participate in local senior nutrition programs,[a] offered at senior congregate feeding sites or home-delivered meals 4. Hire a home health worker (listed under "Home Health Services" in phone book) to cook meals (also make-ahead meals that can be frozen)
Psychological changes that cause poor appetite	1. The following can cause loss of appetite: living alone, having lost a spouse, feeling depressed—participate in senior meal programs, invite family or friends to share a meal, check with a doctor if depression continues 2. If cooking for just one, you may not feel like making meals; invite family or friends for a meal 3. Food may not have much taste, which could be psychological, physiologic, or because of medications; it may help to: a. Eat with family and friends or participate in senior meal programs b. Ask the doctor if drugs could be affecting appetite or taste changes c. Increase the flavor of food by adding spices and herbs

[a]Programs are listed under "County Government" in blue pages of phone book; elder care locator: (800) 677–1116.

Data from Bernstein M, Munoz N. Position of the Academy of Nutrition and Dietetics: Food and nutrition for older adults: Promoting health and wellness. *J Acad Nutr Diet* 2012;112(8):1255–1277.

TABLE 4.1. Dietary Reference Intakes for Older Adults for Macronutrients

Nutrient/Units	Males, 51+ yr	Females, 51+ yr
Energy, kcal	2,204; 1989 RDA	1,978; 1989 RDA
Carbohydrate, g	130	130
Protein, g	56	46
Total fat, g	ND; 1989 RDA: 20%–35%	ND; 1989 RDA: 20%–35%
Linoleic acid, g	14	11
α-Linolenic acid, g	1.6	1.1
Saturated fat, g	As low as possible while consuming a nutritionally adequate diet; 1989 RDA: <10%	As low as possible while consuming a nutritionally adequate diet; 1989 RDA: <10%
Cholesterol, mg	As low as possible while consuming a nutritionally adequate diet; 1989 RDA: <300	As low as possible while consuming a nutritionally adequate diet; 1989 RDA: <300
Fiber, g	30	21

ND, not determined.

Data from large population surveys indicate that up to 6% of people aged 60 are B_{12} deficient (serum vitamin B_{12}, 148 pmol/L), and 20% have marginal depletion (serum vitamin B_{12}, 148 to 221 pmol/L).[13] One reason is that malabsorption from food sources is often the result of the reduction in the production of hydrochloric acid, achlorhydria, as occurs in atrophic gastritis, a common problem in the elderly. In addition, acid-reducing drugs, especially proton pump inhibitors (PPIs), for which use has significantly increased with 14.9 million patients receiving 157 million prescriptions in 2012, may significantly impair B_{12} absorption.[14] The use of PPIs for 2 years or more was associated with a 65% higher risk

TABLE 4.2. Dietary Reference Intakes for Older Adults for Vitamins

Nutrient/Units	Males				Females			
	DRI[a]		Tolerable UL		DRI		UL	
	51–70 yr	70+ yr	51–70 yr	70+ yr	51–70 yr	70+ yr	51–70 yr	70+ yr
Vitamin A, μg	900	900	3,000	3,000	700	700	3,000	3,000
Vitamin D, μg	15	20	100	100	15	20	100	100
Vitamin E, mg	15	15	1,000	1,000	15	15	1,000	1,000
Vitamin K, μg	190	190	ND	ND	120	120	ND	ND
Vitamin B_6, mg	1.7	1.7	100	100	1.5	1.5	100	100
Vitamin B_{12}, μg	2.4	2.4	ND	ND	2.4	2.4	ND	ND
Biotin, μg	30	30	ND	ND	30	30	ND	ND
Choline, mg	550	550	3,500	3,500	425	425	3,500	3,500
Folate, μg	400	400	1,000	1,000	400	400	1,000	1,000
Niacin, mg	16	16	35	35	14	14	35	35
Pantothenic acid, mg	5	5	ND	ND	5	5	ND	ND
Riboflavin, mg	1.3	1.3	ND	ND	1.1	1.1	ND	ND
Thiamin, mg	1.2	1.2	ND	ND	1.1	1.1	ND	ND

[a]DRIs represent RDAs except for vitamins D, K, biotin, choline, and pantothenic acid (AI values).

TABLE 4.3. Dietary Reference Intakes for Older Adults for Minerals

Nutrient/Units	Males				Females			
	DRI[a]		UL		DRI		UL	
	51–70 yr	70+ yr	51–70 yr	70 +yr	51–70 yr	70+ yr	51–70 yr	70+ yr
Chromium, μg	30	30	ND	ND	20	20	ND	ND
Copper, μg	900	900	10,000	10,000	900	900	10,000	10,000
Fluoride, mg	4	4	10	10	3	3	10	10
Iodine, μg	150	150	1,100	1,100	150	150	1,100	1,100
Iron, mg	8	8	45	45	8	8	45	45
Magnesium, mg	420	420	350	350	320	320	350	350
Manganese, mg	2.3	2.3	11	11	1.8	1.8	11	11
Molybdenum, mg	45	45	2,000	2,000	45	45	2,000	2,000
Nickel, mg	ND	ND	1	1	ND	ND	1	1
Phosphorus, mg	700	700	4,000	3,000	700	700	4,000	3,000
Selenium, μg	55	55	400	400	55	55	400	400
Sodium, mg; 1989 RDA	<2,400	<2,400	ND	ND	<2,400	<2,400	ND	ND
Vanadium, mg	ND	ND	1.8	1.8	ND	ND	1.8	1.8
Zinc, mg	11	11	40	40	8	8	40	40

[a]DRIs represent RDAs except for calcium, chromium, fluoride, manganese (AI values).

for B_{12} deficiency.[14] These drugs are also associated with an increased risk for fractures.[15] Vitamin D deficiency is more likely in aging owing to low sun exposure, organ function decline, malabsorption related to chronic diseases such as inflammatory bowel disease, and poor dietary intake. Because of the concern for fractures, the Institute of Medicine revised the DRI for this nutrient in 2011 (Table 4.2).

COMMON PROBLEMS IN AGING

Several problems common in aging affect key aspects of either dietary intake or nutritional needs, and may adversely affect nutritional status. The most notable of these includes dysphagia and pressure ulcers, which, although not unique to the elderly, are highest in this population. The profound and negative effects of these conditions on an elderly patient's nutritional status make nutritional assessment for their presence and/or severity imperative.

Dysphagia

Disease Process

Dysphagia represents both a symptom and a disorder, which affects one or all stages of the swallowing mechanism, making swallowing difficult.[16] The possible causes are varied (Box 4.6), as are the symptoms (Box 4.7). Depending on the cause, dysphagia may be an acute condition that resolves, or it may be chronic. Early identification and intervention is critical not only because of the effect on the quality of life but also because it can lead to serious consequences, such as aspiration pneumonia and malnutrition.

Treatment and Nutrition Intervention

The team approach is important in both assessment and intervention, and can include physician, nurse, speech-language pathologist, registered dietitian nutritionist (RDN), and radiologist.[17] The National Dysphagia Diet (NDD) is the current medical nutrition therapy for the disorder.[18] It

BOX 4.6 Causes of Dysphagia

Achalasia
Aging
Alzheimer disease
Cancer, chemotherapy, radiation
Dementia
Eosinophilic esophagitis
Head and neck surgery
Intubation
Multiple sclerosis
Neurologic disorders
Parkinson disease
Stroke
Diabetic neuropathy
Trauma to esophagus

BOX 4.7 Symptoms of Dysphagia

Absence of gag reflex
Change in vocal quality (gurgling sound)
Choking
Coughing before, during, or after swallowing
Delayed swallow reflex
Drooling, excessive secretions
Frequent throat clearing
Holding pockets of food in cheek
Poor control of tongue movements
"Stuck" feeling in throat
Weight loss

consists of three levels of solid foods (dysphagia pureed, dysphagia mechanically altered, dysphagia advanced) and four levels of fluids (thin, nectar-like, honey-like, spoon thick), each of which modify the texture, consistency, and other attributes of foods and liquids that affect the various stages of swallowing.[17] The stage appropriate for an individual patient depends primarily on the severity of the dysphagia and the stage of swallowing affected (i.e., oral, pharyngeal, or esophageal) (Box 4.8).

BOX 4.8 Overview of the National Dysphagia Diet

Dysphagia Severity	Swallowing Stage Affected	Food Characteristics	Level of Supervision During Meals/Assessment Needed
Level 1: Pureed			
Moderate to severe	Poor oral phase ability; reduced ability to protect airway	Pureed, homogenous, cohesive foods; no course texture; no raw foods (fruits, vegetables, nuts); any foods requiring chewing or bolus formation are excluded	Close or complete supervision
Level 2: Mechanically Altered			
Mild to moderate	Oral and or pharyngeal	Moist, soft-textured foods with some cohesion, which are easily formed into a bolus; meats are ground or minced with pieces no larger than one quarter inch; transition to more solid texture from pureed; chewing ability is required	Assess patient for tolerance to mixed textures; it is expected that some mixed texture foods are tolerated
Level 3: Advanced			
Mild	Oral and or pharyngeal (to a lesser degree than in level 2)	Nearly regular texture with exception of very hard, sticky, or crunchy foods; foods still need to be moist in bite-sized pieces; adequate dentition and mastication needed	Assess patient for tolerance to mixed textures; it is expected that some mixed texture foods are tolerated

Data from National Dysphagia Diet Task Force. *National Dysphagia Diet—Standardization for Optimal Care.* Chicago, IL: American Dietetic Association; 2002:17–19.

Pressure Ulcers

Disease Process

Pressure ulcers, also known as decubitus ulcers or bedsores, represent a point of skin breakdown from continual contact with a surface, such as a bed or wheelchair. Pressure ulcers, or more precisely the complications from them, account for approximately 60,000 deaths every year in the United States and an annual cost of $11 billion.[19] Of significance to health care practitioners is the statistic that 9% of patients admitted to the hospital will develop a pressure ulcer, and of particular significance is the fact that malnutrition is second only to pressure as a cause of pressure ulcers.[20]

Treatment and Nutrition Intervention

Pressure ulcers are assessed as being at one of four stages, relative to depth of tissue involvement and therefore severity (Box 4.9).[21] Inadequate dietary intake and poor nutritional status are major risk factors in both the development of and prolonged healing of pressure ulcers. The goals of the nutrition intervention of pressure ulcers are as follows:

1. Provide adequate energy to maintain or regain lost weight: 30 to 35 kcal/kg increasing to 35 to 40 kcal/kg per day for people who are underweight or losing weight.
2. Provide adequate protein for positive nitrogen and to spare energy: 1.5 to 2.0 g/kg per day.
3. If vitamin and mineral deficiencies are confirmed or suspected, provide a multivitamin/mineral supplement that contains the DRI for micronutrients needed for wound healing.
4. The routine supplementation of zinc in the absence of confirmed or suspected deficiency is not recommended.
5. The use of arginine, glutamine, and HMB (β-hydroxy-β-methylbutyrate) requires further research before any firm conclusions can be drawn.[17]

BOX 4.9 Pressure Ulcer Staging

Stage I: Intact skin with nonblanchable redness of a localized area usually over a bony prominence

Stage II: Partial thickness loss of dermis presenting as a shallow, open ulcer with a red-pink wound bed, without slough. May also present as an intact or open/ruptured, serum-filled blister.

Stage III: Full thickness tissue loss. Subcutaneous fat may be visible, but bone, tendon, or muscle is not exposed. Slough may be present but does not obscure the depth of tissue loss and may include undermining and tunneling.

Stage IV: Full thickness tissue loss with exposed bone, tendon, or muscle. Slough or eschar may be present on some parts of the wound bed. Often includes undermining and tunneling.

Data from National Pressure Ulcer Advisory Panel. 2014 Prevention and Treatment of Pressure Ulcers: Clinical Practice Guideline. Available at: http://www.npuap.org/resources/educational-and-clinical-resources/prevention-and-treatment-of-pressure-ulcers-clinical-practice-guideline. Accessed November 18, 2015.

References

1. Wallace JI. Malnutrition and enteral/parenteral alimentation. In: Hazzard WR, Blass JP, Ettinger WH Jr, et al, eds. *Principles of Geriatric Medicine and Gerontology*. 4th ed. New York: McGraw-Hill; 1999:1455–1469.
2. Ennis BW, Saffel-Shrier S, Verson H. Diagnosing malnutrition in the elderly. *Nurse Pract* 2001;26(3):52–65.
3. Bernstein M, Munoz N. Position of the Academy of Nutrition and Dietetics: Food and nutrition for older adults: Promoting health and wellness. *J Acad Nutr Diet* 2012;112(8):1255–1277.
4. Rush D. Evaluating the nutrition screening initiative. *Am J Public Health* 1993;83(7):944–945.
5. Pepersack T. Outcomes continuous process improvement of nutritional care program among geriatric units. *J Gerontol A Biol Sci Med Sci* 2005;60A(6):787–792.

6. Winter JE, MacInnis RJ, Wattanapenpaiboon N, et al. BMI and all-cause mortality in older adults: A meta-analysis. *Am J Clin Nutr* 2014;99(4):875–890.
7. Frankenfield D. Validation of an equation for resting metabolic rate in older obese, critically ill patients. *JPEN J Parenter Enteral Nutr* 2011;35:264–269.
8. Academy of Nutrition and Dietetics Evidence Analysis Library. Best Method to Estimate RMR. Available at: https://www.andeal.org/worksheet.cfm?worksheet_id=255915. Accessed November 21, 2015.
9. Maday K. Energy estimation in the critically ill: A literature review. *Univ J Clin Med* 2013;1(3):39–43.
10. Bauer J, Biolo G, Cederholm T, et al. Evidence-based recommendations for optimal dietary protein intake in older people: A position paper from the PROT-AGE study group. *J Am Med Dir Assoc* 2013;14(8):542–559.
11. Academy of Nutrition and Dietetics. Healthy Eating for Older Adults. Available at: http://www.eatright.org/resource/food/nutrition/dietary-guidelines-and-myplate/healthy-eating-for-older-adults. Accessed November 21, 2015.
12. Ross AC, Taylor CL, Yaktine AL, et al, eds; Committee to Review Dietary Reference Intakes for Vitamin D and Calcium; Institute of Medicine. *Dietary Reference Intakes for Calcium and Vitamin D*. Washington, DC: National Academies Press; 2011:1103–1116.
13. Allen LH. How common is vitamin B-12 deficiency? *Am J Clin Nutr* 2009;89(Suppl):693S–696S.
14. Lam JR, Schneider JL, Zhao W, et al. Proton pump inhibitor and histamine 2 receptor antagonist use and vitamin B12 deficiency. *J Am Med Assoc* 2013;310(22):2435–2442.
15. Khalili H, Huang ES, Jacobson BC, et al. Use of proton pump inhibitors and risk of hip fracture in relation to dietary and lifestyle factors: A prospective cohort study. *BMJ* 2012;344:1–13.
16. Niedert KC, Dorner B, eds. Nutrition Care *of the Older Adult: A Handbook for Dietetics Professionals Working Throughout the Continuum of Care*. 2nd ed. Chicago, IL: American Dietetic Association; 2004:211.
17. Academy of Nutrition and Dietetics. *Nutrition Care Manual*. Available at: http://nutritioncaremanual.org. Accessed November 8, 2015.

18. National Dysphagia Diet Task Force. *National Dysphagia Diet—Standardization for Optimal Care*. Chicago, IL: American Dietetic Association; 2002:17–19.
19. National Pressure Ulcer Advisory Panel. 2014 World Wide Pressure Ulcer Prevention Day. Available at: http://www.npuap.org/category/press-releases. Accessed November 18, 2015.
20. Straus E, Margolis D. Malnutrition in patients with pressure ulcers: Morbidity, mortality, and clinically practical assessments. *Adv Wound Care* 1996;9(5):37–40.
21. National Pressure Ulcer Advisory Panel. 2014 Prevention and Treatment of Pressure Ulcers: Clinical Practice Guideline. Available at: http://www.npuap.org/resources/educational-and-clinical-resources/prevention-and-treatment-of-pressure-ulcers-clinical-practice-guideline. Accessed November 18, 2015.

NOTES

Notes

Notes

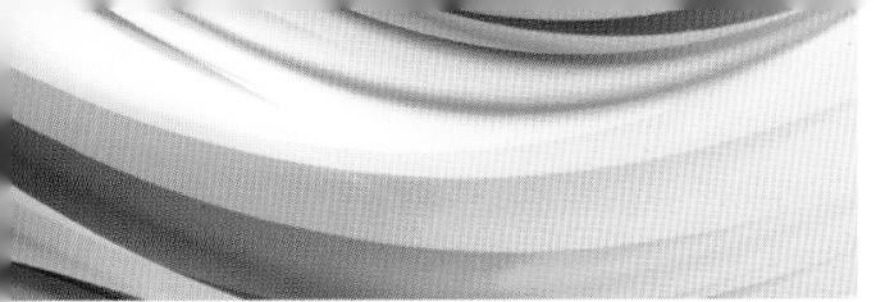

CHAPTER

5

Nutrition Support

Brenda Howell, RDN, CNSC

Patients who are unable to meet nutrition requirements by a conventional oral diet, and aggressive therapies are warranted, need alternative means of nutrition. Alternative means of nutrition are enteral nutrition and parenteral nutrition.

ENTERAL NUTRITION

Indications and Patient Selection

Enteral nutrition (EN) is the preferred route if the gut is functional because of fewer complications, fewer costs, and improved outcomes. Benefits of EN include increased nutrient utilization, maintenance of normal gut pH and flora, inhibiting opportunistic bacterial overgrowth, and support of gut mucosa's immunologic barrier function, which may decrease risk of gut-related sepsis. Examples of clinical situations in which oral intake is deemed unsafe, insufficient, or impossible are patients with altered mentation, severe dysphagia, poor appetite, and respiratory failure requiring vent via endotracheal tube.[1,2] Indications and contraindications for EN can be found in Box 5.1.

Enteral Feeding Route

Route of EN is the next step after determining the patient would benefit from nutrition support (Table 5.1). Long-term access should be considered if anticipated need will be >4

BOX 5.1 Indications and Contraindications for Enteral Nutrition Support

Indications

- Malnourished patient expected to be unable to eat for >5 to 7 days
- Normally nourished patient expected to be unable to eat for >7 to 9 days
- Functional or partially functional gut
- Adaptive phase of short bowel syndrome
- Following severe trauma or burns
- EN initiation within 24 to 48 hours in the critically ill patients whom are unable to maintain volitional intake
- Patients in the ICU setting with acute respiratory distress syndrome/acute lung injury and are expected to have duration of mechanical ventilation greater or equal to 72 hours

Contraindications

- Aggressive intervention not warranted or not desired
- Severe short bowel syndrome
- Nonoperative mechanical GI obstruction
- Intractable vomiting and diarrhea refractory to medical management
- Distal high-output fistulas (too distal to bypass with feeding tube)
- GI ischemia
- Paralytic ileus
- Severe GI bleed
- EN not required for patients whom are at low nutrition risk with normal baseline nutrition status, have low disease severity in the ICU setting, and do not require specialized nutrition therapy over the first week of hospitalization
- Unable to gain enteral access
- Severe coagulopathies (disease related or medication induced) may have potential complication but generally does not preclude placement

Data from (i) Merritt R. *The A.S.P.E.N. Nutrition Support Practice Manual.* 2nd ed. Silver Spring, MD: American Society of Parenteral and Enteral Nutrition; 2005, (ii) Mueller CM. *The A.S.P.E.N. Adult Nutrition Support Core Curriculum.* 2nd ed. Silver Spring, MD: American Society of Parenteral and Enteral Nutrition; 2012, (iii) McClave SA, Taylor BE, Martindale RG, et al; Guidelines for the provision and assessment of nutrition support therapy in the adult critically ill patient: Society of Critical Care Medicine (SCCM) and American Society for Parenteral and Enteral Nutrition (A.S.P.E.N.). *JPEN J Parenter Enter Nutr* 2016;40(2):159–211, and (iv) Kosenecki M, Fritzshall R. Enteral nutrition for adults in the hospital setting. *Nutr Clin Pract* 2015;30(5):634–651.

TABLE 5.1. Enteral Access Devices

	Description	Pros	Cons and Complications
Short-term (<4 wk)			
NGT: prepyloric tube	Used for feeding, decompression of stomach, administration of medications, measurement of gastric pH and residuals. At least 10F needed to avoid clogging from enteral formulas.	• Variety of sizes available (8F–24F) • Generally easy placement • Large-bore tube allows more versatility on feeding regimen • Gastric phase of digestion and nutrient metabolism	• Contraindicated if nasal/facial fractures, severe coagulopathy, severe thrombocytopenia, esophageal obstruction • Complications include clogging, esophageal or sinus perforation, nasal mucosal ulceration, pneumothorax, epistaxis, pulmonary aspiration
Orogastric tube: prepyloric tube	Optional route when tube cannot be placed nasally (facial fracture or head injury)	• Lower incidence of sinusitis	• Tolerated for short periods of time • Complications are the same as with NGT, with exception of nasal-related events

(continued)

TABLE 5.1. Enteral Access Devices (*continued*)

	Description	Pros	Cons and Complications
Nasoenteric tube: postpyloric tube	Tip of tube placed past the pyloric sphincter. Radiologic verification or electromagnetic image of placement needed before use. Not appropriate to check residuals.	• Small-bore tubes are more flexible and more comfortable • Less risk of aspiration as patient is able to lay flat, esophageal reflux, delayed gastric emptying if placement past distal third of duodenum	• Infusion pumps necessary • Difficulty of postligament of Treitz placement • Difficulty of administering some medications
Long-Term Devices (>4 wk)			
Gastrostomy tube: prepyloric	Placed surgically, endoscopically (PEG), or radiologically into the stomach. Available sizes from 10F to 28F.	• Allows bolus feeding • Allows gastric phase of digestion and nutrient metabolism • Low-profile tubes available	• Complications may include dislodgment, bleeding, wound infection, tube occlusion, pneumoperitoneum, stomal leakage

Jejunostomy tube: postpyloric	Placed surgically, endoscopically (PEJ), or radiologically into the jejunum. Size of 9F–12F tube. Not able to check residuals to assess tolerance. Requires infusion via a pump.	• Reduces aspiration risk if the patient is required to lay flat (several studies have demonstrated no difference in aspiration risk between intragastric and small bowel feedings)[5] • Low-profile tubes available	• Not able to bolus enteral feeding • Complications may include wound dehiscence or infection, bowel obstruction, occlusion, bleeding, dislodgment, volvulus
Transgastric jejunostomy	Placed surgically, endoscopically, or radiologically. A jejunal port is placed through gastrostomy tube, allowing to feed into the small bowel while suctioning of gastric contents.	• Can be converted to gastrostomy feeding as tolerated	• Not able to bolus enteral feeding • Complications of both jejunostomy and gastrostomy tubes

PEJ, percutaneous endoscopic jejunostomy.

Data from (i) Merritt R. *The A.S.P.E.N. Nutrition Support Practice Manual*. 2nd ed. Silver Spring, MD: American Society of Parenteral and Enteral Nutrition; 2005, (ii) Mueller CM. *The A.S.P.E.N. Adult Nutrition Support Core Curriculum*. 2nd ed. Silver Spring, MD: American Society of Parenteral and Enteral Nutrition; 2012, (iii) Koseniecki M, Fritzshall R. Enteral nutrition for adults in the hospital setting. *Nutr Clin Pract* 2015;30(5):634–651, and (iv) Miller KR, McClave SA, Kiraly LN, et al. A tutorial on enteral access in adult patients in the hospitalized setting. *JPEN J Parenter Enteral Nutr* 2014;38(3):282–295.

to 6 weeks. Enteral access devices include gastrostomy, jejunostomy, or gastrojejunostomy tubes.

Enteral Formula Selection

Because of the large number of enteral formulas that are available commercially, a comprehensive list is not appropriate for a resource book of this size. A listing of contact information for enteral formula manufacturers is available at the end of this chapter.

Enteral Nutrition Delivery Methods

Once the route of access for EN has been established, dosing and method of delivery can be determined. Box 5.2 shows a sample calculation for determining volume goal and administration methods. Gravity-controlled and pump methods are available. Enteral formulas are provided at full strength because of contamination risk. In critical care patients who are at high nutrition risk, it is recommended to achieve greater than 80% calorie and protein goals within 48 to 72 hours of hospitalization to derive clinical benefit of EN over the first week.[3]

Bowel sounds do not need to be heard before initial feeding. Fluid and air must be present in the intestinal lumen to hear bowel sounds, which may not be heard if there is a nasogastric or percutaneous endoscopic gastrostomy (PEG) tube for suction or decompression.[1] Water flushes should also be added to the EN prescription to provide adequate hydration and decrease constipation. Water flushes can be provided by bolus method, although some infusion pumps can be programmed to provide a timed dose. If refeeding syndrome is a risk, EN should be initiated at 25% to 50% goal rate and slowly advanced to the goal over 5 to 7 days, with daily monitoring of potassium, magnesium, and phosphorus.[1,2] Refeeding syndrome is further discussed in the Parenteral Nutrition section of this book.

Bolus or Intermittent

- Gravity-controlled delivery
- Best suited for gastric feeding

BOX 5.2 Sample Calculation for Determining Goal Enteral Nutrition Volume and Method of Administration

Patient's daily requirements based on nutrition assessment are 80 g protein, 2,000 kcal, and 2,000 mL fluid.

A standard polymeric formula provides 1.2 kcal/mL, 55.5 g protein/L, 820 mL free H_2O/L and meets 100% RDI for vitamins and minerals in 1,000 mL of formula.

- 2,000 kcal needed/1.2 kcal per mL = 1,667 mL formula required (1.7 L)
- 1.7 L × 55.5 g protein/L = 94 g protein provided with formula
- 1.7 L × 820 = 1,394 mL free H_2O provided with formula
- 2,000 mL daily fluid needs – H_2O provided in formula = 606 mL additional H_2O required

If formula to be infused continuously via pump, divide total formula needed by desired duration of therapy: 1,667 mL formula/24 hrs = 69.5 mL/hr, which can round to 70 mL/hr ATC (around the clock) plus additional 200 mL H_2O flush 3×/d to meet daily requirements. Frequent interruptions of enteral feedings in the hospital setting have resulted in delivery of 50% to 60% prescribed daily enteral formula, which has led some institutions to prescribe formula by total volume needs instead of hourly rate.[4,9] An example would be infusing an enteral formula at 70 to 80 mL/hr until goal volume of 1,667 mL/d is reached.

If formula to be infused via intermittent or bolus method, divide total formula needed by desired number of daily feedings: 1,667 mL formula/4 feedings per day = 417 mL formula per feeding. Additional 75 mL H_2O flush before and after each feeding is needed to meet daily fluid requirements. Determine duration of each feeding from 15 to 45 minutes, which depends on individual tolerance.

RDI, recommended daily intake.

- Appropriate for patients who can protect their airway and are neurologically intact
- Most often used in the nonacute care or home care setting
- Advantages include the following: no pump required so more economical; more physiologic because the regimen closely mimics normal meals; allows for increased patient mobility

- Disadvantages include the following: may be poorly tolerated with diagnosis of gastroparesis, uncontrolled gastroesophageal reflux disease, or gastric outlet obstruction
- Administration:
    - Bolus feeding: Infused over approximately 15 minutes via gravity assist or syringe.[4] Tolerated volumes typically range from 240 to 720 mL per bolus, 2 to 6 times daily depending on individual tolerance. Initial bolus of 120 mL is generally tolerated, with advancement by 120 mL increments until goal volume is attained.
    - Intermittent feeding: similar to bolus in total administration volume and frequency, with formula delivery over 30 to 45 minutes by gravity or pump assist[4]

Cyclic

- Pump-assisted delivery
- Can be used in the acute care or home care setting, especially when transitioning to an oral diet
- Advantages include the following: allows for maximal nutrient absorption; allows for gut rest; allows for increased mobility and time away from the pump
- Disadvantages include the following: requires high infusion rates of typically 50 to 250 mL/hr over 8 to 20 hours daily to meet full nutrition and fluid requirements, which can be poorly tolerated by some patients
- Administration: Typically runs for 8 to 20 hours per day, which can be infused either during daytime or nocturnally. Can be initiated at 10 to 40 mL/hr, with advancement by 10 to 20 mL/hr every 8 to 12 hours as tolerated, until goal is reached.
- Cyclic feedings via the jejunum may be limited to ≤90 to 100 mL/hr depending on individual tolerance.

Continuous

- Pump-assisted delivery
- Can be used for gastric and transpyloric feedings
- Commonly used for patients who cannot tolerate bolus or intermittent feedings, for those requiring mechanical ventilation, and for critically ill patients

- Advantages include the following: possible decreased risk of distention as compared with bolus/intermittent infusion
- Disadvantages include the following: requires pump delivery, which is more costly and limits patient mobility
- Administration: Infuses for 24 hours per day, commonly referred to as "around the clock," or ATC. Can be initiated at 10 to 40 mL/hr, with advancement by 10 to 20 mL/hr every 8 to 12 hours as tolerated, until goal is reached.

Monitoring of Enteral Feeding

Monitoring of gastrointestinal (GI) tolerance, hydration status, and nutritional status of patients receiving EN is important. Protocol for monitoring EN may vary by institution; however, Table 5.2 lists some common guidelines for monitoring EN.

TABLE 5.2. Enteral Nutrition Monitoring Guidelines

Parameter	Frequency
Weight	Before initiation and at least twice a week
Intake and output (I/O)	Daily
Stool output and consistency	Daily
Signs/symptoms of edema	Daily
Signs/symptoms of dehydration	Daily
Gastric residuals	q4h–6h when feeding into stomach
Abdominal exam: if soft, firm, or distended	Daily
Serum electrolytes, blood urea nitrogen (BUN), creatinine	Daily until stable, then 2–3 times/wk
Calcium, magnesium, phosphorus	Daily until stable, then weekly
Glucose	Patients with diabetes: q6h Patients without diabetes: daily until stable, then weekly
Nitrogen balance	Weekly, if appropriate

Gastric Residuals

Monitoring gastric residual volume (GRV) has historically been done as an aid in assessing EN tolerance as well as aspiration risk. Gastric residuals are checked by withdrawing and measuring fluid and formula with a syringe via nasogastric tube (NGT) or gastrostomy tube. Normal gastric secretions range from 3,000 to 4,000 mL/d, and residuals of 400 to 500 mL have shown to be tolerated without aspiration.[5] Recommended practice is to avoid holding EN if GRV is ≤500 mL in absence of other signs and symptoms of intolerance.[3] Delayed gastric emptying can be caused by medications like narcotics or paralytics in which initiating a promotility agent such as metoclopramide or erythromycin may be beneficial. Maintaining the head of bed (HOB) >30 to 45 degrees may also aid with enteral feeding tolerance. If high residuals persist, verifying tube placement may be needed. Aspirating syringes must be at least 50 mL for small-bore tubes of 12F or less because of pressure in which the tube may collapse. Residuals should not be checked when feeding via the jejunum.

GI Complications

Tube feeding or GI intolerance may be indicated by abdominal distention, fullness, and pain or cramping. Decreasing infusion rate, ensuring formula is at room temperature, verifying tube placement, and assessing formula osmolarity can help with tolerance. If the patient has delayed gastric emptying or is on medications that slow peristalsis, high-fiber and/or high-fat formulas may not be tolerated and should be adjusted. Nausea and vomiting may indicate tube migration, such as a balloon gastrostomy causing a gastric outlet obstruction.[1] Diarrhea can be defined as >200 mL stool or >3 stools per day. Potential causes of diarrhea are medications, impactions, pathogenic bacteria, pancreatic insufficiency, short bowel syndrome, gut atrophy, and inflammatory bowel disease. If disease-related causes, medications, or pathogen-induced diarrhea has been ruled out, soluble fiber or antimotility agents may be beneficial. Elemental EN formulas may also aid with nutrient absorption.

Transitioning to Discontinue Enteral Nutrition

Temporary EN support is often needed during the critical care process and should be discontinued as patients can adequately tolerate an oral diet. As oral diets are started, enteral feedings should be infused nocturnally via pump, infused between meals via bolus, or stopped more than 1 hour before meals to aid with appetite. When the patient is consuming 60% to 75% of energy and protein needs, the clinician should consider stopping EN and removing the temporary enteral access device.[4] If there is long-term enteral access and suspect of future necessity, the feeding tube may be left in place.

PARENTERAL NUTRITION

Indications and Patient Selection

Parenteral nutrition (PN) is a method of nutrition support in which provision of macronutrients, micronutrients, and some medications is infused directly into the bloodstream via a peripheral or central vein. PN is indicated when patients cannot meet their nutrient needs enterally, via either oral intake or enteral tube feedings, because of the GI tract being compromised. Indications/contraindications for PN are outlined in Box 5.3.

Patient selection for who may benefit from PN relies on thorough nutrition assessment, determination of nutritional status, and the overall clinical condition and prognosis of the patient. Benefits of PN should outweigh the risks. For severely malnourished patients, PN is indicated when an impairment of the GI tract occurs. Patients who are not severely malnourished may tolerate a period of no nutrition for up to 7 to 10 days without adversely affecting their outcome.[2] Postoperative patients who receive PN for >7 to 10 days receive maximal benefit.[2] Many risk factors are related to PN. Intravenous dextrose, lipid, and amino acids provide an optimal host for bacterial and/or fungal infections. Patients are also at risk for catheter-related infections and

BOX 5.3 Indications and Contraindications for Parenteral Nutrition Support

Indications for PN

- Ischemic bowel
- Paralytic ileus
- Short bowel syndrome with malabsorption
- Bowel obstruction
- High-output enterocutaneous fistula with inability to place EN tube distal of the fistula
- Intractable vomiting or diarrhea
- Chylous effusion in which very-low-fat diet/EN not feasible or has failed
- Persistent EN intolerance or inability to gain enteral access

Contraindications for PN

- Catabolic patients expected to have usable GI tract within 5 to 7 days
- Well-nourished patient expected to resume EN/oral diet within 7 to 10 days
- Duration of therapy expected <5 to 7 days
- Aggressive nutrition support not desired by the patient
- Patient's prognosis does not warrant aggressive nutrition support
- Functional GI tract
- Anorexia or inability to ingest enough nutrients orally

Data from (i) Merritt R. *The A.S.P.E.N. Nutrition Support Practice Manual.* 2nd ed. Silver Spring, MD: American Society of Parenteral and Enteral Nutrition; 2005, and (ii) Mueller CM. *The A.S.P.E.N. Adult Nutrition Support Core Curriculum.* 2nd ed. Silver Spring, MD: American Society of Parenteral and Enteral Nutrition; 2012.

complications. Macronutrient, electrolyte, and mineral and fluid abnormalities are risk factors as are hyperglycemia, hepatic steatosis, and compromised renal clearance.

Parenteral Nutrition Access

Central Venous Access

Central venous access allows hypertonic, hyperosmolar medications and nutrition therapy infusion into a large-diameter central vein via a central venous catheter (CVC). Subclavian, cephalic, jugular, femoral, and basilic veins are the most common sites for a CVC. Parenteral nutrition via CVC is indicated if anticipated need is >10 to 14 days and/or peripheral PN (PPN) would not be adequate or medically feasible. Types of CVCs are outlined in Table 5.3.

TABLE 5.3. Central Venous Catheter Types

Type of Access	Definition/Description	Length of Therapy
Nontunneled CVC	Single or multilumen catheter inserted preferable into the subclavian vein. Ease of removal and exchange for short-term therapy in an acute care setting.	Weeks
Tunneled CVC	Single or multilumen catheter inserted into the jugular, subclavian, or cephalic vein, then is tunneled in the subcutaneous tissue (i.e., Hickman/Broviac/Groshong). Secured CVC for long-term use, less infection risk than nontunneled CVC, ease of care.	Months to years
Peripherally inserted central catheter (PICC)	Single or multilumen catheter inserted from peripheral vein into large central vein. Use in acute care or outpatient settings. Routine heparin flushes and site care needed, not ideal for long-term home care.	Several weeks to months
Port	Single or dual lumen subcutaneous port with silicone septum, most commonly placed in anterior chest wall. Venous access via port with noncoring needle.	Months to years

Data from Merritt R. *The A.S.P.E.N. Nutrition Support Practice Manual.* 2nd ed. Silver Spring, MD: American Society of Parenteral and Enteral Nutrition; 2005.

Peripheral Venous Access

PPN is administered into a peripheral vein and is indicated for short-term therapy of up to 14 days. Standard peripheral cannulas require site rotation every 72 to 96 hours to decrease catheter-related complications.[1] Adequate veins are necessary, as well as ensuring PPN solutions do not exceed 900 mOsm/L because of the risk of thrombophlebitis. Formulations for PPN require higher volume and lipid tolerance than central PN, to lower osmolarity and more closely meet caloric and protein requirements. See Box 5.4 for calculating osmolarity of PPN solutions.

Nutrition Requirements: Indirect Calorimetry

Indirect calorimetry is one of several methods in which metabolic requirements of macronutrients are determined in the critically ill. Predictive equations such as those of Penn

BOX 5.4 Calculating Osmolarity of PPN Solutions[a]

1 g amino acid/L = 10 mOsm
1 g dextrose/L = 5 mOsm
1 g lipid (20% stock solution)/L = 1.3 mOsm
1 mEq – calcium gluconate/L = 1.4 mOsm
– magnesium sulfate/L = 1.0 mOsm
– potassium and sodium/L = 2 mOsm

Example calculation: PPN solution provides 1,790 kcal, 80 g lipid, 120 g amino acid, 150 g dextrose, 200 mEq sodium chloride, 8 mEq magnesium sulfate, 40 mEq potassium chloride, 5 mEq calcium gluconate for total volume of 3,000 mL daily.

1. 120 g amino acid ÷ 3.0 L = 40 g/L × 10 = **400 mOsm/L**
2. 150 g dextrose ÷ 3.0 L = 50 g/L × 5 = **250 mOsm/L**
3. 80 g lipid ÷ 3.0 L = 26.7 g/L × 1.3 = **35 mOsm/L**
4. 8 mEq magnesium sulfate ÷ 3.0 L = 2.7 mEq/L × 1 = **2.7 mOsm/L**
5. 5 mEq calcium gluconate ÷ 3.0 L = 1.67 mEq/L × 1.4 = **2.3 mOsm/L**
6. 240 mEq sodium chloride and potassium chloride ÷ 3.0 L = 80 mEq/L × 2 = **160 mOsm/L**

Total osmolarity = 850 mOsm/L[a]

[a]Osmolarity of nutrients may vary slightly among institutions.

State, Mifflin–St. Jeor, and Harris–Benedict are useful but can have significant variance in results. Indirect calorimetry measures energy expenditure and macronutrient utilization by measuring the ratio of CO_2 produced to O_2 consumed, also called the respiratory quotient (RQ). Although RQ does correlate the ratio of calories provided and calorie required, low sensitivity and reduced specificity limit its efficacy as an indicator of under- or overfeeding.[2] The physiologic range for RQ in humans is 0.67 to 1.3; therefore, a RQ outside this range may indicate an invalid study.[2] Box 5.5 reviews technical aspects, which may alter indirect calorimetry results.[1]

Parenteral Formulation: Macronutrients

Carbohydrate

Carbohydrate (CHO) is the primary source of energy for the body, including the brain and central nervous system. Minimum CHO requirements recommended per dietary reference intakes (DRIs) are 130 g/d for healthy adults and children.[6] CHO should not exceed 4 mg/kg/min in critically ill patients and 7 mg/kg/min in stable patients (Box 5.6). Risks

BOX 5.5 Aspects That May Alter Indirect Calorimetry Results

- Mechanical ventilation with $FiO_2 \geq 60\%$ and/or positive end-expiratory pressure (PEEP) >12 cm H_2O
- Acute changes of ventilation (if vent changes, wait 90 minutes to complete study)
- Leak in sampling system
- Inability to collect all expiratory flow (example of air leak via chest tube or bronchopleural fistula)
- Hemodialysis in progress (wait 3 to 4 hours after dialysis to complete the study)
- Error in calibration of indirect calorimeter
- General anesthesia given within 6 to 8 hours prior to the study
- Painful procedure recently completed (wait 1 hour after procedure to complete the study)

Data from Merritt R. *The A.S.P.E.N. Nutrition Support Practice Manual*. 2nd ed. Silver Spring, MD: American Society of Parenteral and Enteral Nutrition; 2005.

BOX 5.6 Calculating Maximum CHO (g) Oxidative Capacity

To calculate maximum dextrose (g):
1. 4–7 mg × wt (kg) × 1,440 min[a] = mg/d
2. mg/d ÷ 1,000 = g dextrose/d

Example: A critically ill patient weighs 73 kg.
1. 4 mg × 73 kg × 1,440 min = 420,480 mg/d
2. 420,480 mg/d ÷ 1,000 = **420 g/d dextrose**

[a]60 min/hr × 24 hr/d = 1,440 min/d

of excessive CHO infusion include hyperglycemia, glucosuria, lipogenesis, hepatic steatosis, and hyperinsulinemia.

Dextrose monohydrate is the CHO source used for PN, which provides 3.4 kcal/g. Stock or base solutions of dextrose range from 5% to 70%. Percentage dextrose concentration is grams of solute per 100 mL of solution. A 10% dextrose solution contains 10 g of dextrose per 100 mL solution, thereby providing 100 g dextrose/L.

Protein

Protein in PN is provided in the form of a crystalline amino acid solution in which standard solutions contain a physiologic mixture of essential and nonessential amino acids. Specialty amino acid formulations should be reserved for patients expected to benefit clinically from their use; indications for these formulations are very limited.[2] Examples of disease-specific solutions are NephrAmine for renal failure and HepatAmine for liver disease. Amino acids are required in PN to minimize lean body mass losses, promote tissue repair, and maintain oncotic pressure in blood plasma. Protein requirements range from 1.2 to 2.0 g/kg/d in critically ill patients and 0.8 to 1.0 g/kg/d in stable patients. Protein needs may exceed >2.0 g/kg if there are extreme losses such as in weeping wounds or large body surface area burns. Amino acids provide 4 kcal/g, with stock or base solutions ranging from 3% to 20%.

Lipid

Intravenous fat emulsions (IVFEs), specifically long-chain fatty acids (LCFAs), are required to prevent essential fatty acid deficiency, which can occur within 1 to 3 weeks of lipid-free nutrition administration. LCFAs are currently the only commercially available form of IVFE in the United States and are available in concentrations of 10%, 20%, and 30%. IVFEs contain egg phosphatides as an emulsifier and glycerol for stability. A 10% IVFE concentration provides 1.1 kcal/mL, whereas a 20% concentration provides 2.0 kcal/mL or 10 kcal/g. Europe has medium-chain fatty acid (MCFA) and LCFA mixtures, which are not available yet in the United States. Minimum LCFA requirements are 3% to 4% total kcal, with a DRI equating to about 10% total kcal. Risks of excessive or too rapid infusion of IV lipids include impairment of clearance as well as compromised reticuloendothelial or immune function. Limiting IV lipid to 1 g/kg/d or 30% of total kilocalorie requirements is recommended. IV lipids in PN can be increased and are tolerated if serum triglycerides are ≤400 mg/dL.

Parenteral Formulation: Total Volume

Formulation of PN includes total volume required to meet estimated fluid needs of 25 to 40 mL/kg/d. Fluid requirements in the critically ill are dependent on total fluid status and organ function. Minimum volume of PN in the critically ill is often required, as there is usually a simultaneous mode of IV fluids that can be adjusted pending the patient's fluid status. Fluids provided by separate IV fluids, medications, and drips should be subtracted from total fluid requirements in determining total volume requirements for PN. Additional fluids may be required if there are excessive losses via diarrhea, vomiting, or fistula drainage. Estimation of total body water (TBW) and TBW deficit can assist with estimating fluid needs in PN formulation (Box 5.7).[2,7]

Types of Parenteral Nutrition

PN solutions comprise protein, CHO, electrolytes, vitamins, minerals, medications, and sterile water. IVFEs infused separately, or "piggy-backed," are referred to as "2-in-1" solutions. IVFEs admixed with other nutrients and additives

BOX 5.7 Estimating Total Body Water and Total Body Water Deficit

TBW Estimation

TBW = 0.6 × wt (kg) males; 0.5 × wt for males ≥80 years of age
= 0.5 × wt (kg) for females; 0.4 × wt for females ≥80 years of age
Subtract 10% for obese, 20% for very obese

TBW Deficit Estimation

Water deficit (L) = TBW × [(Na^1/Na^2) – 1]
Na^1 = actual serum sodium
Na^2 = desired serum sodium

Data from (i) Mueller CM. *The A.S.P.E.N. Adult Nutrition Support Core Curriculum*. 2nd ed. Silver Spring, MD: American Society of Parenteral and Enteral Nutrition; 2012, and (ii) Kingley J. Fluid and electrolyte management in parenteral nutrition. *Support Line* 2005;27(6):13–22.

are "3-in-1" solutions, or total nutrient admixtures (TNAs). Advantages of TNAs are decreased contamination, decreased nursing time, decreased pharmacy preparation time, overall decreased cost, and better fat utilization. Disadvantages of TNAs include decreased stability of the fat emulsion and compatibility with other components. Components of PN must be compounded in a specific sequence for optimal stability.[1] Sample calculations for macronutrients in both 2-in-1 and TNAs are given in Box 5.8. Specifying quantity of needed amino acid (AA), dextrose, and lipid can be ordered in grams or percentage of solution depending on the facility. Ordering nutrients and additives either per day or per liter also varies between facilities, although safe practice guidelines are standardized PN formulations in which nutrients should be in amounts per day.[8] An exception to ordering per day is if the facility has admixed PN solutions in 1-L volumes in which using quantity per liter is supported. Table 5.4 may aid with calculating the PN formulation, as it displays concentrations of dextrose, amino acids, and lipids, as well as what they provide.

BOX 5.8 Sample Calculation for 2-in-1 and TNA PN Formulations

Patient's daily requirements based on nutrition assessment are 80 g protein, 2,000 kcal, 2,000 mL fluid with maximum CHO oxidative capacity of 385 g dextrose/d.

2-in-1: Facility options are:
AA solutions: 10% or 15%
Dextrose solutions: 20%, 30%, 40%, 50%, or ____%
Lipid: 10% (500 mL) or 20% (500 mL) ___ daily or ____ × per week

1. Determine needed lipids/d and what the solution provides:
   a. **10% lipid/d** would provide 500 mL volume, 50 g lipid, and 550 kcal
2. Assess the best AA volume needed to meet AA (g) requirements:
   a. 80 g AA ÷ **10% AA concentration** = 800 mL volume and 320 kcal
3. Calculate needed dextrose (g) by subtracting kcal from daily lipids and AA solutions:
   a. 2,000 kcal – 550 kcal (lipid) – 320 kcal (AA) = 1,130 kcal from dextrose needed
   b. 1,130 kcal ÷ 3.4 = 332 g dextrose needed/d
4. Assess the best dextrose volume needed to meet dextrose (g) requirements:
   a. 332 g dextrose ÷ **50% dextrose concentration** = 664 mL volume
   b. Round to 700 mL volume to provide 350 g dextrose and 1,190 kcal
5. Calculate infusion rate per hour from total AA and dextrose volumes:
   a. 800 mL (AA) + 700 mL (dextrose) = 1,500 mL volume
   b. 1,500 mL ÷ 24 hrs = **62.5 mL/hr** AA and dextrose
   c. Separate 10% lipid infusion (500 mL) * 12 hr = 41.6 mL/hr of lipids
6. PN goal = 62.5 mL/hr * 24 hrs from 800 mL of 10% AA and 700 mL of 70% dextrose. Piggy back 500 mL of 10% lipid at 41.6 mL/hr * 12 hrs. This provides daily total 2060 kcal, 80 g AA, 350 g dextrose, 50 g lipid, and 2,000 mL volume.

TNA: Macronutrients are ordered in grams per day for this facility.

1. Calculate kilocalories provided by goal AA
   a. **80 g AA** × 4 = 320 kcal

(*continued*)

Nutrition Support

BOX 5.8 Sample Calculation for 2-in-1 and TNA PN Formulations (*continued*)

2. Calculate kilocalories provided by desired lipid (g). Typically, initial lipid dose is 30% total kcal requirements.
   a. 2,000 kcal × 30% (0.30) = 600 kcal from lipid
   b. 600 kcal ÷ 10 kcal/g = **60 g lipid**
3. Determine goal dextrose (g) needed by subtracting kilocalories from AA and lipids.
   a. 2,000 kcal – 320 kcal (AA) – 600 kcal (lipid) = 1,080 kcal needed from dextrose
   b. 1,080 kcal ÷ 3.4 kcal/g = 317 g dextrose (round to **320 g dextrose** for 1,088 dextrose kcal)
4. PN goal: 80 g AA, 320 g dextrose, 65 g lipid to provide 2,008 total kcal in 2,000 mL volume

TABLE 5.4. Macronutrient Composition of Solutions

Macronutrient	Concentrations (%)	Grams per Liter	Kilocalories per Liter
Dextrose	5	50	170
	10	100	340
	20	200	680
	30	300	1,020
	40	400	1,360
	50	500	1,700
	70	700	2,380
Amino acids	8.5	85	340
	10	100	400
	15	150	600
	20	200	800
	Concentration	**Kilocalories per Milliliter**	**Kilocalories per Liter**
Lipid emulsions	10	1.1	1,100
	20	2	2,000
	30	3	3,000

Parenteral Formulation: Micronutrients and Additives

Electrolytes

Altered serum electrolyte values are common in the acutely ill, and PN formulations can aid with correcting these abnormalities. Assessing current IV electrolyte administration is needed before developing the PN formulation. Table 5.5 shows the composition of intravenous solutions. Table 5.6 reviews daily electrolyte requirements, what factors may alter electrolyte values, and dosage form.[1,2] Formulation of PN is to maintain electrolyte balance; therefore, repletion of an electrolyte deficiency should be treated with a separate IV bolus. Acetate forms of potassium and sodium are useful when serum CO_2 is low and/or serum Cl^- is elevated in which NaCl or KCl would not be beneficial. Acetate is the precursor to bicarbonate, which is then converted to CO_2 by the liver. Calcium phosphate solubility is a compatibility concern because these precipitated salts have been associated with respiratory distress and death.[2] Various factors influence calcium phosphate solubility (i.e., amino acid type and final pH of the solution); therefore, it is crucial for communication with the compounding pharmacist when formulating a PN solution.

Vitamins, Minerals, and Trace Elements

Standard parenteral multivitamin and multiple–trace element supplements are included in the PN admixture. Multivitamin solutions are based on the U.S. Food and Drug Administration daily requirements. Multivitamin formulations are available with or without vitamin K. Once the multivitamins are added, the solution is stable for 24 hours. Trace elements contain a minimum of chromium, copper, manganese, and zinc. Some trace element additives also contain iodine, molybdenum, and selenium. Trace elements should be held if conjugated bilirubin exceeds >2.0, as copper and manganese toxicity can result. Iron dextran is incompatible with IVFE and can only be added to 2-in-1 PN solutions with caution. Separate

TABLE 5.5. Standard IV Solutions

IV Solution	Glucose (g/dL)	Na^+ (mEq/L)	Cl^- (mEq/L)	K^+ (mEq/L)	Ca^{2+} (mEq/L)	Lactate (mEq/L)	Osmolarity (mOsm/L)
5% dextrose in water	5	—	—	—	—	—	252
10% dextrose in water	10	—	—	—	—	—	505
0.45% NaCl	—	77	77	—	—	—	154
0.9% NaCl (normal saline)	—	154	154	—	—	—	308
5% dextrose in 0.45% NaCl	5	77	77	—	—	—	406
10% dextrose in 0.9% NaCl	5	154	154	—	—	—	560
Lactated Ringer's	—	130	109	4	3	28	273

Data from Mueller CM. *The A.S.P.E.N. Adult Nutrition Support Core Curriculum*. 2nd ed. Silver Spring, MD: American Society of Parenteral and Enteral Nutrition; 2012.

TABLE 5.6. Daily Electrolyte Requirements in Formulation of Parenteral Nutrition

Electrolyte	Daily Requirement (Adult)	Causes of Elevated Levels	Causes of Decreased Levels	Dosage Form
Calcium	10–15 mEq	Vitamin D excess, renal failure, tumor lysis syndrome, hyperparathyroidism, prolonged immobilization and stress, bone cancer	Decreased vitamin D intake, hypoparathyroidism, hypoalbuminemia, hypomagnesemia, citrate binding of calcium with blood product administration	Ca gluconate
Magnesium	8–20 mEq	Excessive Mg intake in renal insufficiency	Refeeding syndrome, alcoholism, diuretic use, nasogastric suction, diabetic ketoacidosis, elevated stool output, Mg wasting medications	Mg sulfate
Phosphorus	20–40 mmol	Excessive phosphate administration, renal failure	Refeeding syndrome, alcoholism, inadequate intake	Na phosphate K phosphate

(*continued*)

TABLE 5.6. Daily Electrolyte Requirements in Formulation of Parenteral Nutrition (*continued*)

Sodium	1–2 mEq/kg	Inadequate free water, excessive water loss, excessive sodium intake, hyperaldosteronism	Excessive hypotonic fluid, nephritis, adrenal insufficiency, congestive heart failure, syndrome of inappropriate antidiuretic hormones (SIADHs), cirrhosis with ascites	Na chloride Na acetate Na lactate
Potassium	1–2 mEq/kg	Renal dysfunction, excessive K^+ intake, metabolic acidosis, K^+-sparing medications	Refeeding syndrome, inadequate K^+ intake, excessive losses with diarrhea or intestinal fluids, diuretic medications, hypomagnesemia, metabolic alkalosis	K phosphate K acetate K chloride

Data from (i) Merritt R. *The A.S.P.E.N. Nutrition Support Practice Manual*. 2nd ed. Silver Spring, MD: American Society of Parenteral and Enteral Nutrition; 2005, and (ii) Mueller CM. *The A.S.P.E.N. Adult Nutrition Support Core Curriculum*. 2nd ed. Silver Spring, MD: American Society of Parenteral and Enteral Nutrition; 2012.

IV infusion of iron dextran is a preferred method of administration, if needed.

Other Additives

Additional additives in PN formulation can also include Sandostatin, insulin, GI prophylaxis such as Famotidine, and heparin. Regular insulin can be added starting at 0.1 units (U) per gram of dextrose per liter of PN solution. Increasing insulin by 0.05 U per gram of dextrose per day may be needed if hyperglycemia continues, until 0.25 U per gram of dextrose is reached.[1,2] Not all insulin provided in PN is utilized, as some will adhere to the plastic bag and tubing. Heparin is often added to PPN in 1 U/mL dose as prophylaxis against peripheral vein thrombophlebitis.

Initiation, Monitoring, and Discontinuation of PN

Initiation

PN can be initiated in adult patients when they are hemodynamically stable and, ideally, if they have satisfactory hydration, electrolyte, and acid–base status.[1] Macronutrients of PN can be advanced to goal by day 2 or 3 if serum glucose is consistently ≤180 mg/dL and electrolytes are satisfactory (Table 5.7).

Monitoring

Monitoring PN tolerance is necessary for achieving caloric and protein goals as well as prevention of metabolic complications. Table 5.8 provides appropriate frequency of lab monitoring.[2] Hypertriglyceridemia >400 mg/dL or a rise of ≥50 mg/dL indicates compromised clearance in which temporary discontinuation or decreased infusion rate of IVFE is warranted. Withholding IVFE is appropriate if triglycerides are >500 mg/dL. Topical linoleic acid via soybean or safflower oil can be an alternative method of preventing essential fatty acid deficiency without exacerbating hypertriglyceridemia.

Elevated or increasing liver function tests (LFTs) from baseline can indicate hepatic steatosis in which provision

TABLE 5.7. Initiation of Parenteral Nutrition

Macronutrient	Initiation Amount	Precautions
Amino acid	• 60–70 g/L	• Infusion of PN should be completed within 24 hr of initiation.
Dextrose	• 100–150 g/L or 10%–15% final concentration with glucose intolerance, risk for hyperglycemia as with steroid therapy, or diabetes • 200 g/L or 15%–20% final concentration as maximum initial amount	• Initiate with caution because of metabolic side effects, including reactive hyperglycemia, hyponatremia, hyperinsulinemia, glucosuria • Infusion of PN should be completed within 24 hr of initiation.
Lipid (IVFE)	• Can initiate full concentration as long as precautions are met	• Administer if baseline serum triglycerides are <200 mg/dL • When infused separately as in a 2-in-1, infusion should be completed within 12 hr.

of dextrose should be reevaluated. Excessive or continuous infusion of dextrose can compromise hepatic function. Decrease of dextrose infusion can ensure that the maximum CHO utilization rate is not being exceeded. Cycling PN is also recommended to provide hepatic rest. Cycling of PN

TABLE 5.8. Monitoring for Adult Patients on Parenteral Nutrition

Parameter	Baseline	Critically Ill Patients	Stable Patients
Chemistry screen (Ca, Mg, LFTs, P)	Yes	2–3×/wk	Weekly
Electrolytes, BUN, creatinine	Yes	Daily	1–2×/wk
Serum triglycerides	Yes	Weekly	Weekly
Complete blood count with differential	Yes	Weekly	Weekly
Prothrombin time (PT), partial thromboplastin time (PTT)	Yes	Weekly	Weekly
Capillary glucose	3×/d	3×/d (until consistently <200 mg/dL)	3×/d (until consistently <200 mg/dL)
Weight	If possible	Daily	2–3×/wk
Intake and output	Daily	Daily	Daily unless fluid status is assessed by physical exam
Nitrogen balance	As needed	As needed	As needed
Indirect calorimetry	As needed	As needed	As needed
Prealbumin or transferrin	Yes	Weekly	Weekly

BUN, blood nitrogen urea.

Data from (i) Merritt R. *The A.S.P.E.N. Nutrition Support Practice Manual*. 2nd ed. Silver Spring, MD: American Society of Parenteral and Enteral Nutrition; 2005, and (ii) Mueller CM. *The A.S.P.E.N. Adult Nutrition Support Core Curriculum*. 2nd ed. Silver Spring, MD: American Society of Parenteral and Enteral Nutrition; 2012.

requires infusion at 50% goal for the first and last hour of infusion. PN can be initially decreased to an 18- to 20-hour infusion and further decreased to 12-hour infusion if there is good glycemic control. Glucose should be monitored before, during, and after PN cycle until glucose tolerance is established.

REFEEDING SYNDROME Metabolic side effects of PN can occur, which may delay reaching nutrition goals. Refeeding syndrome can occur with malnourished patients who have anorexia nervosa, have had extreme weight loss, or have been without nutrition for 7 to 10 days. Refeeding syndrome occurs as the primary fuel source converts from stored fat to CHO because energy is provided after starvation. CHO as the fuel source causes insulin levels to rise, which leads to intracellular shifts of potassium, magnesium, and phosphorus. Rapid decrease of serum potassium, magnesium, and phosphorus may lead to respiratory distress, tetany, cardiac arrhythmias, paresthesia, cardiac arrest, and sudden death. Prevention of refeeding syndrome can be accomplished by correcting electrolyte abnormalities before PN administration, initiating PN at half energy requirements, 15 to 20 kcal/kg, or 1,000 kcal per day.[1,2] Gradually increasing PN to goal nutrients over 5 to 7 days, as well as estimating caloric and protein goals based on actual weight, may also prevent initial overfeeding and refeeding syndrome.

Discontinuation of PN

Discontinuation of PN is the ultimate goal as patients are able to tolerate an oral diet or EN support. Well-nourished individuals prior to PN therapy, who are free of malignancy, not debilitated, or without oral intake for <2 weeks, can have PN stopped as soon as diet tolerance is established.[1] Transitional weaning of PN is necessary in patients who are at higher risk of oral or EN intolerance or suboptimal nutrition intake. PN infusion can suppress appetite if providing >25% of caloric needs. PN can begin to be decreased in comparable amounts as soon as patients are eating 500 kcal daily, with discontinuation of PN when oral or enteral provisions equal >60% of nutrition requirements. Calorie counts can be beneficial to more accurately estimate intake. EN support should be considered if oral intake is inadequate in meeting nutrition requirements within a few days. Transition from PN to EN support should be done gradually. For example, once EN therapy is tolerated and providing approximately 50% of estimated daily nutrition needs, PN therapy can be decreased by 50%. When EN is providing greater than 75% of the patient's requirements, PN can be discontinued. Rebound hypoglycemia can occur if PN is stopped abruptly; therefore, decreasing infusion rate by 50% for 1 to 2 hours before discontinuation is suggested. Blood glucose levels can be checked 30 to 60 minutes after central PN cessation if patient is at risk or has signs of hypoglycemia.

Enteral Formula Manufacturers

Company Name	Phone Number	E-mail/Website
Abbott Nutrition	800-227-5767	http://www.abbottnutrition.com
Hormel Health Labs	800-866-7757	http://www.hormelhealthlabs.com
Mead Johnson Nutritionals	812-429-6399	MJMedicalAffairs@mjn.com http://www.meadjohnson.com/pediatrics/us-en/
Nestle Nutrition	800-247-7893	http://www.nestle-nutrition.com http://www.nestlehealthscience.com

ADIME 5.1 ADIME At-A-Glance

Assessment

- Admission Dx and pertinent PMH, home diet or EN regimen PTA and what nutrients EN was providing, intake from PO diet
- If EN support, tube access and tube patency
- Medications (vitamin/mineral supplements, antinausea, promotility agents, medications in liquid or crushable tablet form)
- Labs (electrolytes, albumin, prealbumin, CRP, hemoglobin A1C)
- Bowel function (Last BM, R/O constipation, diarrhea, ileus or obstruction)
- Physical findings: edema, skin integrity (pressure ulcers, skin around feeding tube site), NFPE findings (loss of muscle mass/fat stores); vitals, functional status
- Anthropometrics (wt history, BMI)

Nutrition Diagnosis

- Inadequate EN infusion RT dislodged gastrostomy feeding tube AEB EN on hold × 2 days with plan for new enteral access within 24 to 48 hours
- Inadequate EN infusion RT increased nutrient requirements with sepsis and skin breakdown AEB current EN regimen meets 80% estimated kcal and 60% estimated protein requirements
- Swallowing difficulty RT oropharyngeal dysphagia s/p CVA AEB + S/S aspiration on all food consistencies per speech pathology findings and recommendation for long-term EN access

Intervention

- State calculated estimated nutrient daily requirements
- EN recommendations
- Addition of multivitamins and minerals
- Nutrition-related medication management (fiber modular, probiotic, promotility agents, anti-emetic agents)
- Instruction for EN administration and requirements
- Communication with multiple medical disciplines (Speech Language Pathology, social work and discharge planning, physicians)

Monitoring and Evaluation

- Patient able to tolerate 100% estimated EN requirements within 3 to 5 days
- No s/s refeeding syndrome
- Consistent BM without abdominal distention, constipation, or diarrhea

ADIME 5.1 ADIME At-A-Glance (*continued*)

- Enteral tube remains functional
- Gradual weight gain of 0.5 to 1 lb weekly, BMI to improve
- Labs to return to normal limits
- Wound healing

References

1. Merritt R. *The A.S.P.E.N. Nutrition Support Practice Manual*. 2nd ed. Silver Spring, MD: American Society of Parenteral and Enteral Nutrition; 2005.
2. Mueller CM. *The A.S.P.E.N. Adult Nutrition Support Core Curriculum*. 2nd ed. Silver Spring, MD: American Society of Parenteral and Enteral Nutrition; 2012.
3. McClave SA, Taylor BE, Martindale RG, et al; Guidelines for the provision and assessment of nutrition support therapy in the adult critically ill patient: Society of Critical Care Medicine (SCCM) and American Society for Parenteral and Enteral Nutrition (A.S.P.E.N.). *JPEN J Parenter Enter Nutr* 2016;40(2):159–211.
4. Koseniecki M, Fritzshall R. Enteral nutrition for adults in the hospital setting. *Nutr Clin Pract* 2015;30(5):634–651.
5. McClave SA, Lukan JK, Stefater JA, et al. Poor validity of residual volumes as a marker for risk of aspiration in critically ill patients. *Crit Care Med* 2005;33(2):324–330.
6. Institute of Medicine, Food and Nutrition Board. *Dietary Reference Intakes: Energy, Carbohydrate, Fiber, Fat, Fatty Acids, Cholesterol, Protein and Amino Acids*. Washington, DC: National Academy Press; 2002.
7. Kingley J. Fluid and electrolyte management in parenteral nutrition. *Support Line* 2005;27(6):13–22.
8. Task Force for the Revision of Safe Practices for Parenteral Nutrition. Safe practices for parenteral nutrition. *JPEN J Parenter Enteral Nutr* 2004;28:S39–S70.
9. Heyland DK, Murch L, Cahill N, et al. Enhanced protein-energy provision via the enteral route feeding protocol in critically ill patients: Results of a cluster randomized trial. *Crit Care Med* 2013;41:2743–2753.

NOTES

Notes

Notes

PART 2

Nutrition Considerations for Specific Diseases

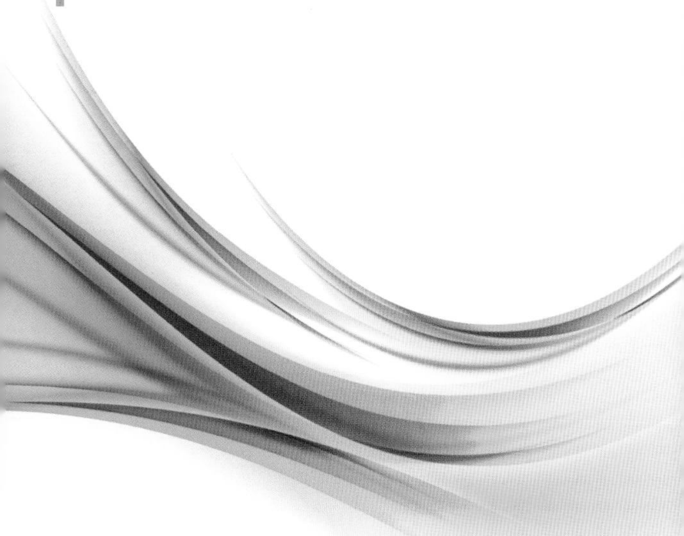

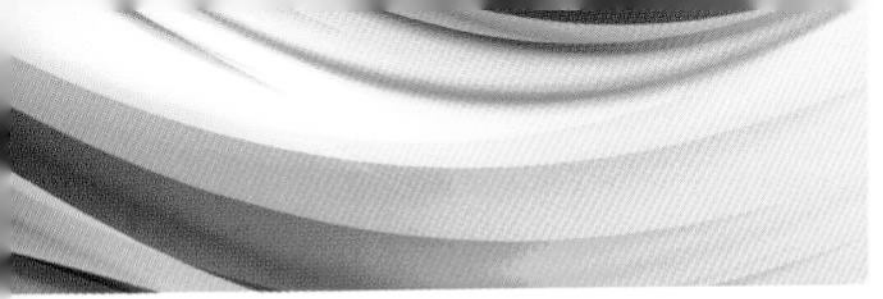

CHAPTER 6

Bariatric Surgery

Lindsey Battistelli, RDN

Obesity has been recognized as a disease entity by the American Medical Association and not simply an issue of overeating and lack of control. The World Health Organization and the Institute of Medicine, as well as other scientific organizations, recognize the metabolic consequences of obesity in high-risk individuals, for whom, depending on the severity of the obesity, they may be life-threatening. Given the strong evidence that a high percentage of people who lose weight using conventional methods will regain it, for high-risk patients, bariatric surgery is considered the most effective treatment for long-term weight loss and maintenance.[1]

BARIATRIC PROCEDURES

When nonsurgical methods have failed to produce weight loss and sustained maintenance, bariatric surgery may be indicated for patients with Class III obesity (body mass index [BMI] ≥ 40) without comorbidities, or Class II obesity (BMI ≥ 35) with at least two specified comorbidities: type 2 diabetes, heart disease, hypertension, dyslipidemia, obstructive sleep apnea, or other respiratory disorders, nonalcoholic fatty liver disease, gastrointestinal (GI) disorders, or osteoarthritis.[2,3] The guidelines include the surgical option for patients with BMI of 30 who have either diabetes or metabolic syndrome, according to the statement "offer bariatric procedure, although current evidence is limited."

Bariatric surgery procedures have evolved and improved over time. The most common procedures performed today include the roux-en-y gastric bypass (RYGB), the sleeve gastrectomy (SG), the adjustable gastric band (AGB), and the biliopancreatic diversion with or without duodenal switch (BPD-DS). Since 2008, the SG has advanced from being an investigative procedure to being comparable to the gastric bypass or gastric band. Most bariatric procedures are performed laparoscopically rather than through a large open incision. This decreases early postoperative complications and enhances recovery. Bariatric surgery is considered a safe and effective treatment for those who meet the criteria. Several procedures are in use, and they vary in regard to the potential nutrient deficiencies that may arise from the specific procedure (Table 6.1).

PREOPERATIVE CARE

All potential bariatric surgery candidates should undergo preoperative evaluation by a multidisciplinary team, including a physician, bariatric surgeon, registered dietitian (RD), psychologist, and an exercise specialist. Box 6.1 includes a preoperative checklist for bariatric surgery.

Preoperative Nutrition Assessment

A complete nutrition assessment should be completed for all patients before any bariatric surgery procedure.[4] This should include assessment of the patient's ability to follow and comply with all pre- and postoperative dietary, behavior, and lifestyle change recommendations, current nutrition intake and history of weight loss attempts, educational needs, as well as micronutrient screening.[3,4] Components of a long-term lifestyle change include the patient's motivation or readiness to change, goal setting, nutrient knowledge, and other factors affecting weight status including behavioral, psychological, cultural, and economic influences.

TABLE 6.1. Bariatric Surgery Procedures

Procedure	Also Known As	How the Procedure Works	Potential Nutrient Deficiencies
Roux-en-y gastric bypass	"Roux-en-y" or "Gastric Bypass," "the Bypass"	Creating a small stomach pouch approximately 30 cc (30 mL) in size and thus bypassing the majority of the stomach and the first portion of the small intestine, including the duodenum	Iron, vitamin B_{12}, calcium, folate, vitamin D, thiamin
Biliopancreatic diversion with (or without) duodenal switch	"the Switch," "BPD-DS" "BPD"	Majority of stomach is removed, and the distal part of the small intestine is connected to the pouch, bypassing the duodenum and jejunum. The bypassed small intestine, which carries the bile and pancreatic enzymes, is reconnected to the last portion of the small intestine to eventually mix with the food. The DS keeps the pylorus intact.	Vitamins A, D, E, K, zinc, iron, calcium, protein
Sleeve gastrectomy	"Gastric Sleeve," "the Sleeve," "Vertical Sleeve Gastrectomy (VSG)"	Approximately 80% of the stomach is removed to leave a long "sleeve" or banana-shaped pouch.	Vitamin B_{12}, calcium, iron, thiamin
Adjustable gastric band	"the Band," "Lap-Band"	Silicone band is placed around the top of the stomach, creating restriction; saline may be injected into the band, making it tighter.	Folate, vitamin B_{12}, calcium, thiamin

Data from Bariatric Surgery Procedures. American Society for Metabolic and Bariatric Surgery web site. Available at: http://asmbs.org/patients/bariatric-surgery-procedures. Accessed January 20, 2016.

BOX 6.1 Preoperative Checklist for Bariatric Surgery

- Complete history and physical examination (H&P) for obesity-related comorbidities, causes of obesity, weight/BMI, weight loss history, commitment, and exclusions related to surgical risk
- Routine labs including fasting blood glucose and lipid panel, kidney function liver profile, urine analysis, prothrombin time/INR, blood type, CBC
- Nutrient screening with thiamin, iron studies, B_{12}, and folic acid, and 25-vitamin D, (vitamins A and E optional)
- Consider more extensive testing in patients undergoing malabsorptive procedures based on symptoms and risks
- Cardiopulmonary evaluation, sleep apnea screening, venous thromboembolism (VTE) risk screening as clinically indicated; ECG, chest x-ray (CXR), echocardiography if cardiac disease or pulmonary hypertension suspected; DVT evaluation if clinically indicated
- GI evaluation (*H. pylori* screening in high-prevalence areas; gallbladder evaluation and endoscopic and radiologic testing if clinically indicated)
- Endocrine evaluation: A1C with suspected or diagnosed prediabetes or diabetes; thyroid-stimulating hormone (TSH) with symptoms or increased risk of thyroid disease; androgens with polycystic ovary syndrome suspicion (total/bioavailable testosterone, DHEAS, D4-androstenedione); screening for Cushing syndrome if clinically suspected
- Clinical nutrition evaluation by RD
- Psychosocial–behavioral evaluation; document medical necessity for bariatric surgery
- Informed consent
- Provide relevant financial information
- Continue efforts for preoperative weight loss
- Optimize glycemic control
- Pregnancy counseling
- Smoking cessation counseling
- Verify cancer screening by primary care physician

Reprinted from Mechanick JI, Youdim A, Jones DB, et al. Clinical practice guidelines for the perioperative nutritional, metabolic, and nonsurgical support of the bariatric surgery patient - 2013 update: Cosponsored by American Association of Clinical Endocrinologists, The Obesity Society, and American Society for Metabolic & Bariatric Surgery. *Surg Obes Relat Dis* 2013;9(2):159–191, Copyright (2013), with permission from Elsevier.

Correction of any insufficient or deficient micronutrient levels should be a primary intervention before bariatric surgery because obesity is a risk factor for nutrient deficiencies, particularly[5]

- Iron
- Vitamin B_{12}
- Zinc
- Vitamin D

The following laboratory studies should be assessed in the presurgical patient:

- Liver function tests
- Lipid profile
- CBC with differential
- Hgb A1C
- Serum iron, ferritin, and TIBC
- Serum calcium, alkaline phosphatase
- Serum vitamin B_{12}
- Serum vitamin B-1 (thiamin)
- Serum folate
- PTH, 25-hydroxyvitamin D

The Mifflin-St. Jeor formula for estimating resting metabolic rate (RMR) is recommended for estimating energy requirements in the obese patient using actual body weight.[6]

$$\text{Men: RMR (kcal/day)} = 10 \times \text{weight (kg)} + 6.25 \times \text{height (cm)} - 5 \times \text{age (years)} + 5$$

$$\text{Women: RMR (kcal/day)} = 10 \times \text{weight (kg)} + 6.25 \times \text{height (cm)} - 5 \times \text{age (years)} - 161$$

Preoperative Diet and Weight Loss

Most programs require that the patient lose weight before bariatric surgery. A weight loss of 5% to 10% is usually recommended to decrease total liver volume and improve ease of a laparoscopic procedure and surgical outcomes.

A high-protein and/or liquid diet may be recommended 2 days or more before the scheduled bariatric surgery, according to program protocols. This allows for adequate protein intake and hydration before surgery, and also gives time for the patient to practice using protein supplements. Presurgery is also an opportune time to include education on lifestyle modification in an effort to improve success after surgery.

All patients are required to be NPO after midnight before their procedure to clear the stomach and bowel before surgery. Some surgeons may require a bowel prep of magnesium citrate or something similar the day before the bariatric procedure to completely clear the bowel. It is also recommended that patients who smoke should stop at least 6 weeks before bariatric surgery.

POSTOPERATIVE CARE

Acute Postoperative Period (Up to 3 Months Following Surgery)

The early postoperative period, typically from immediately after surgery until 3 months later, is a crucial time for meeting nutritional needs that result from the stress of surgery and healing involved (Box 6.2). Protein needs should be met to allow the stomach to heal from surgery and to prevent lean tissue loss. Some patients may require more support and guidance with the progression of their diet, and frequent nutritional follow-up is critical for healthy weight loss. The length and variation of postop diet progression depend on surgeon and dietitian preference, but generally follow the transition listed in Table 6.2.

Patients typically begin a low-sugar, clear liquid diet within 24 hours of surgery, and some surgeons may require an upper GI swallow study before initiating diet to rule out early complications.[3,7] It is important to differentiate between a standard clear liquid diet and a bariatric clear liquid diet related to sugar content. A standard clear liquid diet could cause a postop RYGB patient to experience

BOX 6.2 Early Postoperative Care Checklist

- Monitored telemetry at least 24 hours if high risk for cardiopulmonary complication
- Protocol-derived staged meal progression supervised by RD
- Healthy eating education by RD
- Multivitamin plus minerals (# tablets for minimal requirement)
- Calcium citrate, 1,200 to 1,500 mg/day
- Vitamin D, at least 3,000 units/day, titrate to >30 ng/mL
- Vitamin B_{12} as needed for normal range levels
- Maintain adequate hydration (usually >1.5 L/day PO)
- Monitor blood glucose with diabetes or hypoglycemic symptoms
- Pulmonary toilet, spirometry, DVT prophylaxis, early ambulation
- If unstable, consider pulmonary embolus (PE), intestinal leak (IL)
- If rhabdomyolysis suspected, check CPK

Adapted from Mechanick JI, Youdim A, Jones DB, et al. Clinical practice guidelines for the perioperative nutritional, metabolic, and nonsurgical support of the bariatric surgery patient–2013 update: Cosponsored by American Association of Clinical Endocrinologists, The Obesity Society, and American Society for Metabolic & Bariatric Surgery. *Surg Obes Relat Dis* 2013;9(2):159–191, Copyright (2013), with permission from Elsevier.

TABLE 6.2. Diet Progression Following Bariatric Surgery

Diet	Duration	Goals
Clear liquid	Short-term: 1–2 d; longer requires nutritional supplementation.	Adequate hydration and protein intake, low sugar
Full liquid	10–14 d	Adequate hydration and increased protein intake, low sugar
Pureed/soft foods	7–14 d	Adequate hydration, increased protein intake, addition of fruits and vegetables, low sugar
Modified regular	Ongoing	Adequate hydration, protein, fruits, vegetables, and small amounts of whole grains, low sugar

Data from Cummings S, Ison K. *Pocket Guide to Bariatric Surgery*, 2nd ed. Chicago, IL: Academy of Nutrition and Dietetics; 2015.

dumping syndrome. Straws, carbonation, and caffeine are not recommended in the immediate postop stage. A patient's new stomach can hold only very small amounts owing to the size of the newly created pouch and surgical swelling. As healing progresses, the patient will be able to tolerate thicker consistencies of food. A liquid diet will also allow the stomach to heal properly without added tension to the staple line or stitches. Complete stomach healing is achieved about 6 weeks after surgery.

It is helpful for the dietitian to provide postop discharge instructions to the patient so that questions can be answered. In addition to diet instructions, the patient should be encouraged to walk regularly as part of the treatment plan to lower the risk of deep vein thrombosis (DVT). Patients should be restricted from lifting heavy weights until cleared by the surgeon, usually 2 to 4 weeks after surgery. Laparoscopic surgeries usually only require 1 to 2 days of in-hospital stay before discharge.

Most patients will indicate that they are not hungry after surgery, because of both the surgery anesthesia and the decrease in the hunger hormone, ghrelin. Pancreatic peptide YY (PYY) and glucagon-like peptide-1 (GLP-1), which decrease appetite through different mechanisms, are also shown to be increased in the postprandial period after SG and RYGB procedures.[8] It is important to adhere to the nutrition prescription so as to preserve lean body tissue and to meet nutritional needs. Small, frequent meals are recommended over the course of the day, as is teaching the patient to identify the difference between snacking and grazing on empty calories versus high-quality food sources. Table 6.3 lists specific foods that should be avoided or delayed for reintroduction into the diet.

Dumping Syndrome

Patients are advised to limit the total amount of sugar intake because of the effect of dumping syndrome that can be experienced with a RYGB. Dumping syndrome is considered a complication of surgery where food, particularly food

TABLE 6.3. Recommended Foods to Avoid or Delay Reintroduction

Food Type	Recommendation
Sugar, sugar-containing foods, concentrated sweets	Avoid
Carbonated beverages	Avoid/delay[a]
Fruit juice	Avoid
High-saturated fat, fried foods	Avoid
Soft "doughy" bread, pasta, rice	Avoid/delay[a]
Tough, dry, red meat	Avoid/delay[a]
Nuts, popcorn, other fibrous foods	Delay[a]
Caffeine	Avoid/delay[a] in moderation
Alcohol	Avoid

[a]Foods to delay should be a minimum of 6 weeks, but reintroduction varies by bariatric facility protocol.

Reprinted from Aills L, Blankenship J, Buffington C, et al. ASMBS Allied Health Nutritional Guidelines for the surgical weight loss patient. *Surg Obes Relat Dis* 2008;4(5):S73–S108, with permission from Elsevier.

with a high sugar content, is quickly released or "dumped" into the small bowel owing to the absence of the pyloric sphincter in the bypassed portion of the stomach. Consequently, a hypertonic solution is created in the jejunum that causes distension.[5] Early dumping symptoms include rapid heartbeat, sweating, dizziness, nausea, stomach cramps, and diarrhea. Late dumping occurs 1 to 3 hours afterward with the quick uptake of glucose triggering an insulin release, causing reactive hypoglycemia. Some patients with SG will have dumping syndrome.[9]

Not all patients will experience dumping syndrome, but as a precaution, bariatric patients should receive education on how to avoid excess sugar intake by reading and interpreting nutrition facts labels. There is no specific amount of sugar intake that may cause dumping syndrome, but generally, no more than 25 g of sugar per serving is recommended. Patients are advised to keep a food diary to track any dumping-related symptoms. Fluid intake should be avoided for 30 minutes before, during, and 30 minutes after eating, to avoid the risk of dumping syndrome posed by quick gastric emptying, and to improve satiety. As patients heal after surgery and swelling in the pouch decreases, hydration should continue to be encouraged as patients resume busy and active lifestyles, to avoid dehydration.

Protein

Protein consumption should be individualized and assessed by the dietitian on the basis of age, gender, and body weight of the patient.[3] A factor of 1.5 g/kg of ideal body weight per day (with a minimum of 60 g/day) should provide adequate protein. Owing to the small size of the postoperative stomach, protein needs should be divided throughout the day, with an average of 15 to 30 g of protein per serving to allow for adequate digestion and absorption. Liquid protein supplements are used in the immediate postop period to meet protein requirements, and the patient should be encouraged to sip their protein drinks slowly. Complete protein supplements containing all nine essential amino acids are required. Patients should be given guidance before surgery on the types of high-bioavailability protein supplements to purchase, such as whey, casein, egg white, milk, and soy-based products.

As the diet progresses, some of the liquid protein supplements may be replaced with high-protein food choices such as poultry, fish, meat, low-fat dairy, and soy. One to two ounces may be tolerated at one time, and protein foods must be eaten slowly and chewed well. Behavior modification to support slow eating should be discussed, as eating too much or too quickly or not chewing food well may cause nausea and vomiting. Moist, tender, and juice-containing meats are recommended over dry, rubbery, or dense textures. Patients should be instructed on proper food preparation techniques when cooking foods to avoid rubbery and dry textures. In addition, they should be encouraged to consume protein in small and frequent meals, along with a regular supplement, to consistently meet daily needs.

Alcohol and Tobacco

Alcohol is not recommended after bariatric surgery. Patients are to avoid alcohol intake and continue abstinence 1 year postoperatively and beyond owing to the high-calorie content and low nutritional value. Alcohol may also increase the risk for ulcers and the risk for alcohol abuse, because the patient's tolerance of alcohol is altered. Patients should avoid tobacco use after bariatric surgery owing to the increased risk of anastomotic ulcer and poor wound healing.

Micronutrients

Initially, patients are to consume liquid or chewable vitamin and mineral supplements for maximum digestion and absorption in the early postoperative period. Daily chewable or liquid multivitamins can usually be started when any postsurgical nausea or vomiting has subsided.[3] Supplements are usually recommended to be taken with food because of the highly concentrated formula. Other supplements required may include sublingual vitamin B_{12}, calcium citrate with vitamin D, and iron in the form of ferrous fumarate. Specific micronutrient deficiencies or insufficiencies targeted preop are to continue to be treated depending on the individual's lab results. Table 6.4 lists the suggested vitamin supplementation after specific types of bariatric procedures.

Nutrition Complications in the Postoperative Patient

Every surgery has its own risk for complications. Complications of bariatric surgery are seen in 2% to 10% of all cases and are related to the type of bariatric procedure performed.[5] Acute medical complications following bariatric surgery will usually arise within 30 days of surgery; however, regular follow-up visits with an RD for lifestyle modification are important during the first year after surgery. Acute complications of a bariatric procedure may be anastomotic leak, bleeding, DVT, dysphagia, abscess, stricture, reflux, nausea, vomiting, infection, pulmonary embolism, and cardio/pulmonary complications. Long-term complications include gastrojejunostomy stenosis, ulcer, hernia, gallstones, dumping syndrome, vitamin and/or mineral deficiency, and weight regain.

TABLE 6.4. Suggested Postoperative Vitamin Supplementation

Supplement	AGB	RYGB & SG	BPD/DS	Comment
Multivitamin–multimineral supplement • High potency containing at least 100% DV for 2/3 of nutrients, and 18 mg iron, 400 μg folic acid, and containing selenium and zinc in each serving. • Start with chewable or liquid, and progress to whole tablet/capsule as tolerated. • Avoid children's formulas that are not complete • May separate dosage • May improve GI tolerance when taken close to food intake • Do not mix multivitamin containing iron with calcium, take 2 hr apart	100% of daily value	200% of DV	200% of DV	Begin on day 1 after hospital d/c
Additional cobalamin (B12) • Sublingual tablets, liquid drops, mouth spray, or nasal gel/spray (oral) • Intramuscular (IM) injection • Supplementation after AGB and BPD/DS may be required	None	350–500 μg/day (oral) 1,000 μg/mo (IM)	None	Begin 0–3 mo after surgery

Additional elemental calcium • Calcium citrate and vitamin D_3 • Split into 500–600 mg doses; be mindful of serving size on supplement label • Suggest a brand that contains magnesium, especially for BPD/DS • Do not combine calcium with iron • Promote intake of dairy beverages and/or foods that are significant sources of dietary calcium in addition to recommended supplement, up to 3 servings daily • Combined dietary and supplemental calcium intake >1,700 mg/day may be required to prevent bone loss during rapid weight loss.	1,500 mg/day	1,500–2,000 mg/day	1,800–2,400 mg/day	May begin on day 1 after hospital d/c or within 1 mo after surgery
Additional elemental iron (above that provided by multivitamin) • Recommended for menstruating women and those at risk for anemia (total goal intake = 50–100 mg elemental iron/day) • No enteric coating • Avoid excessive intake of tea owing to tannin interaction • Encourage foods rich in heme iron • Vitamin C may enhance absorption of nonheme sources	None	Add a minimum of 18–27 mg/day elemental	Add a minimum of 18–27 mg/day elemental	Begin on day 1 after hospital d/c

(*continued*)

TABLE 6.4. Suggested Postoperative Vitamin Supplementation (*continued*)

Supplement	AGB	RYGB & SG	BPD/DS	Comment
Fat-soluble vitamins • With all procedures, higher maintenance doses may be required for those with a history of deficiency • Water-soluble preparations of fat-soluble vitamins are available • Retinol sources of vitamin A should be used to calculate dosage • Most supplements contain a high percentage of beta carotene, which does not contribute to vitamin A toxicity • Intake of 2,000 IU vitamin D_3 may be achieved with careful selection of multivitamin and calcium supplements • No toxic effect known for vitamin K_1, phytonadione (phyloquinone) • Vitamin K requirement varies with dietary sources and colonic production • Caution with vitamin K supplementation for patient receiving coagulation therapy • Vitamin E deficiency has been suggested, but is not prevalent in published studies.	None	None	10,000 IU of vitamin A 2,000 IU of vitamin D 300 μg of vitamin K	May begin 2–4 wk after surgery

Optional B complex B-50 dosage • Liquid form is available • Avoid time-released tablets • No known risk of toxicity • May provide additional prophylaxis against B-vitamin deficiencies, including thiamin, especially for BPD/DS procedures as water-soluble vitamins are absorbed in the proximal jejunum. • Note: >1,000 ng of supplemental folic acid, provided in combination with multivitamins, could mask B_{12} deficiency	1 serving/day	1 serving/day	1 serving/day	May begin on day 1 after hospital discharge

AGB, adjustable gastric band; BPD/DS, biliopancreatic diversion with or without duodenal switch; RYGB, roux-en-y gastric bypass; SG, sleeve gastrectomy.

Reprinted from Aills L, Blankenship J, Buffington C, et al. ASMBS Allied Health Nutritional Guidelines for the surgical weight loss patient. *Surg Obes Relat Dis* 2008;4(5):S73–S108, with permission from Elsevier.

Protein malnutrition is not commonly seen in bariatric surgery, but needs to be considered because of the restriction of food and decreased appetite. Enteral and parenteral nutrition should be considered for those at high nutritional risk.[3] Noncritical bariatric surgery patients that are unable to use their GI tract to meet their needs at 5 to 7 days should be considered for parenteral nutrition and at 3 to 7 days in the critical patient, or if severe protein malnutrition is present and enteral nutrition is not shown to be effective. Table 6.5 lists the most common nutritional complications of bariatric surgery along with suggested interventions.

Troubleshooting in the Postoperative Period

Problems can arise in the longer-term postoperative period of more than 3 months, and regular follow-up is imperative (Box 6.3). Common problems can include hair loss and various micronutrient deficiencies. Hair loss after bariatric surgery may or may not be related to nutrition. Stress on the body from a major surgery and rapid weight loss are the common causes of hair loss post bariatric surgery, resulting in telogen effluvium.[10] Hair follicles in the anagen phase are changed into the telogen phase, which only last for about 100 to 120 days before falling out. This is seen most commonly in patients who are 3 to 4 months postsurgery; however, this is temporary and in the absence of a nutritional cause, will grow back normally once the hairs have fallen out. Most patients may not notice, or may only have slight thinning. Patients with severe hair loss may have had thin or receding hair before bariatric surgery.

Hair loss related to a nutritional deficiency after bariatric surgery is usually seen >6 months postoperatively and beyond. Nutritional deficiencies can also contribute to telogen effluvium. Patients whose oral intake is not meeting requirements or whose weight loss is more than what was expected will be at risk for hair loss related to nutritional needs not being met. Iron, zinc, and protein are the nutrients most often correlated with hair loss and should be assessed (Table 6.6).

Once the early postop phase is completed, regular biochemical monitoring is recommended for gauging a patient's micronutrient levels. This also allows the clinician to determine

TABLE 6.5. Common Nutritional Complications After Bariatric Surgery

Complication	Suggested Interventions
Dehydration	Assess fluid intake, IV hydration should be recommended if severe with adequate thiamin (B_1) (See thiamin deficiency)
Nausea/vomiting	Assess PO intake for possible contributors; separate eating/drinking; decrease portion size; sit upright when eating/drinking; take small bites/sips and eat slowly; limit fat, sugar, and highly acidic foods; avoid extreme food temperatures; rule out offending foods; regress diet progression as tolerated
Dysphagia	Assess PO intake for possible contributors including dry, tough, rubbery, doughy, or sticky foods; assess cooking techniques, regress diet progression as tolerated
Diarrhea	Assess PO intake for possible contributors including lactose, whey protein concentrate; high-fat and high-sugar foods
Flatulence	Assess PO intake for possible contributors including lactose, whey protein concentrate; carbonated beverages and straw use
Constipation	Assess PO intake for fluids, fiber
Dumping syndrome	Assess PO intake for concentrated sweets, sweetened beverages, eating and drinking at the same time
Food intolerance/ lactose intolerance	Assess PO intake for lactose, high-fat foods, gas-containing foods. Discontinue offending food, and wait to reintroduce until later; regress diet progression as tolerated
Hair loss	Assess PO intake for protein, fluid, vitamins, and minerals; determine months postop for telogen effluvium

Data from Cummings S, Ison K. *Pocket Guide to Bariatric Surgery*, 2nd ed. Chicago, IL: Academy of Nutrition and Dietetics; 2015.

whether current supplementation is meeting the patient's needs, and whether further supplements are required. Table 6.7 suggests biochemical monitoring tools for nutrition

BOX 6.3 Follow-Up Postoperative Care Checklist

- Initial, interval until stable, once stable (months)
- Monitor progress with weight loss and evidence of complications each visit
- SMA-21, CBC/plt with each visit (and iron at baseline and after as needed)
- Avoid nonsteroidal anti-inflammatory drugs
- Adjust postoperative medications
- Consider gout and gallstone prophylaxis in appropriate patients
- Need for antihypertensive therapy with each visit
- Lipid evaluation every 6 to 12 months based on risk and therapy
- Monitor adherence with physical activity recommendations
- Evaluate need for support groups
- Bone density (DXA), if indicated
- 24-hour urinary calcium excretion, if indicated
- B_{12} (annually; MMA and HCy optional; then q 3–6 months if supplemented)
- Folic acid (RBC folic acid optional), iron studies, 25-vitamin D, iPTH
- Vitamin A (initially and q 6–12 months thereafter)
- Copper, zinc, and selenium evaluation with specific findings
- Thiamin evaluation with specific findings
- Consider eventual body contouring surgery

Data from Mechanick JI, Youdim A, Jones DB, et al. Clinical practice guidelines for the perioperative nutritional, metabolic, and nonsurgical support of the bariatric surgery patient - 2013 update. *Surg Obes Relat Dis* 2013;(9):159–191.

TABLE 6.6. Hair Loss After Bariatric Surgery

Time Frame	Possible Causes	Interventions
<6 mo since surgery	Most likely related to stress from major surgery and rapid weight loss; temporary	Confirm that nutritional needs are being met, and continue to follow-up to access patient >6 mo postop
>6 mo since surgery	Most likely related to nutrient deficiency, disease state, or genetics	Confirm protein needs are being met, as well as zinc, iron, and essential fatty acids

TABLE 6.7. Biochemical Monitoring Tools for Nutrition Status in the Post–Bariatric Surgery Patient

Vitamin/ Mineral	Screening	Additional Laboratory Indexes	Normal Range	Critical Range	Postoperative Deficiency	Comment
B_1 Thiamin	Serum thiamin	↓RBS transketolase ↑ Pyruvate	10–64 ng/mL	Transketolase activity >20% Pyruvate >1 mg/dL	15%–29% more common in AA and Hispanics; often assoc. with poor hydration	Serum thiamin responds to dietary supplementation, but is poor indicator of total body stores
B_6 Pyridoxine	PLP	RBC glutamic pyruvate oxaloacetic transaminase	5–24 ng/mL	<3	unknown	Consider with unresolved anemia; diabetes could influence values
B_{12} cobalamin	Serum B_{12}	↑Serum and urinary MMA, ↑Serum tHcy	200–1,000 pg/mL	<200	10%–13% may occur with older patients and those taking H_2 blockers and PPIs	When symptoms are present and B_{12} 200–250 pg/mL, MMA and tHcy are useful; serum B_{12} may miss 25%–30% of deficiency cases

(continued)

TABLE 6.7. Biochemical Monitoring Tools for Nutrition Status in the Post–Bariatric Surgery Patient (*continued*)

Vitamin/ Mineral	Screening	Additional Laboratory Indexes	Normal Range	Critical Range	Postoperative Deficiency	Comment
Folate	RBC folate, serum folate	Urinary FIGLU Normal serum and urinary MMA ↑Serum tHcy	280–791 ng/mL	<305 nmol/L	Uncommon	Serum folate reflects recent dietary intake rather than folate status; RBC folate is a more sensitive marker; excessive supplementation can mask B_{12} deficiency in CBC; neurologic symptoms will persist.
Iron	Ferritin	↓Serum iron ↑TIBC	Males: 15–200 ng/mL Females: 12–150 ng/mL	<20	9%–16% of adult women in general population are deficient	Low Hgb and Hct are consistent with iron deficiency anemia in stage 3 or stage 4 anemia; ferritin is an acute phase reactant and will be elevated with illness and/or inflammation; oral contraceptives reduce blood loss for menstruating females

Vitamin A	Plasma retinol	RBP	20–80 μg/dL	<10	Uncommon, up to 7% in some studies	Ocular finding may suggest diagnosis
Vitamin D	25(OH)D	↓Serum phosphorus ↑Alkaline phosphatase ↑Serum PTH ↓Urinary calcium	25–40 ng/mL	<20	Common; 60%–70%	With deficiency, serum calcium may be low or normal; serum phosphorus may decrease, serum alkaline phosphatase increase; PTH elevated
Vitamin E	Plasma alpha tocopherol	Plasma lipids	5–20 μg/mL	<5	Uncommon	Low plasma alpha tocopherol to plasma lipids (0.8 mg/g total lipid) should be used with hyperlipidemia
Vitamin K	PT	↑DCP ↓Plasma phylloquinone	10–13 sec	Variable	Uncommon	PT is not a sensitive measure of vitamin K status

(*continued*)

TABLE 6.7. Biochemical Monitoring Tools for Nutrition Status in the Post–Bariatric Surgery Patient (*continued*)

Vitamin/ Mineral	Screening	Additional Laboratory Indexes	Normal Range	Critical Range	Postoperative Deficiency	Comment
Zinc	Plasma zinc	↓RBC Zinc	60–130 µg/dL	<70	Uncommon, but increased risk of low levels associated with obesity	Monitor albumin levels and interpret zinc accordingly, albumin is primary binding protein for zinc; no reliable method of determining zinc status is available; plasma zinc is method generally used; studies cited in this report did not adequately describe methods of zinc analysis
Protein	Serum albumin Serum total protein	↓Serum prealbumin (transthyretin)	4–6 g/dL 6–8 g/dL	<3 <20 mg/dL	Uncommon	Half-life for prealbumin is 2–4 d and reflects changes in nutritional status sooner than albumin, a nonspecific protein carrier with a half-life of 22 d

Reprinted fromAills L, Blankenship J, Buffington C, et al. ASMBS Allied Health Nutritional Guidelines for the surgical weight loss patient. *Surg Obes Relat Dis* 2008;4(5):S73–S108, with permission from Elsevier.

status in the postbariatric patient. Certain nutrients can be particularly problematic if careful attention is not paid to ensuring adequate intake, including thiamin, vitamin B_{12}, iron, calcium, and vitamin D.

Thiamin (Vitamin B1): Part of B-Complex Vitamins

- Reasonable to assume that the daily value (DV) of 1.5 mg should be adequate for most.[10]
- Primary absorption sites are bypassed with some bariatric procedures, and dietary sources may be diminished.
- Include in the multivitamin; gummy vitamins typically do not include thiamin.
- Dietary sources include fortified grains, legumes, nuts, and pork.
- Drug interactions: Lasix and Dilantin.
- Deficiency: Beriberi (dry, wet, cerebral, bariatric).
- Risk factors: poor PO intake, intestinal loss through vomiting, ethyl alcohol (ETOH) intake, eating disorders, dialysis.
- Signs/symptoms: vomiting, loss of appetite, weakness, sleepiness, burning feet, calf and leg pain, abdominal pain, constipation, headache, cramping, peripheral polyneuropathy.
- Treatment: 100 mg of oral thiamin (preferred as thiamin mononitrate), 50 to 100 mg intramuscularly (IM) or intravenously (IV) for several days with emesis; 10 to 20 mg as emesis subsides. Adequate levels of other vitamins and minerals required such as magnesium and B-vitamins.
- With bariatric surgery patients, it is most commonly seen in the early postop phase related to vomiting.

Vitamin B12 (Cobalamin): Part of B-Complex Vitamins

- Include in the multivitamin; separate supplementation may also be required.
- Loss of absorption that results from decrease in gastric acid, HCl, intrinsic factor.
- Dietary sources include meat, eggs, dairy.
- Drug interactions: tetracycline, PPI, and H_2 blockers can reduce B_{12} absorption.

- Deficiency: B_{12} deficiency, pernicious anemia.
- Risk factors: intestinal surgery—loss of HCl, gastric churning, pepsin, and intrinsic factor (IF), atrophic gastritis, *H. pylori* infection, veganism, alcoholism, fad dieting, poor nutrient intake.
- Signs/symptoms: fatigue, weakness, shortness of breath, loss of appetite, paresthesia, sore tongue. Numbness, coldness, cramping and shooting pains, clumsiness and gait abnormality are most common complaints.
- Treatment: oral or sublingual dose of 2,000 μg/day for 2 to 4 weeks; or 1,000 μg IM injection daily for 1 to 2 weeks. Transition to maintenance dose.

Iron

- Consider including in the multivitamin, and additional supplement is recommended in high-risk patients.
- Dietary sources: beef, sardines, turkey, mussels, oysters (heme), lentils, beans, and leafy greens (nonheme).
- Drug interactions: tetracycline, thyroid, bisphosphonates, levodopa, methyldopa, fluoroquinolones, penicillamine. Iron absorption is decreased with acid-reducing medications, calcium, some fiber supplements. Consider absorption of copper, zinc, selenium, and vitamin A with high iron dosages.
- Deficiency: iron deficiency, iron deficiency anemia.
- Risk factors: Menstruating women and those who become pregnant. Preferential absorption site is bypassed in RNYGB and DS (proximal duodenum). Absorption is also dependent upon iron stores. Reduced hydrolysis in the stomach.
- Signs/symptoms: fatigue, leg cramping, pagophagia, pica, hair loss, shortness of breath, pallor, irritability, difficulty swallowing, loss of appetite, sore/swollen tongue, angular cheilitis, brittle nails, koilonychias, headache, rapid pulse, tachycardia, difficulty with concentration, coldness, and decreased immune function.
- Treatment: Oral therapy of 100 to 200 mg elemental iron per day in divided doses. Vitamin C is shown to positively influence absorption. Do not include calcium supplementation with iron; keep at least 2 hours apart

because of the competition for the same absorption site. Iron dextran can also be given intravenously, but monitoring for allergic reaction is very important.

Calcium

- Separate supplementation is required for adequate dosage.
- Dietary sources include dairy products, leafy greens, soybeans, salmon, sardines, and calcium-fortified foods.
- Drug interactions: antibiotics and thyroid hormones and cardiac medications. Other interactions include magnesium, phytate, oxalate, large amounts of sodium and protein, iron, phosphorus, and large amounts of caffeine.
- Deficiency: hypocalcemia, metabolic bone disease (osteoporosis, osteomalacia, hyperparathyroidism).
- Risk factors: low intake, low protein, malabsorption, hypo- or achlorhydria, hypomagnesemia, vitamin D deficiency, steatorrhea.
- Signs/symptoms: paresthesia, numbness, muscle cramping, loss of sensation around the mouth, unexplained GI cramping.
- Treatment: orally 1,000 to 1,500 mg of elemental calcium in divided doses with vitamin D for prevention and maintenance, magnesium may be required. Up to 2,000 mg/day for treatment of chronic or mild hypocalcemia. Low protein levels should be addressed. Calcium citrate is preferred for both prevention and treatment. Bone, dolomite, and shell products should be avoided for possible lead or aluminum.

Vitamin D

- Include with calcium supplementation. Preoperatively, deficiency is seen in 62% of patients.[11]
- Dietary sources are not considered necessary if adequate sunlight is provided. Dietary sources include sardines, dairy products.
- Drug interactions: verapamil, cimetidine, orlistat, bile acid sequestrants, corticosteroids

- Risk factors: fat malabsorption in RNYGB and DS procedures.
- Signs/symptoms: most are related to subsequent calcium deficiency, increased head sweating, burning in the mouth, dysmenorrhea, seasonal affective disorder (SAD), cardiac arrhythmias, seizures, fatigue, loss of balance/falling, hypertension, and poor immune function.
- Treatment: 50,000 IU of D_2 is the typical treatment. Taken daily for up to 2 to 3 weeks is considered for those with levels <8 ng/mL, and in the presence of hypocalcemia.

ADIME 6.1 ADIME At-A-Glance: Bariatric Surgery

Assessment

History of multiple, unsuccessful diets, overweight her whole life. Skips meals and overeats at bedtime (HS). No regimented physical activity reported, and has a sedentary job where she works long hours. Height 65 inches, weight 345 lb.

Nutrition Diagnosis

Excessive energy intake related to unsuccessful attempts at reducing caloric intake as evidenced by BMI of 57.

Intervention

- Increase food frequency to a regular, structured eating pattern of three meals and one to two snacks.
- Avoid skipping meals. Increase physical activity by including a regimented exercise plan of at least 3 days/week of 45 minutes, and increase total steps walked per day by taking regular activity breaks at work for a total of 8,000 to 10,000 steps/day.

Monitoring and Evaluation

Regular follow-up intervals with RD every 2 weeks to evaluate adherence to recommendations, reports of PO intake, and regular weigh-ins. Will monitor the following:

- Energy intake: Caloric intake from food and beverages: food selection and portion consumed.
- Energy expenditure: Caloric output from overall physical activity (steps) and regimented exercises: days per week of exercises and steps per day.

References

1. Livingston EH. The incidence of bariatric surgery has plateaued in the U.S. *Am J Surg* 2010;200(3):378–385.
2. Pentin PL. What are the indications for bariatric surgery. *J Fam Pract* 2005;54(7):633–634.
3. Mechanick JI, Youdim A, Jones DB, et al. Clinical practice guidelines for the perioperative nutritional, metabolic, and non-surgical support of the bariatric surgery patient - 2013 update: Cosponsored by American Association of Clinical Endocrinologists, The Obesity Society, and American Society for Metabolic & Bariatric Surgery. *Surg Obes Relat Dis* 2013;9(2):159–191.
4. Aills L, Blankenship J, Buffington C, et al. ASMBS Allied Health Nutritional Guidelines for the surgical weight loss patient. *Surg Obes Relat Dis* 2008;4(5):S73–S108.
5. Cummings S, Ison K. *Pocket Guide to Bariatric Surgery*, 2nd ed. Chicago, IL: Academy of Nutrition and Dietetics; 2015.
6. Academy of Nutrition and Dietetics Evidence Analysis Library. Adult Weight Management Evidence-Based Practice Guidelines. Available at: http://www.andevidencelibrary.com. Accessed January 7, 2016.
7. Sims TL, Mullican MA, Hamilton EC, et al. Routine upper gastrointestinal gastrografin swallow after laparoscopic roux-en-y gastric bypass. *Obes Surg* 2003;13(1):66–72.
8. Vincent RP, le Roux CW. Changes in gut hormones after bariatric surgery. *Clin Endocrinol* 2008;69(2):173–179.
9. Papamargaritis D, Koukoulis G, Sioka E, et al. Dumping symptoms and incidence of hypoglycemia after provocation test at 6 and 12 months after laparoscopic sleeve gastrectomy. *Obes Surg* 2012;(10):1600–1606.
10. Jacques J. *Micronutrition for the Weight Loss Surgery Patient*. Edgemont, PA: Matrix Medical Communications; 2006.
11. Buffington C, Walker B, Cowan GS Jr, et al. Vitamin D deficiency in the morbidly obese. *Obes Surg* 1993;3(4):421–424.

Notes

Notes

Notes

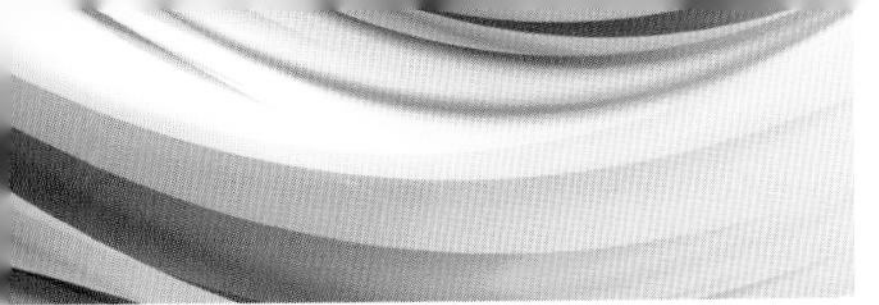

CHAPTER

7 Cancer

Sheri Betz, RD and Damien H. Buchkowski, RD, CSO

Worldwide each year, an estimated 14 million people learn they have cancer and 8 million people die from the disease.[1] By 2030, the global burden is expected to grow to 21.7 million new cancer cases and 13 million cancer deaths, simply because of the growth and aging of the population.[2] Nutrition is important in that it is relevant to both the etiology of many cancers and their treatment. Nearly 33% of annual cancer deaths in the United States have been attributed to nutrition and lifestyle.[3,4] Additionally, protein-calorie malnutrition (PCM) is the most common secondary diagnosis in individuals diagnosed with cancer, stemming from the inadequate intake of carbohydrate, protein, and fat to meet metabolic requirements and/or the reduced absorption of macronutrients.[5]

DISEASE PROCESS

Cancer is not one disease; rather, it represents over 100 diseases. The common characteristics of all cancers are uncontrolled cellular proliferation and the ability of these cells to metastasize, or migrate, from the original site and spread to distant sites throughout the body.

Cancer staging is a system used by physicians and other medical professionals to describe the extent or severity of an individual's cancer. Staging is based on the extent of the primary tumor, as well as on the extent of metastasis. Staging is important when the diagnosis of cancer is made, because it helps the physician plan the course of treatment, estimate the patient's prognosis, and identify any clinical trials that may be suitable for that particular patient.[6] Staging is also important for cancer registries and researchers, as it provides a common language for cancer reporting and for evaluating and comparing the results of clinical trials. Understanding of cancer staging is helpful when working with oncology patients, as the stage of the patient's cancer may correlate with nutritional status and provide insight into possible nutrition interventions.

Staging systems for cancer are constantly evolving, as scientists learn more about the disease. Many staging systems are currently in use. Some cover many different types of cancer, whereas others are specific to a particular type of cancer. The common elements in most staging systems include the following:

- Location of the primary tumor
- Tumor size and number of tumors
- Lymph node involvement
- Cell type and tumor grade
- Presence or absence of metastasis

The Tumor, Node, Metastasis Staging System

The tumor, node, metastasis (TNM) staging system is the most commonly used staging systems by medical professionals around the world.[7] This system was developed and is maintained by the American Joint Committee on Cancer (AJCC), and has been accepted by the Union for International Cancer Control (UICC). The National Cancer Institute (NCI) uses this system in their comprehensive cancer database, and most medical facilities use the TNM system as their main method for cancer reporting.[6]

The TNM system is based on the extent of the tumor (T), the extent of spread to the lymph nodes (N), and the presence of metastasis (M). A number is added to each letter to indicate the size or extent of the tumor and the extent of spread (see Table 7.1).

TABLE 7.1. Tumor, Nodes, Metastasis Cancer Staging System

T = Primary Tumor	
TX	Primary tumor cannot be evaluated
T0	No evidence of primary tumor
Tis	Carcinoma in situ (early cancer that has not spread to neighboring tissue)
T1–T4	Size and/or extent of primary tumor
N = Regional Lymph Nodes	
NX	Regional lymph nodes cannot be evaluated
N0	No regional lymph node involvement
N1–N3	Involvement of regional lymph nodes (number and/or extent of spread)
M = Distant Metastasis	
MX	Distant metastasis cannot be evaluated
M0	No distant metastasis
M1	Distant metastasis

Data from (i) National Cancer Institute, U.S. National Institutes of Health. Cancer staging. Available at: http://www.cancer.gov/about-cancer/diagnosis-staging/staging/staging-fact-sheet#q1. Accessed December 14, 2015, and (ii) American Joint Committee on Cancer. What is cancer staging? Available at: https://cancerstaging.org/references-tools/Pages/What-is-Cancer-Staging.aspx. Accessed December 14, 2015.

An example of the TNM system for staging colon cancer would be T3 N0 M0. This staging would mean a large tumor, located only in the colon, without spread to lymph nodes or any other parts of the body.

Overall Stage Grouping

Overall Stage Grouping is also referred to as Roman Numeral Staging. This system uses numerals I, II, III, and IV (plus the 0) to describe the progression of cancer. Once the TNM staging has been done, the result can then be categorized into one of five stages (see Table 7.2). The criteria for stages differ for different types of cancer, and so a

TABLE 7.2. Overall Stage Grouping

Stage	Definition
Stage 0	Carcinoma in situ (early cancer that is present only in the layer of cells in which it began)
Stages I, II, and III	Higher numbers indicate more extensive disease with greater tumor size, and/or spread of the cancer to nearby lymph nodes and/or organs adjacent to the primary tumor.
Stage IV	The cancer has metastasized.

Data from (i) National Cancer Institute, U.S. National Institutes of Health. Cancer staging. Available at: http://www.cancer.gov/about-cancer/diagnosis-staging/staging/staging-fact-sheet#q1. Accessed December 14, 2015, and (ii) American Joint Committee on Cancer. What is cancer staging? Available at: https://cancerstaging.org/references-tools/Pages/What-is-Cancer-Staging.aspx. Accessed December 14, 2015.

T3 N0 M0 bladder cancer may be a different overall stage than a T3 N0 M0 breast cancer.

Summary Staging

This simple staging system is often used by cancer registries and can be used for all types of cancer.[6]

- **In situ:** Cancer cells are present only in the layer of cells where they developed and have not spread.
- **Invasive:** Cancer cells have spread beyond the original layer of tissue.
- **Localized:** An invasive malignant cancer is confined entirely to the organ of origin.
- **Regional:** Cancer (a) has extended beyond the limits of the organ of origin directly into surrounding organs or tissues and (b) involves regional lymph nodes by way of the lymphatic system.

- **Distant:** Cancer has spread to parts of the body remote from the primary tumor either by direct extension or by discontinuous metastases.
- **Unknown:** Used to describe cases in which there is not enough information to indicate a stage.

TREATMENT AND NUTRITION INTERVENTION

Treatment of cancer with chemotherapy and radiation has significant nutritional consequences. Both types of treatment contribute to nutrient alterations in the cancer patient by reducing food intake, decreasing absorption, and/or altering metabolism.

Chemotherapy

Many chemotherapy medications are used in combination, often referred to as protocols or "cocktails," for treatment of specific cancers. Table 7.3 lists some common antineoplastic agents and their nutritional implications.

Nutrition-Related Side Effects of Chemotherapy (Effects Depend on the Agents Administered)[8,9]

- Anorexia
- Nausea, vomiting
- Mucositis (stomatitis, esophagitis, enteritis, gastritis, proctitis)
- Diarrhea
- Constipation
- Weight loss
- Taste alterations (ageusia—no taste; hypogeusia—little taste; dysgeusia—distorted taste)
- Metallic taste in mouth
- Xerostomia (dry mouth)
- Lactose intolerance
- Thrush
- Fatigue

TABLE 7.3. Chemotherapy Medications

Chemotherapeutic Agent: Generic Name (Trade Name)	Nausea and Vomiting	Diarrhea	Xerostomia	Stomatitis and Esophagitis	Anorexia	Taste Alterations
Anastrozole (Arimidex)	Mild	No	No	No	No	No
Bleomycin (Blenoxane)	Mild to moderate	No	Yes	Yes	Yes	No
Busulfan (Myleran)	Mild	No	No	No	Yes	No
Capecitabine (Xeloda)	Mild	Yes	No	No	No	No
Carboplatin (Paraplatin)	Moderate	Yes	No	No	No	No
Carmustine (BCNU)	Moderate	No	No	Yes	Yes	No
Cisplatin (CDDP)	Severe	Yes	No	No	Yes	Metallic taste
Cyclophosphamide (Cytoxan)	Severe	No	Yes	Yes	Yes	No
Cytarabine (ARA-C)	Severe	Yes	No	Yes	Yes	No
Dacarbazine (DTIC-Dome)	Severe	Yes	No	Yes	No	Metallic taste
Dactinomycin (Actinomycin-D, ACT)	Severe	Yes	Yes	Yes	No	Yes
Daunorubicin citrate (Daunomycin)	Moderate	Yes	Yes	Yes	Yes	Yes
Docetaxel (Taxotere)	Mild	No	No	No	No	No
Doxorubicin (Adriamycin)	Moderate	Yes	Yes	Yes	Yes	No
Epirubicin HCL (Ellence)	Moderate	Yes	No	Yes	No	No
Etoposide (VP-16-23)	Mild to moderate	Yes	No	Yes	Yes	No
Floxuridine (FUDR)	Mild	Yes	No	Yes	Yes	No

5-Fluorouracil (5-FU)	Moderate	Yes	No	Yes	No	Yes
Gemcitabine hydrochloride (Gemzar)	Mild	Yes	No	Yes	No	No
Hydroxyurea (Hydrea)	Mild to moderate	Yes	No	Yes	Yes	No
Irinotecan (Camptosar)	Severe	Yes	No	No	Yes	No
L-Asparaginase (Elspar)	Moderate	No	No	Yes	Yes	No
Mechlorethamine (Mustargen)	Severe	Yes	No	No	Yes	Metallic taste
Methotrexate (MTX)	Mild to moderate	Yes	No	Yes	Yes	Yes
Mitomycin (Mutamycin)	Moderate	Yes	No	Yes	Yes	No
Oxaliplatin (Eloxatin)[a]	Moderate	Yes	No	No	No	No
Paclitaxel (Taxol)	Mild	No	No	Yes	No	No
Procarbazine hydrochloride (Matulane)[b]	Severe	Yes	No	Yes	Yes	No
Streptozocin (Zanosar)	Severe	Yes	No	No	No	No
Tamoxifen citrate (Nolvadex)	Mild	No	No	No	Yes	No
Temozolomide (Temodar)	Moderate	No	No	No	Yes	No
Topotecan hydrochloride (Hycamtin)	Mild	Yes	No	No	Yes	No
Vinblastine sulfate (Velban)	Moderate	Yes	No	Yes	No	No
Vincristine sulfate (Vinscar)	Mild	Yes	No	Yes	Yes	No
Vinorelbine tartrate (Navelbine)	Mild	No	No	No	Yes	No

[a]Sensitivity to cold for 5 or more days following drug administration.
[b]To prevent hypertensive crisis, a low-tyramine diet must be followed while receiving procarbazine hydrochloride and 4 wk after the final dose.
Data from medication product labeling.

Radiation Therapy

Side effects of radiation can be acute or chronic in nature and are dependent on the area of the body that has been irradiated. Changes in taste or saliva caused by radiation to the head or neck can take months to show improvement and sometimes never return to baseline.[8]

Nutrition-Related Side Effects of Radiation Therapy

- General—anorexia, fatigue
- Brain—nausea
- Oropharyngeal
  - Taste alterations (ageusia—no taste, hypogeusia, dysgeusia)
  - Mucositis (stomatitis, esophagitis)
  - Dysphagia, odynophagia (painful swallowing)
  - Xerostomia, thick saliva
  - Dental caries
  - Loss of teeth
  - Swollen, tender gums
  - Change or loss of smell
  - Trismus (restriction or inability to open the mouth)
- Esophagus/chest/thorax
  - Esophagitis
  - Dysphagia
  - Esophageal stricture
- Abdomen/pelvis
  - Nausea, vomiting
  - Diarrhea, steatorrhea
  - Acute colitis and enteritis
  - Fistulas
  - Maldigestion, malabsorption
  - Perforations

Management of Cancer Symptoms and Treatment Side Effects

One of the most severe aspects of cancer is cachexia (often referred to as the "cancer anorexia–cachexia syndrome"), which develops in 80% of patients with advanced-stage cancer and is the cause of death in up to 40% of cancer patients.[5,10] Cachexia is a complex metabolic syndrome associated with underlying illness and characterized by weight loss with or without fat loss and at least three additional criteria for diagnosis, including decreased muscle strength, reduced muscle mass, fatigue, anorexia, or biochemical alterations (anemia, inflammation, low albumin). The etiology of this complex syndrome is not well understood.

Some individuals with cachexia do respond to nutrition therapy, but most will not see a complete reversal of the syndrome, even with aggressive therapy. Therefore, the most advantageous approach to cachexia is the prevention of its initiation through nutrition assessment, intervention, and monitoring.[5]

The symptoms associated with cancer, cachexia, and the side effects of the treatments used to control cancer can have devastating effects on nutritional status. Individualizing treatment plans to help maximize oral intake, and allowing patients to have flexibility in the type, quantity, and timing of their meals and snacks are essential parts of nutrition therapy. Many of these symptoms and side effects cannot be totally alleviated; however, they can be managed through the proper use of medications and through patient education.

Many medications are available to manage the symptoms of cancer and the side effects of cancer treatments. Tables 7.4 through 7.7 list the common medications used to help alleviate the anorexia, oral problems, nausea and vomiting, and diarrhea associated with cancer and its treatments.

The following lists provide tips and techniques that the cancer patients and their family may find useful when managing some of the most common problems associated with cancer/cancer treatments.[11]

Taste Changes

- Eliminate unpleasant odors and food from sight.
- Drink nutritional supplements through a straw (placed in the back of the mouth) in a covered container to decrease odors and contact with taste buds.

TABLE 7.4. Medications to Treat Anorexia

Medication: Generic Name (Trade Name)	Dose	Action	Special Considerations
Dronabinol (Marinol)	2.5 mg BID (up to 20 mg/d)	Increases appetite, decreases nausea	Drug may be habit-forming
Megestrol acetate (Megace)	800 mg daily	Increases appetite, promotes weight gain	May take 8–12 wk to reach maximal weight gain

Data from medication product labeling.

TABLE 7.5. Medications to Treat Oral Problems

Medication	Uses
Benzocaine oral spray (hurricane spray)	Relief of mouth pain, mouth sores
Artificial saliva (Xero-Lube, Salivart)	Used for xerostomia
Nystatin oral suspension	Antifungal used for treating thrush
Mix of Maalox, Benadryl, and lidocaine (often called the "radiation cocktail")	Used orally to swish and swallow for mouth pain and esophagitis
Mix of Maalox, Benadryl, and nystatin (often called "cools solution")	Used orally to swish and swallow for mouth pain associated with, and to treat, thrush
"Magic Mouthwash." Constituents vary by formulation but usually contains a mix of antibiotic, antihistamine, antifungal, corticosteroid, and Maalox (for coating purposes)	Used orally to swish and swallow for mouth pain and discomfort, to kill bacteria, to reduce fungal growth, and to treat inflammation

- Avoid citrus fruits and juices.
- Eat foods high in soluble fiber (oatmeal, barley, bananas, applesauce).
- Avoid foods high in insoluble fiber (whole grains, legumes, cabbage, broccoli, fibrous fruits and vegetables with seeds, skins, or peels).
- Avoid alcohol and caffeine.
- Eat boiled white rice, tapioca, cream of rice cereal, bananas, and peeled potatoes.
- Use low-lactose dairy products such as yogurt and aged cheeses instead of milk and ice cream.

Constipation

- Drink adequate amounts of fluids.
- Increase intake of fiber-rich foods (whole grains, high-fiber cereals, wheat bran, fruits and vegetables, legumes, and popcorn).
- Eat meals at regular intervals on a daily basis.
- Drink a hot beverage in the morning to stimulate a bowel movement.
- If allowed, increase physical activity.

Increasing Kilocalorie and Protein Intake

The nutrition requirements of most cancer patients can be estimated using the following: protein, 1.2 to 2.0 g/kg body weight; energy, 25 to 35 kcal/kg body weight. It is important to note that a patient who has a poor intake needs to consume nutritionally dense foods. Providing your patient with a high-kilocalorie, high-protein diet will help prevent rapid weight loss. The following are some common tips for patients:

- Eat small, frequent meals; keep snacks handy.
- Use nutritional supplements such as Ensure, Boost, etc.
- Add the following to foods to increase caloric and/or protein content: butter, margarine, whipped cream, half and half, cream cheese, sour cream, salad dressings, mayonnaise, honey, jam, sugar, granola, dried fruits, cottage or ricotta cheese, whole milk, powdered milk, ice cream, yogurt, eggs, nuts, seeds, wheat germ, and peanut butter.

NEUTROPENIC DIET

The neutropenic diet has been a mainstay in the oncology setting for decades despite a lack of evidence showing that adherence to this diet provides benefit to individuals with neutropenia. In a randomized controlled trial of 726 hematopoietic stem cell transplantation recipients, half followed a neutropenic diet and half did not. Results from this trial showed that following a neutropenic diet did not reduce infection. Interestingly, following a neutropenic diet was associated with *higher* rates of infection as well as increased rates of *Clostridium difficile* infection.[12] Many institutions have recently shifted from using a neutropenic diet to emphasizing the following safe food handling techniques for healthy and immunocompromised individuals.

General Food Safety Guidelines

- Check expiration dates on all products before buying. Be sure nothing is past its expiration date.
- Wash the following with soap/cleanser and hot water before and after contact with food. Air-dry or use paper towels—do not use cloth towels (using a dishwasher is preferred, if available):
  - Counter tops
  - Cutting boards
  - Cooking utensils
  - Silverware
  - Pots and pans
  - Dishes
- Wash hands frequently with warm soapy water, and dry with paper towels when preparing food. This is important especially after touching raw meat, chicken, eggs, and fish.
- Keep perishable food very hot or very cold. Do not leave perishable items at room temperature for more than 10 to 15 minutes.

- All perishable foods should be cooked thoroughly (no raw or rare meats).
- Thaw frozen foods in the refrigerator overnight or quickly in the microwave. Do not thaw food on the counter.
- Refrigerate leftovers promptly in airtight containers.
- Use leftovers only if they have been stored properly and have been around for no more than 24 hours.

SURVIVORSHIP NUTRITION

Any individual with a cancer diagnosis who is not in need of a specific nutrition intervention should be encouraged to follow dietary guidelines developed for cancer survivors. The American Cancer Society has established guidelines for cancer survivors to follow in order to reduce risk of future disease.[13] The guidelines also apply to individuals wishing to reduce dietary risk for the development of cancer. A summary of these guidelines follows:

- Body weight—achieve and maintain a healthy weight (body mass index [BMI], 18.5 to 25 kg/m^2).
- Physical activity—do 150 minutes of weekly physical activity that includes strength training on at least 2 days.
- Diet—choose a mostly plant-based diet high in fruits, vegetables, and whole grains. Eat at least 2.5 cups of fruits and vegetables daily. Limit red and processed meats, and avoid cooking these and other high-fat protein sources at high temperatures.
- Sugar/fat—limit high-fat foods as well as foods with added sugar.
- Alcohol—advice on alcohol consumption should be tailored to each patient by his or her health care provider, as alcohol may increase risk of specific cancers.
- Supplements—supplements should be considered only if a nutrient deficiency is biochemically or clinically demonstrated.

ADIME 7.1 ADIME At-A-Glance

Assessment

- Diet, appetite, food tolerance, taste alterations, intake history
- Medications (chemo, vitamin/mineral supplements, saliva substitute, antinausea)
- Labs (C-reactive protein, tumor markers, WBC counts)
- Physical findings: GI symptoms (esp. mouth sores, thrush, xerostomia, mucositis, dysphagia, trismus), N&V, diarrhea, constipation; nutrition-focused physical exam findings (loss of muscle mass/fat stores, edema); vitals, functional status
- Anthropometrics (wt/wt history, BMI)

Nutrition Diagnosis

- Predicted Suboptimal Energy Intake RT changes in taste and appetite, and increased nutrient needs due to chronic catabolic illness AEB scheduled therapy predicted to decrease ability to consume sufficient energy or nutrients, side effects of therapy, and nausea/vomiting.
- Inadequate Protein-Energy Intake RT decreased ability to consume sufficient protein and energy and surgery AEB weight loss of >5% × 1 month, BMI-18, bowel resection, NPO × 3 days, and recent Dx of colon cancer.
- Swallowing Difficulty RT pharyngeal/esophageal tumor and esophagitis from radiation therapy AEB dry mucous membranes, pain with swallowing, decreased food intake (eating <50% of meals), and inability to swallow solid foods.

Intervention

- Addition of snacks, nutritional supplements
- Enteral or parenteral recommendations
- Addition of multivitamins and minerals
- Feeding assistance
- Nutrition-related medication management (appetite stimulants, saliva substitute)
- Diet instruction (high kilocalorie and protein, GI symptom management—N&V, dry mouth/throat)
- Communication with Speech Language Pathology, social work, multiple disciplines

ADIME 7.1 ADIME At-A-Glance (*continued*)

Monitoring and Evaluation

- Patient to meet >75% of protein-energy needs PO
- Patient intake to meet 100% of estimated needs
- Enteral nutrition to be initiated
- Patient to follow medication recommendations
- BMI to improve
- No further weight loss with goal for weight gain
- Labs to return to normal limits
- Improvement of GI symptoms or problems
- Wound healing

REFERENCES

1. Centers for Disease Control and Prevention. World Cancer Day. Available at: http://www.cdc.gov/cancer/dcpc/resources/features/worldcancerday/. Accessed December 14, 2015.
2. American Cancer Society. *Global Cancer Facts & Figures*. 3rd ed. Atlanta, GA: American Cancer Society; 2015.
3. American Cancer Society. Nutritional and Physical Activity Research Highlights. Available at: http://www.cancer.org/research/acsresearchupdates/nutrition-and-physical-activity-research-highlights. Accessed November 24, 2015.
4. Anand P, Kunnumakara AB, Sundaram C, et al. Cancer is a preventable disease that requires major lifestyle changes. *Pharm Res* 2008;25(9):2097–2116.
5. National Cancer Institute, U.S. National Institutes of Health. Nutrition in Cancer Care—For Health Professions (PDQ®). Available at: http://www.cancer.gov/about-cancer/treatment/side-effects/appetite-loss/nutrition-hp-pdq#link/_28_toc. Accessed December 14, 2015.
6. National Cancer Institute, U.S. National Institutes of Health. Cancer staging. Available at: http://www.cancer.gov/about-cancer/diagnosis-staging/staging/staging-fact-sheet#q1. Accessed December 14, 2015.
7. American Joint Committee on Cancer. What is cancer staging? Available at: https://cancerstaging.org/references-tools/Pages/What-is-Cancer-Staging.aspx. Accessed December 14, 2015.

8. National Cancer Institute, U.S. National Institutes of Health. Nutrition implications of cancer therapies. Available at: http://www.cancer.gov/about-cancer/treatment/side-effects/appetite-loss/nutrition-hp-pdq#link/_28_toc. Accessed December 14, 2015.
9. Trustees of the University of Pennsylvania. Oncolink.org. Cancer treatment/chemotherapy/side effects. Available at: http://www.oncolink.org/treatment/treatment.cfm?c=145. Accessed December 14, 2015.
10. Argiles JM, Olivan M, Busquets S, et al. Optimal management of cancer anorexia–cachexia syndrome. *Cancer Manag Res* 2010;2:27–38.
11. National Cancer Institute, U.S. National Institutes of Health. Nutritional suggestions for symptom management. Available at: http://www.cancer.gov/about-cancer/treatment/side-effects/appetite-loss/nutrition-hp-pdq#link/_117_toc. Accessed December 15, 2015.
12. Trifilio S, Helenowski I, Giel M, et al. Questioning the role of a neutropenic diet following hematopoietic stem cell transplantation. *Biol Blood Marrow Transplant* 2012;18:1385–1390.
13. Rock CL, Doyle C, Demark-Wahnefried W, et al. Nutrition and physical activity guidelines for cancer survivors. *CA Cancer J Clin* 2012;62:242–274. doi:10.3322/caac.21142.

Notes

Notes

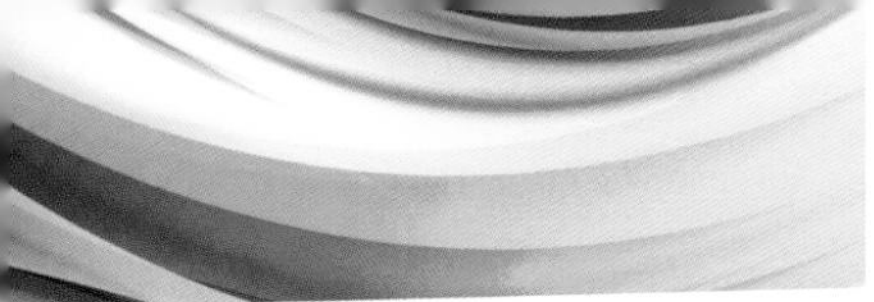

CHAPTER 8

Cardiovascular Disease

Tilakavati Karupaiah, PhD, APD, AN

The cardiovascular system includes the heart and blood vessels linking the heart to other systems to facilitate metabolic functions, nutrient and gas transport, temperature and pH stabilization, maintenance of homeostasis, and initiation of defense mechanisms. Diseases affecting the heart, coronary heart disease leading to myocardial infarction (MI), and the circulatory network, cerebrovascular accident (CVA) or stroke, are collectively grouped as cardiovascular disease (CVD). CVD mortality rates declined by 30.8% between 2001 and 2011, but coronary heart disease at 47.7% and CVA at 16.4% still remain the major causes of mortality in Americans[1,2], with significant racial disparities related to CVD risk factors (Box 8.1). Medical nutrition therapy (MNT) is a crucial intervention component through specific changes in diet to target the signs and symptoms of CVD, particularly managing hypertension and dyslipidemias, as well as potential disease complications (Fig. 8.1).

CORONARY HEART DISEASE

Disease Process

Coronary heart disease (CHD) begins with atherosclerosis, a chronic inflammatory process in response to arterial wall injuries leading to lesion formation.[3] Endothelial injuries can

BOX 8.1 Racial and Gender Disparities for CVD Risk Factors

- In men, the highest **prevalence of obesity** (29.7%) was in Mexican Americans who had completed a high school education. African American women with or without a high school education had a higher prevalence of obesity (48.4%).
- **Hypertension prevalence** was highest in African Americans (41.2%) regardless of sex or educational status.
- **Hypercholesterolemia** was high among white and Mexican American men and white women regardless of educational status.
- **CVD mortality** at all ages was highest in African Americans.

Data from Mozaffarian D, Benjamin EJ, Go AS, et al. Heart disease and stroke statistics—2015 update: A report from the American Heart Association. *Circulation* 2015;131:e29–e322.

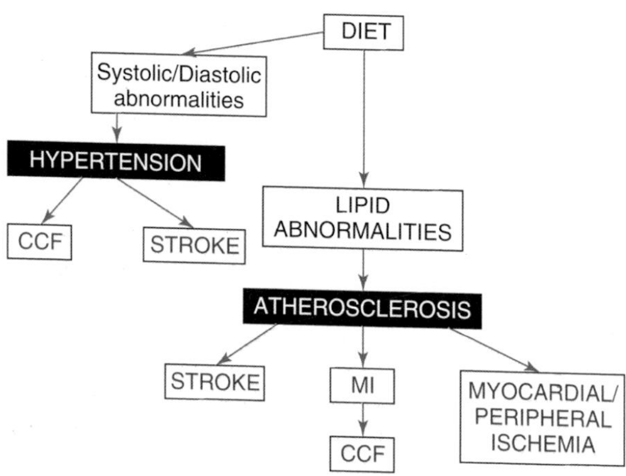

FIGURE 8.1 CVD and nutrition intervention targets. Black box denotes disease condition; blue text denotes endpoints of organ/systemic dysfunction.

be caused by one or more factors such as elevated or oxidized low-density lipoprotein (LDL), free radicals, toxins associated with smoking, infectious microorganisms, high blood pressure (BP), high serum cholesterol, insulin resistance, shear stress, homocysteine, diets high in satura sedentary lifestyle.[4] Atherogenesis results in e dysfunction with abnormal vascular smooth muscle growth, decreased anticoagulant and anti-inflammatory properties, and impaired vasomotor control.[5] Notably, endothelial dysfunction causes reduced nitric oxide production, which adversely affects vasodilation.

The core event in endothelial dysfunction is the trapping of LDLs within the subendothelial space, which subsequently undergo progressive oxidation initiated by free radicals from the intimal wall.[3] Oxidized or modified LDLs induce inflammatory responses, causing lesions in the intima, increased recruitment and adherence of monocytes and T lymphocytes to the atheroma, and penetration of monocytes into the tunica intima.[6] Monocytes convert into macrophages and readily take up oxidized LDLs, which subsequently become transformed into foam cells that eventually form the lipid core of the atherosclerotic plaque.[7] Oxidized LDLs add to endothelium injury, leading to release of platelet-derived growth factor (PDGF), which in turn stimulates the proliferation and migration of smooth muscle cells into intima that take up oxidized LDL to form foam cells.[8]

The high lipid- or cholesterol-enriched atheromatous plaque is prone to rupture, as the lesion is not stable. The ruptured fatty plaque is exposed to blood flow, attracting the deposition of small dense LDL, which subsequently leads to thrombus formation and platelet activation. The continuous deposition or accumulation of LDL and foam cells will progressively occlude the lumen of the blood vessel and slowly induce thrombosis, a proximate cause for a CVD event which, depending on the site, may be angina pectoris, ischemic heart disease, or MI.[5] Lipoprotein particles vary in size, with small, dense LDL particles proposed to be more atherogenic than larger- or normal-sized LDL particles, and are considered to be an independent risk factor for CVD (Table 8.1).[9]

Previous guidelines from the American Heart Association (AHA) advocated treating individual patients to risk-based

TABLE 8.1. Lipoprotein Subclasses and Atherogenic Risk

Lipoprotein Subclasses	Size in Nanometer (nm)	Atherogenicity
Large LDL	21.2–23.0	↓
Small LDL	18.0–21.2	↑
Large HDL	8.8–13.0	↓
Medium HDL	8.2–8.8	↓
Small HDL	7.3–8.2	↑

HDL, high-density lipoprotein; LDL, low-density lipoprotein; ↓, decreases risk; ↑, increases risk.

Data from Mora S, Szklo M, Otvos JD, et al. LDL particle subclasses, LDL particle size, and carotid atherosclerosis in the Multi-ethnic Study of Atherosclerosis (MESA). *Atherosclerosis* 2007;192:211–217.

LDL goals as the principle target of therapy. But, the Adult Treatment Panel IV (ATP IV) 2013 Guideline, jointly developed by the American College of Cardiology (ACC) and AHA, set no specific primary LDL-C goals for treatment.[10] Instead, the new ACC/AHA guideline emphasizes treating four specific patient groups with statin therapy, identified as patients with known atherosclerotic CVD (ASCVD), diabetes mellitus, untreated LDL-C >190 mg/dL, or a 10-year estimated ASCVD risk of >7.5%.

In addition, the ACC/AHA Task Group opted to not use the Framingham 10-year Risk Score (FRS) algorithm, because the FRS algorithm was derived exclusively from a white sample population and the scope was limited to only determining outcome related to CHD alone. Rather, the Task Group derived risk equations for 10-year estimated ASCVD risk of >7.5% based on pooled cohorts representative of the US population of whites and African Americans (Box 8.2).[10] The Task Group focused on estimation of the first hard ASCVD events (defined as the first occurrence of nonfatal MI, CHD death, or fatal or nonfatal CVA) as the outcome of interest. The *Risk Estimator* is intended for use in those without ASCVD and with an LDL-C <190 mg/dL. The information required to estimate ASCVD risk includes age,

BOX 8.2 Calculation Steps for 10-Year Risk Estimate for Hard ASCVD

Step 1—The natural log of age, total cholesterol, HDL-C, and systolic BP (treated or untreated value) are first calculated.
Step 2—Interaction terms between the natural log of age are multiplied with values for total cholesterol, HDL-C, and treated or untreated systolic BP.
Step 3—Calculated values are then multiplied by the coefficients from equation parameters ("Coefficient" column) for the specific race–sex group of the individual derived from pooled cohort equations for estimation of 10-year risk of ASCVD[a].
Step 4—The "Coefficient × Value" calculation provides the results of the multiplication for the risk profile for each parameter.
Step 5—The sum of the "Coefficient × Value" column is then calculated for the individual, shown as "Individual Sum" for each race and sex group.
Step 6—The estimated 10-year risk[a] of a first hard ASCVD event is formally calculated as 1 minus the survival rate at 10 years ("Baseline Survival"), raised to the power of the exponent of the "Coefficient × Value" sum minus the race- and sex-specific overall mean "Coefficient × Value" sum; or, in equation form: $1 - S10^{(IndX'B - MeanX'B)}$.

[a]A spreadsheet enabling estimation of 10-year and lifetime risk for ASCVD and a Web-based calculator are available at http://my.americanheart.org/cvriskcalculator and http://www.cardiosource.org/science-and-quality/practice-guidelines-and-quality-standards/2013-prevention-guideline-tools.aspx.

Data from Goff DC, Lloyd-Jones DM, Bennett G, et al. 2013 ACC/AHA guideline on the assessment of cardiovascular risk—A report of the American College of Cardiology/American Heart Association Task Force on Practice Guidelines. *Circulation* 2014;129(Suppl 2):S49–S73.

sex, race, total cholesterol, high-density lipoprotein (HDL) cholesterol, systolic BP, blood pressure-lowering medication use, diabetes status, and smoking status.

Treatment and Nutrition Intervention

The 2013 ACC/AHA guidelines focus on treatment of blood cholesterol to reduce ASCVD risk (Table 8.2).[10] The Task Group emphasized that intensive lifestyle modification (LM)

TABLE 8.2. LDL-C Targets for Statin Therapy Combined with Lifestyle Modification

Patient Groups	Statin Therapy	Intensive Lifestyle Modification
Individuals aged 40–75 years without clinical ASCVD or diabetes and with LDL-C 70–189 mg/dL (recalculate estimated 10-year ASCVD[a] risk every 4–6 years)	These individuals will not receive cholesterol-lowering drug therapy.	Heart healthy lifestyle habits are the foundation of ASCVD prevention.
Individuals >21 years with clinical ASCVD	**Age ≤75 years** **High-intensity statin** (moderate-intensity statin if not candidate for high-intensity statin)	Counsel on intensive healthy lifestyle habits: • Regularly monitor adherence to lifestyle management. • Reinforce healthy lifestyle during follow-ups 3–12 mo.
• Secondary causes of severe elevations of LDL-C ≥190 mg/dL and triglycerides ≥500 mg/dL should be evaluated and treated appropriately.	Age >75 years or if not candidate for high-intensity statin **Moderate-intensity statin**	*Evaluate diet as a secondary cause of hyperlipidemia:* • Elevated LDL-C—saturated or trans fats, weight gain, anorexia • Elevated TG—weight gain, very low-fat diets, high intake of refined carbohydrates, excessive alcohol intake

Individuals >21 years with primary elevations of LDL-C ≥190 mg/dL	**High-intensity statin** (moderate-intensity statin if not candidate for high-intensity statin)	All individuals receiving statins should be counseled on healthy lifestyle habits.
Individuals 40–75 years of age with diabetes and with LDL-C 70–189 mg/dL	**Moderate-intensity statin** **High-intensity statin if** estimated 10-year ASCVD risk ≥7.5%[a]	If a statin-treated individual develops diabetes, he or she should be counseled to adhere to a heart healthy dietary pattern, engage in physical activity, achieve and maintain a healthy body weight, cease tobacco use, and continue statin therapy to reduce his or her risk of ASCVD events.
Individuals without clinical ASCVD or diabetes who are 40–75 years of age with LDL-C 70–189 mg/dL and an estimated 10-year ASCVD risk of 7.5% or higher[a].	**Moderate- to high-intensity statin**	Statins modestly increase the excess risk of type 2 diabetes in individuals with risk factors for diabetes.

High-intensity statin: Atorvastatin (40)–80 mg; Rosuvastatin 20 (*40*) mg; for history of hemorrhagic stroke and Asian ancestry.
Moderate-intensity statin: Atorvastatin 10 (*20*) mg; Rosuvastatin (*5*) 10 mg; Simvastatin 20–40 mg; Pravastatin 40 (*80*) mg; Lovastatin 40 mg; Fluvastatin XL 80 mg; Fluvastatin 40 mg BID; pitavastatin 2–4 mg.

[a]A spreadsheet enabling estimation of 10-year and lifetime risk for ASCVD and a Web-based calculator are available at http://my.americanheart.org/cvriskcalculator and http://www.cardiosource.org/science-and-quality/practice-guidelines-and-quality-standards/2013-prevention-guideline-tools

Data from Stone NJ, Robinson JG, Lichtenstein AH, et al. ATP IV: 2013 ACC/AHA guideline on the treatment of blood cholesterol t atherosclerotic cardiovascular risk in adults—A report of the American College of Cardiology/American Heart Association Task F Practice Guidelines. *Circulation* 2013;129(2):S1–S45.

remains a critical component of health promotion and ASCVD risk reduction, both prior to, and in concert with, the use of cholesterol-lowering drug therapies.[11] The Task Group proposed a population-based approach as part of multifaceted health management to improve cardiovascular health of Americans.[12]

The goal of this approach is "ideal cardiovascular health" and identifies seven metrics for assessing individual and community health behaviors in individuals aged 40 to 75 years and children without clinical ASCVD or diabetes and with LDL–C <190 mg/dL (Box 8.3). To meet this goal, lifestyle treatments target schools and workplaces in local communities throughout the nation, providing health coaching at the community level for both children and adults in specific diet and lifestyle management (Box 8.4). For adults aged 40 to 75 years with or without ASCVD or diabetes and with LDL–C >190 mg/dL, the Task Group developed dietary recommendations for lowering LDL–C and provided evidence ratings for each recommendation (Box 8.5). In addition, the AHA/ACC proposed dietary patterns to promote as healthy diets for individuals and communities to target modifiable CVD risk factors of BP and lipids (Box 8.6).[12]

BOX 8.3 Ideal Cardiovascular Health: 7 Metrics to Assess Population Behaviors

- Current smoking status
- BMI
- Physical activity
- Healthy Diet Score
- Total cholesterol
- Blood pressure
- Fasting plasma glucose

"The metrics with the greatest potential for improvement are health behaviors, including diet quality, physical activity, and body weight."

BMI, body mass index.

Data from Eckel RH, Jakicic JM, Ard JD, et al. 2013 AHA/ACC guideline on lifestyle management to reduce cardiovascular risk: A report of the American College of Cardiology/American Heart Association Task Force on Practice Guidelines. *Circulation* 2013;129(2):S76–S99.

BOX 8.4 2013 AHA/ACC Lifestyle Management Guideline for Diet and Lifestyle: Key Recommendations of AHA/ACC Task Group for Lifestyle Modification

Healthy Diet	Physical Activity
Adults and Children In the context of a DASH-type dietary pattern, to achieve at least four of five key components of a healthy diet: 1. Fruits and vegetables: >4.5 cups/d 2. Fish: more than two, 3.5-oz servings/wk (preferably oily fish) 3. Fiber-rich whole grains (>1.1 g of fiber per 10 g of carbohydrates): three 1-oz-equivalent servings/d 4. Sodium: <1,500 mg/d 5. Sugar-sweetened beverages: <450 kcal (36 oz)/wk	**Children** *Ideal:* ≥60 minutes of moderate to vigorous physical activity per day *Intermediate:* 1 to 59 minutes of moderate to vigorous physical activity per day *Poor:* No physical activity
Children/Adults • *Ideal:* Diet Score 4 to 5 • *Intermediate:* Diet Score 2 to 3 • *Poor:* Diet Score 0 to 1	**Adults** *Ideal:* At least 150 minutes of moderate or 75 minutes of vigorous physical activity each week *Intermediate:* 1 to 149 min/wk moderate or 1 to 74 min/wk vigorous activity *Poor:* No physical activity

Data from Eckel RH, Jakicic JM, Ard JD, et al. 2013 AHA/ACC guideline on lifestyle management to reduce cardiovascular risk: A report of the American College of Cardiology/American Heart Association Task Force on Practice Guidelines. *Circulation* 2013;129(2):S76–S99.

BOX 8.5 Dietary Recommendations for Lowering LDL-C

Diet Recommendations	Evidence Rating
1. Consume a dietary pattern that emphasizes intake of vegetables, fruits, and whole grains; includes low-fat dairy products, poultry, fish, legumes, nontropical vegetable oils, and nuts; and limits intake of sweets, sugar-sweetened beverages, and red meats. • Adapt this dietary pattern to appropriate calorie requirements, personal and cultural food preferences, and nutrition therapy for other medical conditions (including diabetes mellitus). • Achieve this pattern by following plans such as the DASH dietary pattern, the USDA Food Pattern, or the AHA Diet.	NHLBI Grade: A (Strong); *ACC/AHA COR: I, LOE: A*
2. Aim for a dietary pattern that achieves 5% to 6% of calories from saturated fat.	NHLBI Grade: A (strong); *ACC/AHA COR: I, LOE: A*
3. Reduce percentage of calories from saturated fat.	NHLBI Grade: A (strong); *ACC/AHA COR: I, LOE: A*
4. Reduce percentage of calories from trans fat.	NHLBI Grade: A (strong); *ACC/AHA COR: I, LOE: A*
5. In general, advise adults to engage in aerobic physical activity to reduce LDL-C and non-HDL-C: 3 to 4 sessions a week, lasting on average 40 minutes per session and involving moderate to vigorous intensity physical activity.	NHLBI Grade: B (moderate); *ACC/AHA COR: IIa, LOE: A*

For adults aged 40 to 75 years with or without ASCVD or diabetes and with LDL-C >190 mg/dL.

NHLBI, The National Heart, Lung, and Blood Institute; USDA, U.S. Department of Agriculture; COR, class of recommendation; LOE, level of evidence.

Data from Eckel RH, Jakicic JM, Ard JD, et al. 2013 AHA/ACC guideline on lifestyle management to reduce cardiovascular risk: A report of the American College of Cardiology/American Heart Association Task Force on Practice Guidelines. *Circulation* 2013;129(2):S76–S99.

BOX 8.6 Healthy Dietary Patterns to Target Both BP and LDL-C Lowering

Type of Diet	Description	Clinical Targets
MED Pattern	• Higher in fruits (particularly fresh), vegetables (emphasizing root and green varieties), whole grains (cereals, breads, rice, or pasta), fatty fish (rich in omega-3 fatty acids) • Lower in red meat (and emphasizing lean meats) • Substitute lower-fat or fat-free dairy products for higher-fat dairy foods • Use oils (olive or canola), nuts (walnuts, almonds, or hazelnuts), or margarines blended with rapeseed or flaxseed oils in lieu of butter and other fats • Overall moderate in total fat (32% to 35% of total calories), relatively low in saturated fat (9% to 10% of total calories), high in fiber (27 to 37 g/d), and high in polyunsaturated fatty acids (particularly omega-3s)	• May benefit BP management • No consistent effect on plasma LDL-C, HDL-C, and TG

(*continued*)

BOX 8.6 Healthy Dietary Patterns to Target Both BP and LDL-C Lowering (*continued*)

Type of Diet	Description	Clinical Targets
DASH Dietary Pattern	• High in vegetables, fruits, low-fat dairy products, whole grains, poultry, fish, and nuts • Low in sweets, sugar-sweetened beverages, and red meats • Low in saturated fat, total fat, and cholesterol • Rich in potassium, magnesium, and calcium, as well as protein and fiber	• Evidence strong for BP lowering in all and subgroups (men and women, African and non-African groups, hypertensive and nonhypertensive adults) • Evidence strong for lowering of LDL-C and HDL in all and similar effect for all subgroups • No effect on TG
DASH Variations/ Glycemic Index/ Load Dietary Approaches	Two variations of the DASH dietary pattern: replacement of 10% of total daily carbohydrate calories with calories from either protein or unsaturated fat	• May benefit BP management • May benefit lowering of LDL-C and TG with marginal increase in HDL-C

TG, triglyceride.

Data from Eckel RH, Jakicic JM, Ard JD, et al. 2013 AHA/ACC guideline on lifestyle management to reduce cardiovascular risk: A report of the American College of Cardiology/American Heart Association Task Force on Practice Guidelines. *Circulation* 2013;129(2):S76–S99.

HYPERTENSION

Hypertension (HTN) is a significant contributor (8.3%) to CVD mortality in the US population, and an estimated 78 million adults are affected by HTN, with a higher prevalence in African Americans (41.2%).[13] Only 81.5% of adults with HTN have been diagnosed, and of those seeking treatment (74.9%), only 52.5% are under control. Untreated HTN significantly increases risk of CVA, with 77% of those with a first CVA have BP >140/90 mm Hg and diabetics with BP <120/80 mm Hg have half the lifetime CVA risk than those with just HTN.[14]

Disease Process

Blood is pumped to the body by the left ventricle of the heart, imparting a pressure that is opposed by the resistance of blood vessels through which it flows. The balance of these two opposing forces produces BP, which rises and falls as the heart contracts and relaxes. The peak, when the heart contracts, is known as the systolic pressure and the minimum, when the heart relaxes, as diastolic pressure. Homeostatic regulation of BP via the kidney and the sympathetic nervous system (SNS) also has a role in controlling BP peripherally.[15,16] Maintenance of BP within certain limits enables adequate blood flow to the brain and other tissues. Systolic-diastolic abnormalities lead to the development of essential HTN and event endpoints.[17]

Resistance of blood vessels increases when the diameter of arterial vessels narrows with progressive atherosclerosis. Regulatory mechanism failure from a hyperactive SNS or renin–angiotensin system also contributes to vasoconstriction and HTN. In the short term, elevated BP damages the endothelial lining of the arteries, allowing increased entry of LDL–C. In the long term, arterial stiffening and end-stage kidney disease develop with untreated BP. Left ventricular hypertrophy develops over time with uncontrolled HTN leading to heart failure, sometimes referred to as congestive heart failure. Occlusion of blood vessels in the heart can cause MI, retinopathy of the eyes, or in the brain, a CVA.

The AHA made HTN a primary focus area of its strategic plan, seeking to reduce the death rate from CVD and CVA by 20% by 2020.[18] Similarly, *Million Hearts*, spearheaded by the Centers for Disease Control and Prevention (CDC) to prevent a million heart attacks and strokes by 2017, has focused on actions to improve and achieve control of HTN.[19] The AHA identified BP as one of the seven metrics of cardiovascular health.[14] Because a high percentage of the population is undiagnosed, identification and diagnosis is a key step in achieving control of HTN. The Eighth Joint National Committee (JNC 8) designated normal BP to be a systolic level <120 mm Hg and a diastolic level <80 mm Hg and HTN diagnosis based on BP levels at three stages: prehypertension, stage 1 HTN, and stage 2 HTN (Box 8.7).[20]

Treatment and Nutrition Intervention

The ACC/AHA Task Group developed a HTN treatment algorithm as part of a multifactorial approach to improve BP control (Box 8.8). In addition, the Task Group strongly recommended LM as an additional therapeutic approach to prevent or control HTN (Box 8.9).[13] For people with

BOX 8.7 JNC 8 Classification of Blood Pressure

Category	Systolic		Diastolic
Normal	<120	And	<80
Prehypertension	120 to 139	Or	80 to 89
Stage 1 HTN	140 to 159	Or	90 to 99
Stage 2 HTN	≥160	Or	≥100

Data from James PA, Oparil S, Carter BL, et al. 2014 Evidence-based guideline for the management of high blood pressure in adults: Report from the panel members appointed to the Eighth Joint National Committee (JNC 8). *JAMA* 2014;311(5):507–520.

BOX 6.6 Hypertension Treatment Algorithm

Patient Groups	Antihypertension Therapy		Lifestyle Modification
	Type	Monitoring	
Stage 1 hypertension with systolic BP 140 to 159 mm Hg or diastolic BP 90 to 99 mm Hg	Consider adding thiazide	*Recheck and review reading in 3 months* *If BP goal not met:* • Consider ACEI, ARB, CCB, or combo	Start lifestyle modification as a trial
Stage 2 hypertension with systolic BP >160 mm Hg or diastolic BP >100 mm Hg	Two drug combination[a] preferred: • Thiazide with ACEI, ARB, or CCB • ACEI and CCB	*Review in 2 to 4 weeks* *If BP goal not met:* • Optimize dose or add medications • Address adherence, self-monitoring • Consider secondary causes • Consider referral to HTN specialist *If BP goal is met:* • Encourage self-monitoring and adherence to medication • Alert if BP elevation or side effects occur • Continue clinical follow-up	Intensive lifestyle modification

[a]Suggested medications for hypertension treatment if with comorbidities:
Coronary artery disease/post-MI: BB, ACEI
Systolic heart failure: ACEI or ARB, BB, ALDO ANTAG, thiazide
Diastolic heart failure: ACEI or ARB, BB, thiazide
Diabetes: ACEI or ARB, thiazide, BB, CCB
Kidney disease: ACEI or ARB
Stroke or TIA: thiazide, ACEI

ACEI, angiotensin-converting enzyme inhibitor; ALDO ANTAG, aldosterone antagonist; ARB, angiotensin II receptor blocker; BB, β-blocker; BP, blood pressure; CCB, calcium channel blocker; HTN, hypertension.

Data from Go AS, Bauman MA, Coleman King SM, et al. An effective approach to high blood pressure control: A science advisory from the American Heart Association, the American College of Cardiology, and the Centers for Disease Control and Prevention. *Hypertension* 2014;63:87-8–885.

BOX 8.9 Lifestyle Modification for Adults Who Would Benefit From BP Lowering

	Target	Recommendations for BP Lowering	Evidence Rating
1.	Community action to adopt healthful behaviors • Health coaching to modify diets	Consume a dietary pattern that emphasizes intake of vegetables, fruits, and whole grains; includes low-fat dairy products, poultry, fish, legumes, nontropical vegetable oils, and nuts; and limits intake of sweets, sugar-sweetened beverages, and red meats. • Adapt this dietary pattern to appropriate calorie requirements, personal and cultural food preferences, and nutrition therapy for other medical conditions (including diabetes mellitus). • Achieve this pattern by following plans such as the DASH dietary pattern, the USDA Food Pattern, or the AHA Diet.	*NHLBI Grade: A (strong); ACC/AHA COR: I, LOE: A*
2.	Community action to adopt healthful behaviors • Health coaching to read food labels • Understand fresh vs. processed food choices	Lower sodium intake.	*NHLBI Grade: A (strong); ACC/AHA COR: I, LOE: A*

3.	Individual health management • [a]African Americans	a. Consume no more than 2,400 mg/d of sodium. b. Further reduction of sodium intake to 1,500 mg/d[a] is desirable since it is associated with an even greater reduction in BP. c. Reduce sodium intake by at least 1,000 mg/d since that will lower BP, even if the desired daily sodium intake is not yet achieved.	*NHLBI Grade: B (moderate); ACC/AHA COR: IIa, LOE: B*
4.	Individual health strategy	Combine the DASH dietary pattern with lower sodium intake.	*NHLBI Grade: A (strong); ACC/AHA COR: I, LOE: A*
5.	Individual health strategy	In general, advise adults to engage in aerobic physical activity to lower BP: 3 to 4 sessions a week, lasting on average 40 minutes per session and involving moderate to vigorous intensity physical activity.	*NHLBI Grade: B (moderate); ACC/AHA COR: IIa, LOE: A*

NHLBI, The National Heart, Lung, and Blood Institute; USDA, U.S. Department of Agriculture; COR, class of recommendation; LOE, level of evidence.

Data from Go AS, Bauman MA, Coleman King SM, et al. An effective approach to high blood pressure control: A science advisory from the American Heart Association, the American College of Cardiology, and the Centers for Disease Control and Prevention. *Hypertension* 2014;63:878–885.

HTN aged 18 years or older, BP goals are systolic <140 and diastolic <90, with a higher limit for those aged 60 or older at 150 and 90, respectively.[20] Depending on a patient's race and status with regard to the presence of diabetes and/or chronic kidney disease, the choice of initial medication varies, but all patients are recommended to implement LM. Of the various drugs used to treat HTN, some have nutrition implications. Antihypertensives are grouped according to mechanistic function and may interact with specific foods or nutrients, or cause gastrointestinal distress, fluid retention, or dehydration (Box 8.10).

The Dietary Approaches to Stop Hypertension (DASH) eating plan has been shown to lower BP when managing patients with HTN (Table 8.3).[21] The DASH eating plan can be incorporated into any diet, including those with diabetes. It emphasizes an eating plan lower in sodium content that is also low in saturated fat, cholesterol, and total fat, and higher in fruits, vegetables, and low-fat dairy foods compared with other dietary patterns. Higher potassium intake through increasing fruit and vegetable intakes can also help lower BP. Sodium chloride or salt reduction is the core of LM, with nutrition coaching targeting several approaches to supporting healthful behaviors (Box 8.11).[22,23]

ACUTE CARE FOR CARDIOVASCULAR EVENTS

Myocardial Infarction

Disease Process and Nutrition Intervention

An MI cuts off blood supply to the heart, causing an oxygen deficit to cells of the heart muscle, leading to necrosis; therefore, the more prolonged the time to treatment to restore blood flow, the greater the damage to heart muscle.[24] The critical stage for an MI patient is within the first 48 hours, followed by the acute stage that lasts between 3 and 14 days, and convalescence for the next 15 days to 3 months. Post-MI arrhythmias, nausea and vomiting, and fatigue are common symptoms.[25]

BOX 8.10 Medications Used in HTN Management with Nutritional Implications

Antihypertensive Class	Mechanism of Action	Nutritional Implications
Diuretics	Promote excretion of excess sodium and water, thus helping control BP. Likely use in combination therapies.	May cause hyperkalemia if potassium-sparing • Monitor mineral salts/ supplements. May increase urinary potassium, zinc, calcium, or magnesium excretion (e.g., thiazides) • Weakness, leg cramps, or being tired may result. • Eating potassium-rich foods may offset significant potassium loss.
β-Blockers	Reduce heart rate, the heart's workload, and the heart's output of blood, which lowers BP.	Gastrointestinal side effects, including heartburn, gas, diarrhea, vomiting, or constipation • Monitor dehydration.
ACE inhibitors	Angiotensin causes arteries supplying the kidney as well as the rest of the body to become narrow in uncontrolled hypertension. Angiotensin-converting enzyme (ACE) inhibitors help the body produce less angiotensin, which helps blood vessels vasodilate, which, in turn, lowers BP.	May cause increased mineral retention (potassium, calcium, or magnesium) • Monitor mineral salts/supplements.

(*continued*)

BOX 8.10 Medications Used in HTN Management with Nutritional Implications (*continued*)

Antihypertensive Class	Mechanism of Action	Nutritional Implications
Angiotensin II receptor blockers (ARBs)	Blocks the effects of angiotensin. ARBs block the angiotensin receptors so the angiotensin fails to constrict the blood vessel. This means blood vessels stay open and BP is reduced.	—
Calcium channel blockers (CCBs)	Prevent calcium from entering the smooth muscle cells of heart and arteries, thus preventing hardening and reduced contractility of the vessels. CCBs relax and open up narrowed blood vessels, reduce heart rate, and lower BP.	• Grapefruits and grapefruit juice can affect the action of many CCBs. • Alcohol interferes with the effects of CCBs and increases side effects. Common side effects: edema, constipation, diarrhea, gastroesophageal reflux disease
α-Blockers	Reduce arteries' resistance, relaxing the muscle tone of the vascular walls.	Side effects: weight gain
α-2 Receptor agonist	Reduce BP by decreasing the activity of the sympathetic (adrenaline-producing) portion of the involuntary nervous system.	—

Combined α- and β-blockers	Combined α- and β-blockers are used as an IV drip for those patients experiencing a hypertensive crisis and at risk for heart failure.	—
Central agonists	Decrease blood vessels' ability to tense up or contract via a different nerve pathway than the α- and β-blockers, but accomplish the same goal of BP reduction.	Side effects: dry mouth, constipation
Peripheral adrenergic inhibitors	Reduce BP by blocking neurotransmitters in the brain, which block the smooth muscles from getting the "message" to constrict. Rarely used unless other medications do not help.	Side effects: diarrhea or heartburn
Vasodilators	Cause the muscle in the walls of the blood vessels (especially the arterioles) to relax, allowing the vessel to dilate (widen). This allows blood to flow through better, thus reducing BP.	Side effects: may cause fluid retention (marked weight gain)

TABLE 8.3. DASH Eating Plan Based on Energy Level

Food Group	Serving Size	Calories per Serving[a]	Servings as per Daily Calorie Plan			
			1,600 kcal	2,000 kcal[b]	2,600 kcal	3,100 kcal
Grains	1 slice bread 1 cup ready-to-eat cereal[c] 1/2 cup cooked rice, pasta, or cereal	75	6–7	7–8	9–10	11–12
Vegetables	1 cup raw leafy vegetable 1/2 cup cooked vegetable 6-oz vegetable juice	Estimated as ~25 kcal	3–4	4–5	5–7	6–8
Fruits	1 medium fruit 1/4 cup dried fruit 1/2 cup fresh, frozen, or canned fruit 6-oz fruit juice	60	3–4	4–5	5–7	6–8
Low-fat or fat-free dairy	8-oz milk 1 cup yogurt 1 1/2-oz cheese	125 if low fat or 90 if fat-free	2	2–3	3–4	3–5
Meats, poultry, fish	3-oz cooked lean meat, skinless poultry, or fish	158 if meat/poultry, but 85 if fish	≤2	2 or fewer	3 or fewer	4 or fewer

Nuts, seeds, dry beans, and peas	1/3 cup or 1 1/2-oz nuts 1 Tbsp or 1/2-oz seeds 1/2 cup cooked dry beans	45	3–4/wk	4–5/wk	5–7/wk	6–8/wk
Fats and oils[d]	1 tsp soft margarine 1 Tbsp low-fat mayonnaise 2 Tbsp light salad dressing 1 tsp vegetable oil	45	2	2–3	3–4	3–5
Sweets	1 Tbsp sugar 1 Tbsp jelly or jam 1/2-oz jelly beans 8-oz lemonade	60	4/wk	5/wk	7/wk	8/wk
Sodium	*Check food labels for sodium content per serving size.*		2,300 mg *1,500 mg for high risk*[e]			

[a]Calories estimated from website: http://glycemic.com/DiabeticExchange/The%20Diabetic%20Exchange%20List.pdf
[b]Gray area is the recommended DASH eating plan. Servings are calculated for a 2,000 kcal diet. http://www.nhlbi.nih.gov
[c]Serving sizes vary between 1/2 cup and 1 1/4 cups. Check the product's nutrition label.
[d]Fat content changes serving counts for fats and oils: For example, 1 Tbsp of regular salad dressing equals 1 serving, 1 Tbsp of low-fat salad dressing equals 1/2 serving, and 1 Tbsp of fat-free salad dressing equals 0 servings.
[e]For African Americans at high risk for hypertension. Lower sodium goal effective at lowering BP.
Data from National Heart, Lung, and Blood Institute. *Your Guide to High Blood Pressure with DASH*. NIH Publication No. 06-4082. Washington, DC: U.S. Department of Health and Human Services; 2006.

BOX 8.11 Education Topics for Achieving Sodium Reduction

Topics	Tips	Why?
But, I *never* use the salt shaker—so I must be eating a low-sodium diet	Where does sodium come from? 43% of sodium consumed by children comes from pizza, bread/ rolls, cold cuts/meats, savory snacks, sandwiches, cheese, chicken patties/nuggets, pasta mixed dishes, Mexican mixed dishes, soups.[21]	77% of salt consumed comes from processed foods and meals eaten away from home. Only 11% comes from salt added during cooking and at the table. Average intake = 3,466 mg/d (excludes table and cooking salt)[22]
Label language	**Sodium-Free/Salt-Free** Less than 5 mg sodium per serving **Very Low Sodium** 35 mg or less per serving **Low Sodium** 140 mg or less sodium per serving **Unsalted or No Added Salt** No salt added during processing does not necessarily mean "sodium-free"	Label reading—best way to avoid excess sodium

	Reduced/Less Sodium At least 25% less sodium per serving than the same food with no sodium reduction **Light in Sodium/Lightly Salted** At least 50% less sodium **Low-Sodium Meal** 140 mg or less sodium per 100 g (3½ oz)	
Salt substitution	Compare products within food categories: Oats, deli foods, tomato products, cereals, sauces, canned goods	Label reading—best way to avoid excess sodium by substituting "high" for "low" sodium content products in each food class
Eating out	**Forming the sodium budget** Plan a sodium allowance for meals eaten outside.	Being aware of the sodium content of food can make a *big* difference in sodium intake.
Meal planning	**Fresh vs. processed**	Using whole unprocessed foods in low-sodium meals can save more than *3,130 mg* of sodium.

(*continued*)

BOX 8.11 Education Topics for Achieving Sodium Reduction (*continued*)

Topics	Tips	Why?
Cooking skills	**Flavor without salt** **Beef:** dry mustard, nutmeg, onion, sage, pepper, ginger, garlic **Lamb:** garlic, curry, mint, rosemary **Chicken:** paprika, thyme, sage, parsley, curry, ginger, garlic **Fish:** dry mustard, paprika, curry, lemon juice, dill, basil **Eggs:** pepper, dry mustard, paprika, tarragon **Asparagus:** lemon juice, caraway seed **Green beans:** lemon juice, nutmeg, onion **Broccoli:** lemon juice, oregano **Cabbage:** mustard, caraway seed, vinegar **Carrots:** allspice, ginger, cloves **Cauliflower:** nutmeg, celery, seed **Peas:** onion, mint **Potatoes:** parsley, chives **Squash:** ginger, basil, oregano **Tomatoes:** basil, oregano, sage, thyme	Flavors are taste substitutes for low sodium. Flavor enhancers are inexpensive and delicious.

ADIME 8.1 ADIME At-A-Glance: Coronary Heart Disease and Hypertension

Assessment

- BMI ≥25, recent wt gain, waist circumference >40 in men and >35 in women
- Sedentary lifestyle
- Excess dietary intake of energy, trans and saturated fatty acids, proinflammatory foods, salt/sodium, alcohol
- Inadequate dietary intake of fruits and vegetables—anti-inflammatory foods and antioxidants
- BP levels: TG, LDL-C, HDL-C, inflammatory markers
- Diabetes, hx of previous CVD event
- Food and nutrition knowledge deficit, beliefs/attitudes, or practices about food, nutrition

Nutrition Diagnosis

- Overweight RT sedentary lifestyle AEB BMI of 27 and recent wt gain of 10% x 1 year
- Class 1 obesity RT excessive energy intake AEB BMI of 31 and diet hx of 2,600 kcal/d
- Excessive SFA/TFA RT knowledge deficit AEB diet hx and elevated LDL-C of 190 mg/dL
- Intake of PUFA inconsistent with needs RT undesirable food choices AEB LDL-C of 190 mg/dL
- Excessive sodium intake RT knowledge deficit AEB diet hx and elevated BP
- Inadequate potassium intake RT undesirable food choices AEB diet hx of low fruit/veg intake
- Limited adherence to recommendations RT low interest in change AEB diet hx of low compliance

Intervention

- Decrease energy (1,800 kcal) and increase physical activity (20 minutes, 3x/wk)
- Decrease SFA/TFA to <6% total energy and increase PUFA/MUFA to 15% total energy
- Decrease sodium intake to 1,500 mg/d
- Increase potassium intake to 3 to 5 g/d by following DASH diet pattern
- Referral to outpatient nutrition counseling for decreased SFA/energy and increased PUFA diet

Monitoring and Evaluation

- Body weight
- Dietary intake
- BP, blood lipids, inflammatory markers (if available)

MNT in the acute stage focuses on reducing stress on the heart and preventing arrhythmias (Box 8.12).[26] As the patient moves to the next stage, a liquid diet is progressed as tolerated to soft, easily digested foods offered in small, frequent meals, with the exclusion of potential stimulants, such as caffeine, to reduce the potential for arrhythmias. In addition, serving foods at body temperature may also help in this regard. Prior to discharge, patient education should include the ACC/AHA recommendations for dietary modification and encouragement to follow up with a cardiac rehabilitation program and outpatient nutrition counseling.[12] Potential nutrition implications for medication used in the treatment of acute MI and other acute CVD events are shown in Box 8.13.

BOX 8.12 MNT Strategies in Acute MI

Treatment Phase	MNT Approach	Assess and Monitor
Post-MI/critical stage *Rest to reduce heart strain*	To reduce heart strain: • *Use clear to full liquid diets* • *Small volume feeding*	I/O charts, LDH, CPK, BP, BUN, Pco_2, Po_2, triglycerides, PT • Aspiration • Vomiting • Abdominal distention • Flatulence • Constipation
Prevent arrhythmias	To minimize arrhythmias: • *Food must be at body temperature* • *Exclude stimulants such as coffee*	
Acute stage/ recovery	• Liquid diet progress to soft easily digested foods • Small frequent meals • Exclude gas-forming foods • Exclude stimulants to minimize arrhythmias	• Abdominal distention • Constipation
Convalescence/ stable stage	Either Med or DASH diet as per ACC/AHA guidelines	• Optimize weight by using calorie plan • Sodium control

BOX 8.13 Nutritional Implications of Medications Used in Acute CVD Events

Acute Event	Drugs	Nutritional Implications
Myocardial infarction	CCBs	Common side effects: edema, constipation, diarrhea, gastroesophageal reflux disease
	β-Blockers	Gastrointestinal side effects, including heartburn, gas, diarrhea, vomiting, or constipation
		Monitor dehydration
	Anticoagulant and thrombolytic therapy—Warfarin (Coumadin) or heparin	Excessive intake of vitamin K foods alters PT values.
		Also dong quai, fenugreek, gingko, ginseng
		Vitamin E and CoQ10 contraindicated
	Mexitil, Rythmol, Procan	Nausea, vomiting, or constipation
		Bitter taste, nausea, anorexia, or diarrhea with Procan

(continued)

BOX 8.13 Nutritional Implications of Medications Used in Acute CVD Events (*continued*)

Acute Event	Drugs	Nutritional Implications
Heart failure	Thiazide diuretics	Deplete urinary potassium, zinc, calcium, or magnesium excretion (e.g., thiazides)
	Furosemide (Lasix)	Weakness, leg cramps, or being tired may result.
	KCl	Side effect: hyperkalemia
	Digitalis	Deplete potassium when taken with Lasix
		Side effect: anorexia or nausea
	Arterial vasodilators	Side effect: nausea and vomiting
	Anticoagulant and thrombolytic therapy—Warfarin (Coumadin) for bedridden patients	As above
	ACE inhibitors	Side effect: nausea and vomiting, abdominal pain, hyperkalemia
Cerebrovascular accident	Anticoagulant and thrombolytic therapy—Warfarin (Coumadin) or heparin	As above
	Reserpine	Cramping and diarrhea

ACE, angiotensin-converting enzyme; CCBs, calcium channel blockers.

ADIME 8.2 ADIME At-A-Glance: Acute Myocardial Infarction[a]

Assessment

- Oral intake
- Changes in digestion, absorption, or elimination (check for constipation, flatulence, abdominal distention)
- Impaired or difficult movement of food and liquid from oral cavity to stomach (check for swallowing ability, vomiting, choking/gagging, aspiration)

Nutrition Diagnosis

- Altered GI function RT medications AEB abdominal distention and constipation
- Swallowing difficulty RT impaired movement of food/liquid AEB vomiting and aspiration

Intervention

- Liquid diet, progress as tolerated from clear to full liquid to soft food
- Small volume, frequent feedings
- Exclude gas-forming foods
- Referral to outpatient nutrition counseling

Monitoring and Evaluation

- I&Os
- PO intake (food, fluid)
- Swallowing function, abdominal distention

[a]see CHD and HTN for post-MI/discharge ADIME.

Heart Failure

Disease Process and Nutrition Intervention

Heart failure (HF) or congestive heart failure (CHF) occurs when the heart muscle is unable to pump blood efficiently in the lower ventricles. This failure commonly arises from narrowing of arteries resulting from coronary artery disease, HTN, chronic pulmonary disease, or heart damage from a previous MI, gradually leaving the heart too weak or stiff to fill and pump efficiently. An estimated 5.7 million Americans are affected by HF, and prevalence is projected to increase by 46% by 2030, resulting in more than eight million people ≥18 years of age with the disease.[14,24,27] Right-sided HF causes pitting edema in all extremities, whereas left-sided HF results in pulmonary edema, rales, and dyspnea. Decreased renal blood flow causes elevated blood urea nitrogen (BUN), and cardiac cachexia presents in advanced-stage HF.

Treatments can improve the signs and symptoms of HF and increase life span. Short-term management focuses on reducing edema and preventing cachexia, whereas long-term management emphasizes lifestyle changes, including dietary salt restriction, weight loss if indicated, and physical activity (Box 8.14).[28–31]

BOX 8.14 MNT Strategies for HF

Treatment Phase	MNT Approach	Assess and Monitor
Restoration of hemodynamic stability	NPO with IV fluids for first 24 hours	• Monitor: I/O charts, electrolytes, BP, BUN, oliguria, Pco_2, Po_2, triglycerides, PT, albumin, prealbumin • Avoid overhydration
Elimination or reduction of edema	Sodium restriction—<1,000 mg if severe or 2,000 to 3,000 mg if less severe Fluid restriction—500 to 1,000cc depending on severity of HF	• Daily I/O charting • Daily weight monitoring • Fluid plan—75% for meals, 25% for mediations and in between sipping
Distention and elevation of diaphragm	Small frequent meals Rest before and after meals High calorie diet—low-volume supplements needed Indications for tube feeding—small bowel feeding ideal	• Poor appetite • Excessive refeeding • Aspiration • Gastric ileus

BOX 8.14 MNT Strategies for HF (*continued*)

Treatment Phase	MNT Approach	Assess and Monitor
Prevent cardiac cachexia	Small frequent meals Rest before and after meals High-calorie protein—low-volume supplements needed Indications for tube feeding (small bowel feeding) or even parenteral nutrition	• Poor appetite • Fatigue • Muscle depletion • Aspiration
Prevent pressure ulcers	Calorie and protein optimization to promote wound healing	• Improving mobility in the bedbound patient • Improving circulation • Weight optimization
Long-term goals	Assess functional status Attain ideal body weight to decrease O_2 needs Replete lean body mass Limit cardiac stimulants Fluid and sodium goals Moderate aerobic activity	• Calorie and protein optimization essential • Weight gain or loss should be monitored. • Adequate fiber from food or supplementation is necessary to prevent constipation.

ADIME 8.3 ADIME At-A-Glance: Heart Failure

Assessment

- BMI, UWL, decrease in appetite and food intake
- Muscle wasting, loss of adipose tissue
- BP, SOB, pitting edema, oliguria
- Excessive dietary sodium intake

Nutrition Diagnosis

- Inadequate oral intake RT decreased appetite, AEB recent UWL of 5% × 3 weeks, poor PO intake of 40%
- Unintended weight loss RT inadequate oral intake AEB UWL of 5% × 3 weeks, poor PO intake of 40%
- Chronic disease-related malnutrition RT HF AEB UWL of 5% × 3 weeks, poor PO intake of 40%, muscle wasting
- Excessive sodium intake RT knowledge deficit AEB exacerbation of edema, diet hx

Intervention

- Small, frequent feedings
- Provision of commercial beverage product
- Insert enteral feeding tube
- Feeding assistance
- Referral to Home Delivered Meals Program

Monitoring and Evaluation

- Body weight
- PO intake (food, fluid)
- Hydration status, BUN, edema

Cerebrovascular Accident (Stroke)

Disease Process and Nutrition Intervention

An estimated 6.6 million Americans ≥20 years of age had a stroke, with an overall stroke prevalence of 2.6%.[14,32] Stroke is the fifth leading cause of death in the United States, with 130,000 deaths annually. High-risk segments of the population include older adults, African Americans, individuals of lower socioeconomic status, and those living in the southeastern United States.

CVA types include ischemic stroke (IS), which accounts for 87%, intracranial hemorrhage (ICH) at 10%, and subarachnoid hemorrhage (SAH) contributing 3%. BP is a powerful risk determinant for both IS and ICH. Transient ischemic attacks

(TIAs), which block blood flow to the brain for no more than 5 minutes, may serve as an early warning for severe CVA.

Depending on the site of the CVA and extent of brain damage, unconsciousness or paralysis may occur. Left CVA affects sight and hearing, whereas right CVA, bilateral or brain stem CVA, causing significant feeding and swallowing food problems with associated speech problems.[33] Neurogenic deficits are motor related, causing muscle weakness of tongue and lips, and sensory and cognitive deficit. Patients with right CVA typically are unable to coordinate food from plate to mouth, taste, chew, or coordinate swallowing of food, causing dysphagia.

If dysphagia is present, which may be temporary or permanent, the food matrix or texture becomes critical.[33,34] Liquids may be aspirated or may cause drooling, and chewing difficulties with normal texture foods may lead to choking. Patients may require enteral nutrition consisting of nasogastric feeding for the short term and percutaneous endoscopic gastrostomy feeding in the long term, if the speech and swallowing reflexes are not rehabilitated. MNT focuses on the specific stage of CVA and feeding problems related to type of stroke and area of the brain affected in order to prevent dehydration and malnutrition (Box 8.15).[35–38]

BOX 8.15 MNT Strategies for CVA

Treatment Phase	MNT Approach	Assess and Monitor
Initial	NPO with IV fluids for first 24 hours	• Monitor: I/O charts, electrolytes, BP, BUN, triglycerides, PT • Avoid overhydration
If patient is comatose	Transit from NPO to liquids Tube feeding required (nasogastric, gastrostomy, or jejunostomy)	• Elevation of bed-head to prevent aspiration • Monitoring of gastric residual volumes

(continued)

BOX 8.15 MNT Strategies for CVA (*continued*)

Treatment Phase	MNT Approach	Assess and Monitor
If patient is not comatose, dysphagia assessment required	Sip feeding or tube feeding may be required depending on short- or long-term needs.	• Aspiration prevention • Hydration adequacy • Pressure sores increase nutritional requirement.
Those with lower category of dysphagia assess saliva secretion	For those not requiring liquids, transition to thick pureed liquids or to mechanical soft diet.	• Eating slowly • Easy-to-chew foods necessary • Identify foods that trigger choking (dry) or coughing (tart) or drooling (sweet).
Stable long-term goals • Assess functional status	If dysphagia is permanent, patient may be dependent totally or partially on enteral supplements or modified textured foods. • Use thickeners to make semisolids of liquid foods (soups, beverages, juices, and shakes). • Syringe or training cups useful For first stroke patients with mild disabilities and return to good quality of life, a preventive approach to the second event is critical. • Lifestyle modification emphasizing adherence to the DASH dietary pattern and adoption of the 1,500 mg sodium limit are important.	• Hospital readmission for aspiration-related pneumonia • 6 to 8 cups of fluid to prevent dehydration • Calorie and protein optimization essential • Adequate fiber from food or supplementation is necessary to prevent constipation. Consider prune juice as stool softener (add to tube feeding). • Weight gain or loss should be monitored.

ADIME 8.4 ADIME At-A-Glance: Cerebrovascular Accident

Assessment

- BMI, UWL, decrease in appetite and food intake, dehydration
- Swallowing difficulty
- Self-feeding ability
- Ability to prepare foods/meals

Nutrition Diagnosis

- Swallowing difficulty RT CVA AEB coughing and choking, poor PO intake of 60%
- Inadequate fluid intake RT CVA AEB high BUN, high serum osmolality, high Na, thirst
- Inadequate protein-energy intake RT CVA and decreased appetite AEB UWL of 6% × 3 weeks, poor PO intake of 60%
- Self-feeding difficulty RT CVA AEB dropping of utensils, and decreased PO intake of 60%
- Unintended weight loss RT CVA, swallowing difficulty, and poor PO intake of 6% x 3 weeks AEB UWL of 6% × 3 weeks
- Impaired ability to prepare foods/meals RT recent CVA AEB reduced mobility

Intervention

- Provision of commercial beverage product
- Increased fluid diet
- Dysphagia diet/liquid consistency—nectar thick liquids
- Feeding assistance
- Referral to Home Delivered Meals Program

Monitoring and Evaluation

- Body weight, BUN, serum osmolality
- PO intake (food, fluid)
- Swallowing function, self-feeding ability

References

1. Centers for Disease Control and Prevention, National Center for Health Statistics. Compressed Mortality File 1999–2011. Series 20 No. 2P. CDC WONDER Online Database (database online). Released January 2013. Available at: http://wonder.cdc.gov/cmf-icd10.html. Accessed October 12, 2015.
2. National Center for Health Statistics. Mortality Multiple Cause Micro-data Files, 2011. Public-use data file and documentation.

NHLBI tabulations. Available at: http://www.cdc.gov/nchs/products/nvsr.htm. Accessed October 14, 2015.
3. Stoll G, Bendszus M. Inflammation and atherosclerosis. *Stroke* 2006;37:1923–1932.
4. Ross R. Atherosclerosis—An inflammatory disease. *N Engl J Med* 1999;340(2):115–126.
5. Berliner JA, Navab M, Fogelman AM, et al. Atherosclerosis: Basic mechanisms, oxidation, inflammation, and genetics. *Circulation* 2000;91:2488–2496.
6. Libby P, Ridker PM, Maseri A. Inflammation and atherosclerosis. *Circulation* 2002;105:1135–1143.
7. Spagnoli LG, Bonanno E, Sangiorgi G, et al. Role of inflammation in atherosclerosis. *J Nucl Med* 2007;48:1800–1815.
8. Chaabane C, Coen M, Bochaton-Piallat ML. Smooth muscle cell phenotypic switch: Implications for foam cell formation. *Curr Opin Lipidol* 2014;25:374–379.
9. Mora S, Szklo M, Otvos JD, et al. LDL particle subclasses, LDL particle size, and carotid atherosclerosis in the Multi-ethnic Study of Atherosclerosis (MESA). *Atherosclerosis* 2007;192:211–217.
10. Goff DC, Lloyd-Jones DM, Bennett G, et al. 2013 ACC/AHA guideline on the assessment of cardiovascular risk—A report of the American College of Cardiology/American Heart Association Task Force on Practice Guidelines. *Circulation* 2014;129(Suppl 2):S49–S73.
11. Stone NJ, Robinson JG, Lichtenstein AH, et al. ATP IV: 2013 ACC/AHA guideline on the treatment of blood cholesterol to reduce atherosclerotic cardiovascular risk in adults—A report of the American College of Cardiology/American Heart Association Task Force on Practice Guidelines. *Circulation* 2013;129(2):S1–S45.
12. Eckel RH, Jakicic JM, Ard JD, et al. 2013 AHA/ACC guideline on lifestyle management to reduce cardiovascular risk: A report of the American College of Cardiology/American Heart Association Task Force on Practice Guidelines. *Circulation* 2013;129(2):S76–S99.
13. Go AS, Bauman MA, Coleman King SM, et al. An effective approach to high blood pressure control: A science advisory from the American Heart Association, the American College of Cardiology, and the Centers for Disease Control and Prevention. *Hypertension* 2014;63:878–885.
14. Mozaffarian D, Benjamin EJ, Go AS, et al. Heart disease and stroke statistics—2015 update: A report from the American Heart Association. *Circulation* 2015;131:e29–e322.

15. Oparil S, Zaman MA, Calhoun DA. Pathogenesis of hypertension. *Ann Intern Med* 2003;139(9):761–776.
16. Carretero OA, Oparil S. Essential hypertension. Part I: Definition and etiology. Circulation 2000;101(3):329–335.
17. Hall JE, Guyton AC. *Textbook of Medical Physiology*. St. Louis, MO: Elsevier Saunders; 2006:216–223.
18. Lloyd-Jones DM, Hong Y, Labarthe D, et al; American Heart Association Strategic Planning Task Force and Statistics Committee. Defining and setting national goals for cardiovascular health promotion and disease reduction: The American Heart Association's Strategic Impact Goal through 2020 and beyond. *Circulation* 2010;121:586–613.
19. Frieden TR, Berwick DM. The "Million Hearts" initiative—Preventing heart attacks and strokes. *N Engl J Med* 2011;365:e27.
20. James PA, Oparil S, Carter BL, et al. 2014 Evidence-based guideline for the management of high blood pressure in adults: Report from the panel members appointed to the Eighth Joint National Committee (JNC 8). *JAMA* 2014;311(5):507–520.
21. National Heart, Lung, and Blood Institute. *Your Guide to High Blood Pressure with DASH*. NIH Publication No. 06-4082. Washington, DC: U.S. Department of Health and Human Services; 2006.
22. *What We Eat in America*, National Health and Nutrition Examination Survey, United States, 2009–2010.
23. Ayala C, Kuklina EV, Peralez J, et al. Application of lower sodium intake recommendations to adults—United States, 1999–2006. *MMWR Morb Mortal Wkly Rep* 2009;58(11):281–283.
24. Thygesen K, Alpert JS, Jaffe AS, et al. Third universal definition of myocardial infarction. *Circulation* 2012;126:2020–2035.
25. Medscape. Myocardial Infarction Medication. Available at: http://emedicine.medscape.com/article/155919-medication. Accessed November 12, 2015.
26. Gaby AR. Nutritional treatments for acute myocardial infarction. *Altern Med Rev* 2010;15(2):113–123.
27. Heidenreich PA, Albert NM, Allen LA, et al; American Heart Association Advocacy Coordinating Committee, Council on Arteriosclerosis, Thrombosis and Vascular Biology, Council on Cardiovascular Radiology and Intervention, Council on Clinical Cardiology, Council on Epidemiology and Prevention, and Stroke Council. Forecasting the impact of heart failure in the United States: A policy statement from the American Heart Association. *Circ Heart Fail* 2013;6:606–619.

28. Escott-Stump S. *Nutrition and Diagnosis-Related Care.* 8th ed. North American Edition. Baltimore, MD: Wolters Kluwer; 2015:373–375.
29. Nelms M, Roth SL. Medical Nutrition Therapy: A Case Study Approach. 4th ed. Stamford, CT: Cengage Learning; 2014:59–63.
30. Yancy CW, Jessup M, Bozkurt B, et al. 2013 ACCF/AHA guideline for the management of heart failure: Executive summary. A report of the American College of Cardiology Foundation/American Heart Association Task Force on Practice Guidelines. *Circulation* 2013;128:1810–1852.
31. Albert NM, Barnason S, Deswal A, et al. Transitions of care in heart failure: A scientific statement from the American Heart Association. *Circ Heart Fail* 2015;8:384–409.
32. Go AS, Mozaffarian D, Roger VL, et al; American Heart Association Statistics Committee and Stroke Statistics Subcommittee. Heart Disease and Stroke Statistics—2013 update: A report from the American Heart Association. *Circulation* 2013;127:e6–e245.
33. Wirth R, Smoliner C, Jäger M, et al. Guideline clinical nutrition in patients with stroke. *Exp Transl Stroke Med* 2013;5:14.
34. Vivanti AP, Campbell KL, Suter MS, et al. Contribution of thickened drinks, food and enteral and parenteral fluids to fluid intake in hospitalised patients with dysphagia. *J Hum Nutr Diet* 2009;22:148–155.
35. Foley NC, Martin RE, Salter KL, et al. A review of the relationship between dysphagia and malnutrition following stroke. *J Rehabil Med* 2009;41:707–713.
36. Whelan K. Inadequate fluid intakes in dysphagic acute stroke. *Clin Nutr* 2001;20:423–428.
37. Milne AC, Potter J, Vivanti A, et al. Protein and energy supplementation in elderly people at risk from malnutrition. *Cochrane Database Syst Rev* 2009;(2):CD003288.
38. Corrigan ML, Escuro AA, Celestin J, et al. Nutrition in the stroke patient. *Nutr Clin Pract* 2011;26(3):242–252.

Notes

Notes

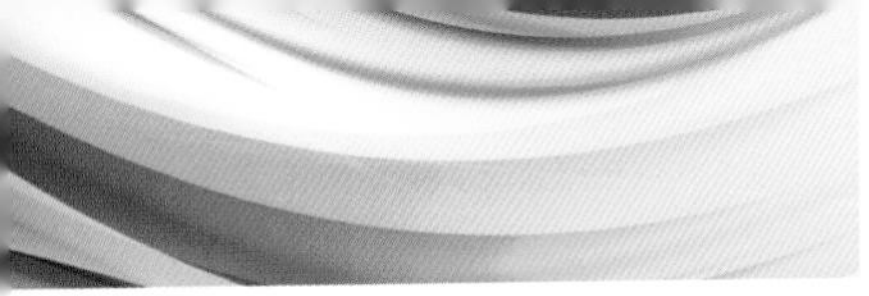

CHAPTER

9 Diabetes

Diabetes mellitus is a disease known since ancient times, cited by both the Greeks and Egyptians in as early as 1500 BC. In its various forms, it affects over 29 million Americans every year, and another 86 million people have prediabetes. It is the seventh leading cause of death and a major cause of complications, such as heart disease, kidney disease, blindness, and amputations.

DIABETES: CLASSIFICATION, SCREENING, AND DIAGNOSIS

Classification of Diabetes

To provide comprehensive and effective medical and nutritional care for patients with diabetes, we must first understand the definitions and classifications of diabetes, which are issued by the American Diabetes Association (ADA). Table 9.1 includes the four clinical classes of diabetes.[1] It should be noted that the traditional standards of type 1 diabetes occurring only in children and type 2 diabetes only in adults are no longer accurate, as both diseases occur in both cohorts.[2] Assigning a type of diabetes to an individual often depends on the circumstances present at the time of diagnosis, with individuals not always fitting clearly into a single category.

TABLE 9.1. Classification of Diabetes Mellitus

Type 1 diabetes	Results from autoimmune destruction of pancreatic β-cells, usually leading to absolute insulin deficiency. Accounts for 5%–10% of diagnosed diabetes in the United States.
Type 2 diabetes	Results from a progressive insulin secretory defect on the background of insulin resistance. Accounts for 90%–95% of diagnosed diabetes in the United States.
Other specific types of diabetes	Specific types of diabetes as a result of other causes: monogenic diabetes syndromes (such as neonatal diabetes and maturity-onset diabetes of the young [MODY]); diseases of the exocrine pancreas (e.g., cystic fibrosis); genetic defects of the β-cell; genetic defects in insulin action; endocrinopathies; drug- or chemical-induced; infections; uncommon forms of immune-mediated diabetes; other genetic syndromes associated with diabetes.
Gestational diabetes mellitus	Diagnosed during pregnancy

Data from American Diabetes Association. Diagnosis and classification of diabetes mellitus. *Diabetes Care* 2014;37(Suppl 1):S81–S90.

Screening for Diabetes

Adults

Dietitians and other health care providers should encourage regular screening for diabetes, especially for individuals in high-risk groups. Box 9.1 lists the recommendations for screening for type 2 diabetes and prediabetes in asymptomatic adults.

Children

Because of the dramatic increase of type 2 diabetes in children, the ADA recommends screening for children at increased

BOX 9.1 Screening for Diabetes or Prediabetes in Asymptomatic Adults

1. Testing should be considered in all individuals at age 45 years and above, particularly in those who are overweight or obese (body mass index [BMI] $\geq$25 kg/m^2 or $\geq$23 kg/m^2 in Asian Americans).
2. Testing should be considered *before* age 45 in individuals who are overweight (BMI $\geq$25 kg/m^2 or $\geq$23 kg/m^2 in Asian Americans) and have additional risk factors:
   - Physical inactivity
   - First-degree relative with diabetes
   - Members of a high-risk ethnic population (African American, Asian American, Latino, Native American, Pacific Islander)
   - Have delivered a baby weighing >9 lb or have been diagnosed with GDM
   - Hypertensive ($\geq$140/90 mm Hg or on therapy for hypertension)
   - HDL cholesterol level <35 mg/dL and/or triglyceride level >250 mg/dL
   - Women with polycystic ovary syndrome
   - A1C > 5.7%, IGT or IFG on previous testing
   - History of vascular disease
   - Have other clinical conditions associated with insulin resistance (severe obesity, acanthosis nigricans)
3. If results are normal, repeat at a minimum of 3-year intervals, with consideration of more frequent testing depending on initial results (e.g., those with prediabetes should be tested yearly) and risk status.

Data from American Diabetes Association. Classification and diagnosis of diabetes. *Diabetes Care* 2015;38(Suppl 1):S8–S16.

risk for the presence of type 2 diabetes and prediabetes.[3] Box 9.2 shows the testing criteria for type 2 diabetes and prediabetes in asymptomatic children.

Pregnant Women

The ADA recommends that all pregnant women with risk factors for type 2 diabetes be screened at the first prenatal

BOX 9.2 Testing for Type 2 Diabetes or Prediabetes in Asymptomatic Children (Persons Aged ≤18 Years)

Age of initiation: 10 years of age or at onset of puberty, if puberty occurs at a younger age
Frequency: Every 3 years
Criteria: Overweight (BMI >85th percentile for age and sex, weight for height >85th percentile, or weight >120% of ideal for height).
Plus any two of the following risk factors:

- Family history of type 2 diabetes in first- or second-degree relative
- Race/ethnicity (African American, Asian American Latino, Native American, Pacific Islander)
- Signs of insulin resistance or conditions associated with insulin resistance (acanthosis nigricans, dyslipidemia, hypertension, or polycystic ovary syndrome, or small-for-gestational-age birth weight)
- Maternal history of diabetes or GDM during the child's gestation

BMI, body mass index.
Data from (i) American Diabetes Association. Diagnosis and classification of diabetes mellitus. *Diabetes Care* 2014;37(Suppl 1):S81–S90 and (ii) American Diabetes Association. Classification and diagnosis of diabetes. *Diabetes Care* 2015;38(Suppl 1):S8–S16.

visit, using standardized diagnostic criteria. Women with diabetes in the first trimester would be classified as having type 2 diabetes versus gestational diabetes mellitus (GDM). GDM is diabetes diagnosed in the second or third trimester of pregnancy that is not clearly overt diabetes. The current recommendations for screening for GDM in pregnant women come from the U.S. Preventive Services Task Force (USPSTF), who recommends that all asymptomatic pregnant women after 24 weeks of gestation be tested for diabetes.[4] Box 9.3 lists the risk factors that increase a woman's risk for developing GDM. Further information on diabetes in pregnancy can be found in Chapter 2.

BOX 9.3 Screening for Gestational Diabetes Mellitus

Recommendation: Screen for GDM in all asymptomatic pregnant women after 24 weeks of gestation

Risk factors that increase a woman's risk of developing GDM:

- Obesity
- Increased maternal age
- History of GDM
- Family history of diabetes
- Belonging to an ethnic group with increased risk for type 2 DM (African American, Asian American Latino, Native American, Pacific Islander)

DM, diabetes mellitus.

Data from International Expert Committee. International Expert Committee report on the role of the A1C assay in the diagnosis of diabetes. *Diabetes Care* 2009;32:1327–1334.

Diagnosis of Diabetes

Children and Nonpregnant Adults

Diabetes may be diagnosed using fasting plasma glucose (FPG), hemoglobin A1C (A1C), or a 2-hour plasma glucose during an oral glucose tolerance test (OGTT). A1C was not previously recommended for the diagnosis of diabetes in part because of lack of standardized assays. However, assays are now highly standardized, and the ADA supports the use of A1C as a diagnostic test for diabetes, as recommended by an International Expert Committee.[3] A1C has several advantages to the FPG and OGTT, including greater convenience (no fasting required), greater preanalytical stability, and less day-to-day perturbations during illness and stress.[2] These advantages must be balanced by greater cost, limited availability of A1C testing in certain regions of the developing world, and the incomplete correlation between A1C and average glucose in certain individuals. Box 9.4 lists the laboratory testing methods currently recommended for the diagnosis of diabetes.

BOX 9.4 Testing Methods Used to Diagnose Diabetes[a]

1. **A1C > 6.5%**
   - The test should be performed in a laboratory using a method that is NGSP-certified and standardized to the DCCT assay.

or

2. **FPG ≥ 126 mg/dL**
   - Fasting is defined as no caloric intake for at least 8 hours.

or

3. **2-hour plasma glucose ≥200 mg/dL during an OGTT**
   - The test should be performed as described by the World Health Organization, using a glucose load containing the equivalent of 75-g anhydrous glucose dissolved in water.

or

4. **Classic symptoms of diabetes and a random plasma glucose ≥200 mg/dL**
   - Random is defined as any time of day without regard to time since last meal.
   - Classic symptoms of diabetes include polyuria, polydipsia, and unexplained weight loss.

[a]In absence of unequivocal hyperglycemia, result to be confirmed by repeat testing.

NGSP, National Glycohemoglobin Standardization Program; DCCT, diabetes control and complications trial.

Data from American Diabetes Association. Classification and diagnosis of diabetes. *Diabetes Care* 2015;38(Suppl 1):S8–S16.

Prediabetes

An intermediate group of subjects has been recognized whose glucose levels do not meet the criteria for diabetes but are too high to be considered normal.[1,2] Individuals who fall into this category have impaired fasting glucose (IFG) and/or impaired glucose tolerance (IGT), and are referred to as having "prediabetes." These individuals are considered at risk for the future development of diabetes and cardiovascular disease.[2] IFG and IGT are associated with obesity (especially abdominal or visceral obesity), dyslipidemia with high triglycerides and/or low high-density lipoprotein (HDL) cholesterol, and hypertension. Table 9.2 lists the

TABLE 9.2. Diagnostic Criteria for Diabetes and Prediabetes[a]

	Fasting Plasma Glucose (mg/dL)	A1C (%)	2-Hour Plasma Glucose in the OGTT (mg/dL)
Normal	<100	≤5.6	≤139
Prediabetes	100–125	5.7–6.4	140–199
Diabetes	≥126	≥6.5	≥200

[a]Each criterion must be confirmed by repeat testing unless unequivocal symptoms of hyperglycemia are present.

Data from American Diabetes Association. Classification and diagnosis of diabetes. *Diabetes Care* 2015;38(Suppl 1):S8–S16.

diagnostic criteria for types 1 and 2 diabetes and prediabetes using the three diagnostic tests mentioned earlier.

Gestational Diabetes

Screening for GDM can be accomplished with either of two strategies: the "one-step" strategy is supported by the International Association of the Diabetes and Pregnancy Study Groups (IADPSG), an international consensus group with representatives from multiple obstetrical and diabetes organizations, including the ADA; and the "two-step" strategy, which is a recommendation from the National Institutes of Health (NIH) consensus panel of experts in obstetrics/gynecology, maternal–fetal medicine, pediatrics, diabetes research, and biostatistics.

The strategies are summarized in Table 2.9 in Chapter 2 of this book.[1]

MEDICAL NUTRITION THERAPY

Medical nutrition therapy (MNT) is an integral component of diabetes prevention, management, and self-management.[4]

The recommendations by the ADA for MNT in diabetes are based in part on the Dietary Guidelines and the recommended daily allowances (RDAs) from the Institute of Medicine of the National Academy of Sciences.

- Provide regular, individualized meal planning advice and guidelines, preferably by a registered dietitian skilled in diabetes MNT.
- Maintain a reasonable weight through therapeutic lifestyle change, including a reduction in energy intake and an increase in physical activity. Weight loss of 2 to 8 kg may provide clinical benefits in those with type 2 diabetes, especially early in the disease process.
- Evidence suggests that there is not an ideal percentage of calories from carbohydrate, protein, and fat for all people with diabetes. Therefore, macronutrient distributions should be based on individualized assessment of current eating patterns, preferences, and metabolic goals.
- A variety of eating patterns have been shown to be effective in managing diabetes, including Mediterranean style, Dietary Approaches to Stop Hypertension (DASH) style, and plant-based (vegan or vegetarian), lower-fat, and lower-carbohydrate patterns.
- Monitoring carbohydrate intake, whether by carbohydrate counting or experience-based estimation, remains critical in achieving glycemic control.
- The amount of dietary saturated fat, cholesterol, and trans fat recommended for people with diabetes is the same as that recommended for the general population.
- The recommendation for the general population to reduce sodium to less than 2,300 mg/d is also appropriate for people with diabetes. For individuals with both diabetes and hypertension, further reduction in sodium intake should be individualized.

ADIME 9.1 ADIME At-A-Glance: Type 1 Diabetes

Assessment

- Ht, wt, BMI
- Labs: Blood pressure, fasting plasma glucose, A1C (quarterly), lipid profile, serum creatinine, BUN, GFR, microalbuminuria (annually)
- Blood glucose self-monitoring log, food history/logs, vitamin/mineral/supplement use

Nutrition Diagnosis

- Altered nutrition-related laboratory values for blood glucose RT insufficient or inappropriate insulin administration AEB A1C of 7.5% and consistent preprandial hyperglycemia per blood glucose logs despite good eating habits.

Intervention

- Review insulin regimen and timing of food intake with patient.
- Recalculate insulin-to-carbohydrate ratio (ICR) and sensitivity factor (SF).
- Consult with physician regarding adequacy of current insulin prescription.

Monitoring and Evaluation

- Improvements in blood glucose levels; have patient submit blood glucose log results for 1 week
- Recheck A1C in 3 months; goal level <7%

Carbohydrate Counting

Carbohydrate counting is a meal planning approach for people with diabetes that focuses on balancing carbohydrate food choices throughout the day. It places emphasis on the total amount of carbohydrate consumed, rather than on the source or type of carbohydrate consumed, and is based on two ideas:

1. Carbohydrate, whether from sugars or starches, has the greatest impact on postprandial blood glucose levels compared with protein and fat.

2. Eating equal amounts of sugar, starch, or milk will raise blood glucose level about the same amount.

Two levels of carbohydrate counting have been defined: basic and advanced.

Basic Carbohydrate Counting

This approach promotes consistency in the timing and amount of carbohydrate intake. Patients should learn about the relationship among food, physical activity, diabetes medications, and blood glucose levels. In addition, education on how to identify carbohydrate foods, appropriate portion or serving sizes, weighing and measuring foods, and how to read food labels should be included.[5]

Carbohydrate counting is based on the principle that one carbohydrate serving (or carb choice) is equal to 15 g of carbohydrate and can be a starch, fruit, milk, or sweet/dessert. Patients can use basic carbohydrate counting with type 1 or type 2 diabetes. Although the type of carbohydrate consumed is not as important as the amount and timing in this method, carbohydrate intake from vegetables, fruits, whole grains, legumes, and dairy products should be emphasized over intake from other carbohydrate sources, especially those that contain added fats, sugars, or sodium.

Advanced Carbohydrate Counting

This approach is for those patients who have mastered basic carb counting and wish to have more freedom in their carbohydrate choices and/or tighter blood glucose control, such as those with type 1 diabetes who use a basal-bolus insulin regimen or an insulin pump. For patients using this method, the following skills are recommended:[5,6]

- Understanding target blood glucose levels
- Ability to quantify food intake and use basic math skills
- Understanding the action of insulin and the basal-bolus insulin concept
- Ability to carry out pattern management and keep adequate records

- Ability to calculate a bolus insulin dose using the ICR
- Willingness to check blood glucose before and after meals
- Ability to correct blood glucose using insulin SF

Advanced carbohydrate counting involves calculating an individual's ICR and insulin SF.

ICR is the number of grams of carbohydrate counteracted by 1 unit (U) of rapid-acting or short-acting (bolus) insulin. The method used to calculate the ICR is the 450/500 Rule (Box 9.5). The ICR allows flexibility in food choices because any number of carbohydrates can be covered with a matching dose of insulin.

BOX 9.5 The 450/500 Rule for Calculating the ICR

- If using rapid-acting insulin (i.e., Humalog or Novolog), use the 500 Rule. If short-acting (regular) insulin is used (i.e., Humulin R or Novolin R), use 450.
- Divide 450 or 500 by the total daily dose (TDD) of insulin.

Example: A man uses Humalog insulin at 50 U per day. His ICR would be 1:10 based on the equation:

500/50 U (TDD) of insulin = 10 g of carbohydrate covered by 1 U of insulin, or a **1:10 ICR**

- The TDD includes all basal plus bolus insulin.
- It should be noted that the 450/500 Rule works best for patients with type 1 diabetes with *no* insulin production, using the basal/bolus approach to insulin therapy. People with type 2 diabetes who require insulin injections often produce some insulin naturally, so a TDD cannot be calculated reliably.
- ICR can vary from person to person, and for the same person during different times of the day, based on their physical activity, insulin needs, body weight, hormonal changes, and other variables. As always, self-monitoring of blood glucose is imperative.

Data from (i) American Diabetes Association. Getting started with an insulin pump. Available at: http://www.diabetes.org/living-with-diabetes/treatment-and-care/medication/insulin/getting-started.html. Accessed February 16, 2016 and (ii) BD Worldwide. The diabetes learning center. How to calculate in insulin-to-carb ratio. Available at: http://www.bd.com/us/diabetes/page.aspx?cat=7001&id=7303. Accessed February 18, 2016.

When a patient's blood glucose level goes unexpectedly high, a correction bolus of insulin can be given to lower the level back to baseline. This correction value is referred to as the insulin sensitivity factor (can also be referred to as correction factor). The 1500/1800 Rule is a commonly accepted formula for estimating the drop in a person's blood glucose per unit of short-acting or rapid-acting insulin (Box 9.6).[7] Knowing their SF can help a person with type 1 diabetes to determine the correct dose of bolus insulin to correct an elevated blood glucose level.

The calculations of ICR and SF should be monitored and adjusted frequently based on the patient's blood glucose levels, because the values can change based on many factors such as hormonal changes, physical activity, body weight, and others.[7]

BOX 9.6 Calculating Insulin Sensitivity Using 1500/1800 Rule for Blood Glucose Correction

- Use the 1500 Rule for patients using short-acting (regular) insulin (i.e., Humulin R or Novolin R). Use the 1800 Rule for those using rapid-acting insulin (i.e., Humalog or NovoLog).
- Determine the total daily dose (TDD) of all basal and bolus insulin.
- Divide 1,500 or 1,800 by the TDD to find the SF.
- *Example:* 1,800 divided by 50 U (TDD) of insulin = 36. So, it would be estimated that 1 U of rapid-acting insulin would lower the blood glucose by 36 mg/dL.
- This rule works best when basal insulin makes up about 50% of TDD.
- SF can vary from person to person, and for the same person during different times of the day, based on their physical activity, insulin needs, body weight, hormonal changes, and other variables. As always, self-monitoring of blood glucose is imperative.

Data from (i) American Diabetes Association. Getting started with an insulin pump. Available at: http://www.diabetes.org/living-with-diabetes/treatment-and-care/medication/insulin/getting-started.html. Accessed February 16, 2016 and (ii) BD Worldwide. The diabetes learning center. How to calculate in insulin-to-carb ratio. Available at: http://www.bd.com/us/diabetes/page.aspx?cat=7001&id=7303. Accessed February 18, 2016.

ADIME 9.2 ADIME At-A-Glance: Type 2 Diabetes

Assessment

- Ht, wt, BMI, waist circumference
- Labs: Blood pressure, fasting plasma glucose, A1C (quarterly), lipid profile, serum creatinine, BUN, GFR, microalbuminuria (annually)
- Blood glucose self-monitoring log, food history/logs, vitamin/mineral/supplement use

Nutrition Diagnosis

- Inconsistent carbohydrate intake RT lack of knowledge and confusion regarding carb counting and portion sizes AEB food records with excessive carb choices at meals/snacks and postprandial glucose levels above desired targets.

Intervention

- Nutrition prescription: 18 carb choices with 3 to 4 choices per meal and 2 to 3 choices per snack
- Review carb-containing foods and appropriate portion sizes, particularly when dining out
- Review label reading and meal planning

Monitoring and Evaluation

- Improvements in blood glucose levels; have patient submit blood glucose log results for 1 week
- Food intake logs to show more consistent carb intake at meals and snack; have patient submit logs for 1 week

Exchange Lists

The Exchange Lists for Meal Planning (Table 9.3) were one of the first meal planning systems used to help patients with diabetes control their blood glucose levels. This system separates foods into six categories (or lists) based on their macronutrient content. Depending on the energy level, an exchange pattern consists of a set number of exchanges from each group. Within each list, foods can be exchanged, but the serving size may vary.

Although most health professionals prefer to use carbohydrate counting as the method of choice for managing blood glucose because of its ease of use, many patients still rely

TABLE 9.3. Exchange Lists for Meal Planning

Food Groups	Kilocalories	Carbohydrate	Protein	Fat
Carbohydrates				
Starch	80	15	3	0–1
Milk—skim and low-fat	90	12	8	0–3
2%	120	12	8	5
Whole	150	12	8	8
Fruit	60	15	—	—
Vegetables	25	5	2	—
Meat and Meat Substitutes				
Very lean	35	—	7	1
Lean	55	—	7	2–3
Medium-fat	75	—	7	5
High-fat	100	—	7	8
Fat	45	—	—	5

on the Exchange system to help keep their diabetes under control. In addition, because some patients with type 2 diabetes would benefit from even a modest weight loss, the Exchange lists can be a useful tool for the registered dietitian in planning a weight loss regimen. This system can be used to plan a more Mediterranean-style eating plan, which has been shown to not only aid with weight loss, but also help patients with diabetes decrease their cardiovascular disease risk by improving their lipid profiles.[8] The Mediterranean-style diet has also been shown to reduce the incidence of type 2 diabetes, which can be helpful in the prediabetes population.[9]

PHARMACOLOGIC MANAGEMENT OF DIABETES

Oral Hypoglycemic Medications

See Table 9.4 for a listing of oral medications for diabetes.

TABLE 9.4. Oral Medications for Type 2 Diabetes

Mode of Action	Class Brand Name (Generic Name)	When to Take?
Insulin secretagogues	**First-generation sulfonylureas**	
Stimulate insulin secretion from the pancreas	Diabinese (chlorpropamide)	Take with first meal of day
	Second-generation sulfonylureas	
	Glucotrol (glipizide)	30 min before meal
	Glucotrol XL (glipizide)	Take with first meal of day
	Micronase/DiaBeta (glyburide)	Take with first meal of day
	Glynase (micronized glyburide)	Take with first meal of day
	Amaryl (glimepiride)	Take with first meal of day
	Meglitinide–Benzoic acid derivative	
	Prandin (repaglinide)	Take with meals
	Meglitinide–d-phenylalanine derivative	
	Starlix (nateglinide)	1–30 min before meals

(*continued*)

TABLE 9.4. Oral Medications for Type 2 Diabetes (*continued*)

Mode of Action	Class Brand Name (Generic Name)	When to Take?
Insulin sensitizers	**Biguanides**	
Improve insulin sensitivity via the liver and peripheral tissue	Glucophage (metformin HCL)	Take with meals
	Glucophage XR, Fortamet, Glumetza (metformin HCL extended-release)	Once daily with evening meal
	Riomet (metformin HCL liquid)	Take with meals
	Thiazolidinediones	
	Avandia (rosiglitazone)	Take without regard to meals
	Actos (pioglitazone)	Take without regard to meals
Delay glucose absorption in GI	**α-Glucosidase inhibitors**	
	Precose (acarbose)	Take with first bite of main meals
	Glyset (miglitol)	Take with first bite of main meals

Increase insulin secretion and decrease glucagon secretion	**DPP-4 inhibitors**	Once daily without regard to meals
	Januvia (sitagliptin)	
	Onglyza (saxagliptin)	
	Tradjenta (linagliptin)	
	Nesina (alogliptin)	
Blocks glucose reabsorption in the kidney	**SGLT-2 inhibitors**	
	Invokana (canagliflozin)	Once daily before first meal
	Farxiga (dapagliflozin)	Once daily, in morning, with or without food
	Jardiance (empagliflozin)	Once daily, in morning, with or without food
Mechanism of action in diabetes is unknown	**Bile acid sequestrants**	
	Welchol (colesevelam HCL)	6 tablets once daily or 3 tablets twice daily, with a meal and liquid

DPP, dipeptidyl peptidase; SGLT, sodium glucose transporter.

Data from (i) Shaikh N, Goldman J. Current therapy in diabetes. *On The Cutting Edge*. Diabetes Care and Education Dietetic Practice Group 2015;36(2):4–7, (ii) RxList. The Internet Drug List. Available at: http://www.rxlist.com. Accessed February 18, 2016, and medication product labeling.

Insulin

See Table 9.5 for a listing of insulin and insulin analogs and their action.

Other Injectable Medications for Diabetes

Glucagon-Like Peptide-1 Agonists

Incretin mimetics are a class of medication for the treatment of type 2 diabetes. In individuals with type 2 diabetes, the naturally occurring incretin hormones (such as glucagon-like peptide-1 [GLP-1]) are blunted. An incretin mimetic works to mimic the antidiabetic or glucose-lowering actions of incretins by enhancing glucose-dependent insulin secretion and several other glucoregulatory actions. These medications suppress inappropriately elevated glucagon levels, promote satiety, reduce food intake, and slow the rate of gastric emptying.[10]

Amylin Analogs

Amylin analogs can mimic the actions of amylin, a hormone cosecreted with insulin that helps to slow gastric emptying and reduces elevated glucagon levels postprandially. Amylin, like insulin, is absent or deficient in patients with diabetes. When used with insulin, amylin analogs can help patients achieve improved glycemic control.[10] See Table 9.6 for a listing of noninsulin injectable medications for the control of diabetes.

BLOOD GLUCOSE, BLOOD PRESSURE, AND LIPID GOALS FOR ADULTS WITH DIABETES

Blood Glucose and Hemoglobin A1C

A1C is considered the primary target for glycemic control. The A1C test measures a patient's average glycemia over the preceding 2 to 3 months and can help health providers to determine whether a patient's metabolic control had been reached and maintained within a target range.[11] The ADA is recommending the use of the term *estimated average glucose* (eAG) in reference to A1C levels.[12] Health care providers can now report A1C results to patients using the

TABLE 9.5. Insulin and Insulin Analogs

Type of Insulin: Brand Name (Generic Name)	Onset	Peak	Duration (hr)	When to Administer?
Rapid-acting	15 min	30–90 min	3–5	0–15 min before meals
Humalog (insulin lispro)				
NovoLog (insulin aspart)				
Apidra (insulin glulisine)				
Rapid-acting by inhalation				
Afrezza (regular human insulin)	12–15 min	60 min	2–3	
Short-acting (regular)	30–60 min	2–4 hr	5–8	30–45 min before meals
Humulin R (Regular [R])				
Novolin R (Regular [R])				
Intermediate-acting	1–3 hr	6–10 hr	12–16	Before a.m. and p.m. meal or before am meal and at bedtime
Humulin N (NPH [N])				
Novolin N (NPH [N])				

(continued)

TABLE 9.5. Insulin and Insulin Analogs (*continued*)

Type of Insulin: Brand Name (Generic Name)	Onset	Peak	Duration (hr)	When to Administer?
Long-acting				
Lantus (insulin glargine U-100)	1 hr	No peak	Up to 24	In a.m. *or* at bedtime
Toujeo (insulin glargine U-300)	6 hr			Once daily
Levemir (insulin detemir)	1 hr	No peak	Up to 24	Once or twice daily
Tresiba (insulin degludec)			Up to 42	Once daily
Combinations				
Humulin 50/50 (NPH/Regular)	30–60 min	2.5–5	14–18	Before breakfast and dinner
Humulin 70/30 (NPH/Regular)	30–60 min	2–12	14–24	Before breakfast and dinner
Novolin 70/30 (NPH/Regular)	30–60 min	2–12	14–24	Before breakfast and dinner
Humalog Mix 75/25 (lispro protamine/lispro)	10–15 min	1–6.5	22–24	Before breakfast and dinner
NovoLog Mix 70/30 (aspart protamine/aspart)	5–15 min	1–4	18–24	Before breakfast and dinner
Ryzodeg 70/30 (degludec/aspart)			Beyond 24	

Data from (i) Shaikh N, Goldman J. Current therapy in diabetes. *On The Cutting Edge*. Diabetes Care and Education Dietetic Practice Group 2015;36(2):4–7, (ii) RxList. The Internet Drug List. Available at: http://www.rxlist.com. Accessed February 18, 2016, and product labeling.

TABLE 9.6. Injectable (Noninsulin) Antihyperglycemic Medications

Type of Medication *Brand Name* *(Generic Name)*	When to Inject	Indications for Use
GLP-1 Agonists:		
Byetta (exenatide) Used only in Type 2 patients	1–60 min *prior* to the main morning and evening meals (at least 6 hr apart). Do not take after meals.	• Not for use in patients with type 1 diabetes or for the treatment of diabetic ketoacidosis • Not a substitute for insulin, in insulin-requiring individuals • Not recommended as first-line therapy for patients who have inadequate glycemic control on diet and exercise
Bydureon (exenatide extended-release)	Once weekly, any time of day without regard to meals	
Victoza (liraglutide) Used only in Type 2 patients	Once daily, without regard to meals	
Tanzeum (albiglutide)	Once weekly, any time of day, without regard to meals	
Trulicity (dulaglutide)	Once weekly, any time of day, without regard to meals	
Amylin Analogs:		
Pramlintide Acetate (Symlin) Used only in type 1 or type 2 patients treated with insulin	Immediately prior to each major meal[a]	Indicated for use in type 1 or type 2 diabetes, as an adjunct treatment in patients who use mealtime insulin therapy who have failed to achieve desired glucose control despite optimal insulin therapy.

[a]Major meal is defined as containing at least 250 kcal or at least 30 g carbohydrate

Data from (i) Shaikh N, Goldman J. Current therapy in diabetes. On The Cutting Edge. Diabetes Care and Education Dietetic Practice Group 2015;36(2):4–7 and (ii) RxList. The Internet Drug List. Available at: http://www.rxlist.com. Accessed February 18, 2016.

same units (mg/dL or mmol/L) that patients see routinely in blood glucose measurements. Table 9.7 shows the correlation between A1C and eAG levels. The ADA recommends the following for A1C testing:[11]

- Perform the A1C test at least two times per year in patients who are meeting treatment goals and who have stable glycemic control.
- Perform the A1C test every 3 months in patients whose therapy has changed or who are not meeting glycemic goals.
- The A1C goal for *patients in general* is <7%.
- Providers might reasonably suggest more stringent A1C goals for selected individual patients (such as <6.5%) if this can be achieved without significant hypoglycemia or other adverse effects of treatment.

TABLE 9.7. Correlation Between A1C Level and eAG

A1C (%)	eAG (mg/dL)
6	126
7	154
8	183
9	212
10	240
11	269
12	298

The relationship between A1C and eAG is described by the formula 28.7 × A1C – 46.7 = eAG

A calculator for converting A1C results into eAG is available at http://professional.diabetes.org/diapro/glucose_calc.

Data from (i) American Diabetes Association. Standards of Medical Care in Diabetes—2015. *Diabetes Care* 2015;38(Suppl 1):S1–S93 and (ii) American Diabetes Association. eAG/A1C Conversion Calculator. Available at: http://professional.diabetes.org/diapro/glucose_calc. Accessed February 19, 2016.

Pre- and postprandial plasma glucose testing is an important part of diabetes management. Table 9.8 lists current recommendation for glycemic control.

Blood Pressure and Lipids

Hypertension and dyslipidemia are common comorbid conditions for patients with diabetes, and evidence indicates that the control of these coexisting conditions is essential in the treatment of diabetes. The American Association for Endocrinologist (AACE) recommendations for blood pressure and lipids for patients with type 2 diabetes are included in Table 9.9.

TABLE 9.8. Recommendations for Glycemic Control for Nonpregnant Adults with Diabetes

Glycemic Control	ADA Goals	AACE[a] Goals
A1C	<7%	≤6.5%
Preprandial plasma glucose	80–130 mg/dL	110 mg/dL
Peak postprandial plasma glucose	<180 mg/dL[b]	140 mg/dL

More or less stringent targets may be appropriate for individual patients if achieved without significant hypoglycemia or adverse events. Individualize targets based on:

- Age/life expectancy
- Comorbid conditions
- Diabetes duration
- Hypoglycemia status
- Individual patient considerations
- Known CVD[c]/advanced microvascular complications

[a]American Association of Clinical Endocrinologists.
[b]Postprandial glucose measurements should be made 1–2 hr after the beginning of the meal.
[c]Cardiovascular disease.
Data from American Diabetes Association. Standards of Medical Care in Diabetes—2015. *Diabetes Care* 2015;38(Suppl 1):S1–S93.

TABLE 9.9. AACE Lipid and Blood Pressure Targets for Patients with Type 2 Diabetes

Lipids	High-Risk Patients (T2D but No Other Major Risk and/or Age <40 yr)	Very-High-Risk Patients (T2D Plus >1 Major ASCVD Risk[a] or Established ASCVD)
LDL cholesterol (mg/dL)	<100	<70
Non-HDL cholesterol (mg/dL)	<130	<100
Triglycerides (mg/dL)	<150	<150
Total cholesterol/ HDL cholesterol	<3.5	<3.0
Apo B (mg/dL)	<90	<80
LDL-particle	<1,200	<1,000
Blood Pressure	<130/80 mm Hg	

[a]Hypertension, family history of ASCVD, low HDL-C, smoking.

LDL, low-density lipoprotein; HDL, high-density lipoprotein; ASCVD, atherosclerotic cardiovascular disease.

Data from Garber AJ, Abrahamson MJ, Barzilay JI, et al. Consensus statement by the American Association of Clinical Endocrinologists and American College of Endocrinology on the comprehensive type 2 diabetes management algorithm—2016 executive summary. *Endocr Pract* 2016;22(1):84–113.

SICK DAY MANAGEMENT

Educating patients on sick day management is important. Illnesses such as viral colds or flu, infections, injuries, fever, vomiting, and diarrhea all increase the need for insulin. Emotional stress or crises, physical injury, and surgery can also affect blood glucose levels.

General Guidelines for Sick Days

- Test blood glucose every 4 hours and record in logbook.
- Test for urine ketones every 4 hours and record in log book (type 1 diabetes).

- Continue taking insulin and diabetes medications.
- Supplemental doses of rapid- or short-acting insulin may be needed because of elevated blood glucose levels or the presence of large or persistent ketones.
- Adjustments need to be individualized and based on tested blood glucose levels.
- Drink 8 oz of fluid every hour. If blood glucose is high, drink water or other calorie-, caffeine-free fluids. If blood glucose is low, drink sugar-based liquids.
- Eat at least 15 g of carbohydrate every hour or 45 to 50 g every 3 to 4 hours (Box 9.7).
- Soft foods or liquids may be easier to consume.

When to Call the Doctor?

- Persistent hyperglycemia (blood glucose >240 mg/dL) even after extra insulin called for in patient's sick plan
- Persistent vomiting and/or diarrhea (more than 6 hours)
- Sick or have fever for more than 2 days and are not getting better

BOX 9.7 Foods for Sick Day Management (~15 g Carbohydrate Each)

½ cup (4 oz) fruit juice	1 cup (8 oz) milk (nonfat)[a]
1 cup (8 oz) Gatorade or sports drink	½ cup (4 oz) regular, nondiet soft drink
½ cup unsweetened applesauce	3 squares graham cracker
1 slice toast	1 cup soup
½ cup regular gelatin	6 saltine crackers
½ cup oatmeal	1 popsicle (single)
⅓ cup rice or pasta	½ cup ice cream
¼ cup sherbet	½ cup frozen yogurt
3 glucose tablets	8 Lifesavers
2 tablespoons raisins	

[a]Avoid food high in fat content as it may slow gastric emptying and absorption of carbohydrate.

- Symptoms that might signal ketoacidosis of dehydration (chest pains, difficulty breathing, breath smells fruity, lips or tongue dry and cracked)
- Moderate to large amounts of ketones in urine

ACUTE COMPLICATIONS OF DIABETES

Hypoglycemia

Hypoglycemia, or low blood glucose, occurs when the blood glucose level drops too low to provide enough energy for the body's activities (Box 9.8). In adults or children older than 10 years, hypoglycemia is uncommon except as a side effect of diabetes treatment, but it can result from other medications or diseases, hormone or enzyme deficiencies, or tumors.[11]

BOX 9.8 Hypoglycemia

Definition	Plasma glucose <70 mg/dL
Signs and symptoms	Hunger, sweating, shakiness, dizziness, lightheadedness, difficulty speaking, sleepiness, confusion and disorientation, anxiety, weakness, unconsciousness
Causes	• Excessive insulin or oral medications • Inappropriate timing of insulin in relation to food intake • Inadequate food intake (not eating enough or skipping meals/snacks) • Prolonged duration or increased intensity of exercise • Alcohol intake without food

Treatment	**Mild hypoglycemia: 15/15 rule**
	1. Check blood glucose (BG).
	  • If BG is 50–69 mg/dL, give **15 g** carbohydrate[a].
	  • If BG is <50, give 30 g carbohydrate.
	2. Wait **15 minutes** and recheck BG.
	  • If BG <70, repeat step 1.
	  • If BG >70, monitor for signs/symptoms of low BG.
	  • Eat next meal or snack within 1 hour.
	Severe hypoglycemia:
	1. If able to swallow without risk of aspiration, offer juice or regular, nondiet soft drink or place glucose gel, honey, syrup, or jelly inside the person's cheek.

BOX 9.8 Hypoglycemia (*continued*)

2. If unable to swallow without risk of aspiration, give glucagon injection as recommended:
   - Older children and adults: 1 mg
   - Children under age 5: 0.5 mg
   - Infants: 0.25 mg

Special note People who take acarbose (Precose) or miglitol (Glyset) should know that only pure glucose (dextrose), available in tablet or gel form, will raise the blood glucose level during a hypoglycemic episode. Other quick-fix food and drinks will not raise the level quickly enough because these medications slow the digestion of other forms of carbohydrate.

[a]Pure glucose is the preferred treatment, but any form of carbohydrate that contains glucose will raise blood glucose. Examples of 15 g carbohydrate include 4 oz fruit juice, 2 Tbsp raisins, 3 glucose or 4 dextrose tablets, 5–6 oz regular soda, 7–8 Lifesavers, 1 Tbsp sugar, honey, corn syrup, or jelly.

Data from (i) American Diabetes Association. Standards of Medical Care in Diabetes—2015. *Diabetes Care* 2015;38(Suppl 1):S1–S93, (ii) American Diabetes Association. Hypoglycemia. Available at: http://www.diabetes.org/living-with-diabetes/treatment-and-care/blood-glucose-control/hypoglycemia-low-blood.html. Accessed February 19, 2016, and (iii) National Institute of Diabetes and Digestive and Kidney Diseases. Hypoglycemia. Available at: http://www.niddk.nih.gov/health-information/health-topics/Diabetes/hypoglycemia/Pages/index.aspx. Accessed February 18, 2016.

Diabetic Ketoacidosis and Hyperosmolar Hyperglycemic State

Hyperglycemia can lead to diabetic ketoacidosis (DKA) or hyperosmolar hyperglycemic state (HHS), both of which are life-threatening conditions. DKA is a state of severe metabolic decompensation manifested by the overproduction of ketone bodies and keto acids, resulting in metabolic acidosis.[13] DKA is characterized by severe disturbances in carbohydrate, protein, and fat metabolism, and is most frequently seen in those with type 1 diabetes. HHS is a metabolic derangement most frequently seen in type 2 diabetes and is usually precipitated by illness or infection that leads to profound dehydration. HHS is similar to DKA except that insulin deficiency is not as prevalent.[14] Table 9.10 gives a comparison of DKA and HHS.

TABLE 9.10. Comparison of DKA and HHS

	DKA	HHS
Age	Under 40 years of age	Over 60 years of age
Hallmark features	• More common in patients with type 1 diabetes • Ketosis, ketonuria, metabolic acidosis, dehydration	• Most commonly occurs in patients with type 2 diabetes • Markedly elevated blood glucose, hyperosmolality, profound dehydration, no significant ketosis
Signs and symptoms	Polyuria, polydipsia, hyperventilation, dehydration, fruity odor of ketones, fatigue, blurred vision, weakness, abdominal pain, nausea, vomiting, disorientation, confusion	Fatigue, blurred vision, dry mouth, mental status changes, coma
Causes	Absolute or relative insulin deficiency, typically caused by underlying infection, disruption of insulin treatment, and new onset of diabetes	Illness, infection, noncompliance, and undiagnosed diabetes are common precipitating factors.
Plasma glucose	250–600 mg/dL	600–2,000 mg/dL
Ketones	4+	<2+
Arterial pH	Low (<7.3)	Normal
Serum osmolality	<320 mOsm/kg	>320 mOsm/kg
Bicarbonate concentration	Low	Normal

TABLE 9.10. Comparison of DKA and HHS (*continued*)

	DKA	HHS
Treatment	Insulin administration, fluid resuscitation, correction of electrolyte imbalance, monitoring for complications of treatment	Fluid and electrolyte replacement and insulin administration

Data from (i) Mahan LK, Escott-Stump S, Raymond JL. *Krause's Food and the Nutrition Care Process*. 13th ed. St. Louis, MO: Elsevier Saunders; 2012:703–704, (ii) Hemphill R. Hyperosmolar hyperglycemic state. Available at: http://emedicine.medscape.com/article/1914705-overview#a4. Accessed February 19, 2016, and (iii) Hamdy O. Diabetic ketoacidosis. Available at: http://emedicine.medscape.com/article/118361-overview#a4. Accessed February 19, 2016.

REFERENCES

1. American Diabetes Association. Diagnosis and classification of diabetes mellitus. *Diabetes Care* 2014;37(Suppl 1):S81–S90.
2. American Diabetes Association. Classification and diagnosis of diabetes. *Diabetes Care* 2015;38(Suppl 1):S8–S16.
3. International Expert Committee. International Expert Committee report on the role of the A1C assay in the diagnosis of diabetes. *Diabetes Care* 2009;32:1327–1334.
4. Moyer VA. Screening for gestational diabetes mellitus: U.S. Preventive Services Task Force recommendation statement. *Ann Intern Med* 2014;17(6):414–422.
5. Kulkarni KD. Carbohydrate counting: A practical meal-planning option for people with diabetes. *Clin Diabetes* 2005;23:120–122.
6. Hall M. Understanding advance carbohydrate counting—A useful tool for some patients to improve blood glucose control. *Today's Dietitian* December 2013;15(12). Available at: http://www.todaysdietitian.com/newarchives/120913p40.shtml. Accessed February 15, 2016.

7. American Diabetes Association. Getting started with an insulin pump. Available at: http://www.diabetes.org/living-with-diabetes/treatment-and-care/medication/insulin/getting-started.html. Accessed February 16, 2016.
8. Estruch R, Ross R, Salas-Salvado J, et al. Primary prevention of cardiovascular disease with a Mediterranean diet. *N Engl J Med* 2013;368:1279–1290.
9. Salas-Salvado J, Bullo M, Babio N, et al. Reduction in the incidence of type 2 diabetes with the Mediterranean diet: Results of the PREDIMED-Reus nutrition intervention randomized trial. *Diabetes Care* 2011;42(1):14–19.
10. Shaikh N, Goldman J. Current therapy in diabetes. *On The Cutting Edge*. Diabetes Care and Education Dietetic Practice Group 2015;36(2):4–7.
11. American Diabetes Association. Standards of Medical Care in Diabetes—2015. *Diabetes Care* 2015;38(Suppl 1):S1–S93.
12. American Diabetes Association. eAG/A1C Conversion Calculator. Available at: http://professional.diabetes.org/diapro/glucose_calc. Accessed February 19, 2016.
13. Mahan LK, Escott-Stump S, Raymond JL. *Krause's Food and the Nutrition Care Process*. 13th ed. St. Louis, MO: Elsevier Saunders; 2012:703–704.
14. Hemphill R. Hyperosmolar hyperglycemic state. Available at: http://emedicine.medscape.com/article/1914705-overview#a4. Accessed February 19, 2016.

Notes

Notes

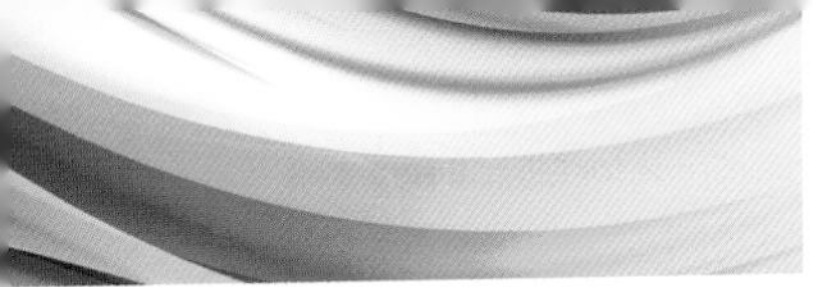

CHAPTER 10

Gastrointestinal Disease

Considering the importance of the gastrointestinal (GI) tract's key roles in maintaining life and health, it becomes clear as to how profoundly GI diseases can affect nutritional status, and ultimately overall health. Nutritional problems can arise from both upper gastrointestinal tract (UGI) and lower gastrointestinal tract (LGI) diseases. These problems can be caused by the underlying disease process, disease symptoms, interventions, and/or self-imposed dietary restrictions. For these reasons, a comprehensive nutritional assessment is essential, with particular focus on a detailed diet history, as is highly individualized interventions.

DISEASES OF THE UPPER GASTROINTESTINAL TRACT

Gastroesophageal Reflux Disease

Disease Process

Gastroesophageal reflux is the process in which acid from the stomach refluxes up through the lower esophageal sphincter (LES) into the esophagus, with inflammation of the sensitive tissue, resulting in esophagitis. Acute esophagitis can be caused by ingesting a caustic compound, often a medication, such as nonsteroidal anti-inflammatory drugs (NSAIDs), and it can arise from repeated vomiting, especially when self-induced as in anorexia and bulimia. Chronic reflux is termed *gastroesophageal reflux disease* (GERD) and increases risk for Barrett esophagus, a precancerous condition.[1] Inappropriate relaxation of the LES can be caused by many factors, some of which are related to diet and lifestyle (Box 10.1). Medications and substances that slow gastric emptying can also cause or exacerbate reflux (Box 10.2).

A common cause of GERD is hiatal hernia, particularly type 1 (sliding), which accounts for 95% of all hiatal hernias, with studies reporting that over half of GERD diagnoses were associated with hiatal hernia.[2] Another potential cause of GERD is eosinophilic esophagitis, esophageal

BOX 10.1 Factors Affecting LES Pressure in GERD

Reduce Pressure (Open)

Alcoholic Beverages
Caffeine
Chocolate
Cigarettes
Dietary fat
Mint oils

High Pressure on Stomach

- Overeating, drinking

Hormone Level

- Progesterone (pregnancy, late phase of menstrual cycle)

Medications

- Anticholinergics: Atropine, Bentyl, Robinul, Scopolamine
- Bronchodilators: Albuterol (Proventil, Ventolin), metaproterenol (Alupent), montelukast (Singulair), terbutaline (Brethine), theophylline (Aerolatte, Slo-Bid, Slo-Phyllin, Theo-24, Theo-Dur, Theolair, Uniphyl), zafirlukast (Accolate)

Increase Pressure (Close)

Dietary Protein

Medications

- Bethanechol
- Metoclopramide

BOX 10.2 Medications and Substances That Slow Gastric Emptying

Medications

Calcium Channel Blockers

Adalat, Calan, Cardene, Cardizem, DynaCirc, Isoptin, Nimotop, Norvasc, Plendil, Posicor, Procardia, Sular, Vascor, Verelan

Opiates/Opioids

Alfenta, Buprenex, codeine, Dalgan, Darvon, Demerol, Dilaudid, Dolophine, Levo-dromoran, Nubain, Roxicodone, Sublimaze, Sufenta, Talwin, Ultiva

Tricyclic Antidepressants

Anafranil, Adapin/Sinequan, Aventyl/Pamelor, Janimine/Tofranil, Vivactil, Norpramin/Pertofrane

Other Substances

Alcohol
Marijuana
Tobacco

inflammation resulting from allergy, most often food allergy, with up to 20% of patients experiencing GERD.[3] In achalasia, a neurologic disorder of the lower esophagus in which the LES fails to relax causing dysphagia (see Chapter 4), the disease process itself and treatments can also result in GERD.[4]

Treatment and Nutrition Intervention

Treatment for GERD includes diet and lifestyle changes, medications, and, failing these, surgery. Medications to reduce gastric acidity include antacids, H_2 receptor antagonists, and proton pump inhibitors (PPIs). Reducing acidity of the gastric contents renders the reflux fluid less caustic. Chronic and long-term use of acid-reducing medications may cause malabsorption or interference with several nutrients, especially PPIs, including folic acid, vitamin B_{12}, iron, calcium, zinc, and magnesium.[5]

Dietary considerations for GERD focus on prevention of reflux and reduction of gastric acidity, which involves manipulating dietary constituents that affect LES pressure, reducing gastric acid secretion, and avoiding tart or acidic foods and irritating spices in a flare-up[6] (Box 10.3). Smoking exerts a wide range of GI effects, most of which worsen GI problems, including reduced LES pressure and increased acid secretion.[7]

BOX 10.3 Dietary and Other Recommendations for GERD

Diet to Prevent Reflux	Other Treatment Aspects	Diet in Acute Esophagitis
Eat small, frequent meals, avoid large meals	• Do not lie down after eating (wait 3 hours)	• Avoid acidic foods (citrus fruits, tomatoes)
Avoid single high-fat meals	• Elevate the head of the bed, if needed	• Avoid spicy foods (red, black pepper)
Eat low-fat, higher protein meals	• Limit or avoid smoking	• Follow a bland, soft diet
Limit alcohol	• Use antacids to lower gastric acidity • Weight loss, if indicated • Wear loose-fitting clothing	• Eat small, frequent meals
Avoid foods that lower LES[a] pressure: chocolate, coffee, mints, garlic, onions, cinnamon		
Avoid drinking liquids with meals; drink between meals		

[a]Based on individual experience.

ADIME 10.1 ADIME At-A-Glance: GERD

Assessment

- High BMI/high WC
- Epigastric pain, erosions/ulceration, UGI bleeding
- Diet Hx; meal pattern, high fat intake, alcohol intake
- Laboratory: hgb, hct; if long-term use PPIs, B_{12}, folate, Ca, Mg

Nutrition Diagnosis

- Food–medication interaction of PPI use × 3 years and B_{12} R/T GERD Dx, AEB low serum B_{12} level
- Class 1 Obesity R/T xs intake and sedentary lifestyle, AEB BMI 32, diet Hx

Intervention

- Small, frequent meals; avoid large meals, esp high-fat meal
- Fat 30% or less, higher protein (esp if GI bleed)
- Limit alcohol, smoking, foods that lower LES pressure (caffeine, chocolate, mint oils)
- Modest wt loss, if indicated
- Supplementation w/ cited nutrients if PPI use

Monitoring and Evaluation

- Body weight, WC
- Laboratory values
- Control of GI symptoms

Peptic Ulcer Disease

Disease Process

Peptic ulcer disease (PUD) is the collective term for ulcers, eroded areas of tissue in either the stomach or the duodenum. The erosion arises from the stomach's own acid and pepsin, most commonly instigated by *Helicobacter pylori* (*H. pylori*), which secretes proteins and toxins that attract macrophages, resulting in irritation and inflammation in gastric epithelial cells.[8,9] Another major cause of PUD is the chronic use of medications that irritate the mucosa, most commonly NSAIDs and corticosteroids, which are associated with a relative risk of 4.7 for bleeding and perforation.[10] The stress of severe illness or trauma can produce ulcers, termed *stress ulcers*, which is the reason for prophylactic use of acid-reducing drugs in some acute care patients.

Of nutritional concern, PUD often results in self-imposed dietary restriction and concomitant reduction in essential nutrients. In addition, pain and other GI symptoms may affect food intake and compromise nutritional status. PUD can lead to life-threatening complications, including perforation, bleeding, and obstruction.

Treatment and Nutrition Intervention

The history of PUD treatment reflects various regimens that were not evidence based, therefore ineffective, and often nutrient deficient.[11] Treatment for PUD involves determining the cause of the disease and, when it exists, eradicating *H. pylori*. The foods and substances to avoid are those that may irritate the mucosa or increase acid secretion[6] (Box 10.4).

BOX 10.4 Goals and Nutrition Intervention for PUD

Goals

1. Optimize nutritional intake to correct any deficiencies (iron, B_{12} most common) and to meet nutritional needs
2. Adopt dietary and lifestyle factors to minimize symptoms and pain and promote healing

Nutrition Intervention

1. Avoid foods that increase gastric acid secretion or irritate gastric mucosa Alcohol, pepper, caffeine-containing products (energy drinks, soft drinks), tea and coffee (including decaffeinated), chocolate
2. Avoid eating at least 2 hours before bedtime
3. Individualize the diet for any foods not tolerated
4. Avoid large meals (distend the stomach); small, frequent meals may be helpful
5. Ensure adequate intake of protein and vitamin C to promote healing

Other Recommendations

1. Avoid cigarette smoking
2. Avoid NSAIDs

Avoiding smoking is another important aspect of lifestyle change for treating PUD.[7]

Other aspects of treatment include a variety of medications to accomplish the objectives of eradicating *H. pylori* if present, reducing acid secretion and gastric acidity, and promoting ulcer healing (Box 10.5). Gastric surgery is sometimes needed because of complications such as perforation, obstruction, or cancer. After surgery, nutritional problems can arise, such as nutrient malabsorption, poor food intake, and weight loss, depending on the type and extent of the surgery (Box 10.6). The most common complication of gastric surgery is dumping syndrome, which often leads to many of these nutritional problems.

BOX 10.5 Common Medications in Peptic Ulcer Disease

Antacids
Antibiotics (if *H. pylori* present)
Ulcer drugs

- H_2 antagonists (cimetidine/Tagamet, famotidine/Pepcid, ranitidine/Zantac, Nizatidine/Axid)
- Omeprazole/Prilosec, lansoprazole/Prevacid
- Sucralfate/Carafate
- Misoprostol/Cytotec

BOX 10.6 Surgery for Peptic Ulcer Disease

Truncal Vagotomy and Pyloroplasty

The truncal vagotomy cuts the main trunks of the vagus nerve on each side of the distal esophagus; it eliminates nerve-induced secretion of acid; it also reduces contractions and delays gastric emptying. To offset these effects, the pyloroplasty is also done. In the pyloroplasty, the pylorus is surgically altered so that it can act as a barrier to contents of the stomach as it empties. The result is that liquids empty more quickly, but solids take longer.

(continued)

BOX 10.6 Surgery for Peptic Ulcer Disease (*continued*)

Truncal Vagotomy and Antrectomy

This procedure is more aggressive, because the antrectomy connects the antrum and pylorus. When the antrum is altered, the portion of the stomach that secretes gastrin (hormone which stimulates all gastric secretions) is removed. The two surgical procedures for attaching the remaining stomach to the intestine are Billroth I and Billroth II.

Highly Selective Vagotomy (Proximal Gastric Vagotomy)

This procedure reduces gastric acid secretion but does not interfere with motility (i.e., the stomach's movement). This prevents problems related to gastric emptying (i.e., dumping syndrome).

ADIME 10.2 ADIME At-A-Glance: Peptic Ulcer Disease

Assessment

- Low BMI, UWL, anorexia/decrease in appetite and food intake
- Abdominal pain, fatigue, nausea and vomiting
- Epigastric pain, UGI bleeding
- Laboratory: hgb, hct; if long-term use PPIs, B_{12}, folate, Ca, Mg

Nutrition Diagnosis

- Inadequate oral intake RT decreased appetite from abdominal pain and nausea with PUD Dx, AEB recent UWL of 6% × 2 months, and PO intake of <50%

Intervention

- Protein 1.0 g to 1.2/kg for repletion
- NGS, individualize per tolerance
- Avoid eating 2 hours before bedtime
- Avoid large meals
- Supplementation w/ cited nutrients if PPI use

Monitoring and Evaluation

- Body weight
- Laboratory values for specific nutrients
- Control of GI symptoms

Dumping Syndrome

Disease Process

The major nutritional complication, dumping syndrome, is a group of symptoms that result from rapid emptying of undigested food into the jejunum from the stomach and proceeds through distinct phases of early, intermediate, and late.[12] Some patients experience only early phase dumping syndrome, whereas others have both early and late. The rapid movement of the hyperosmolar load into the small intestine pulls fluid from vascular compartment into the intestine, producing gastrointestinal and vasomotor symptoms of pain, nausea, dizziness, sweating, and tachycardia. These symptoms occur within 10 to 20 minutes of eating, referred to as early phase dumping syndrome. Within 20 to 30 minutes of eating, the undigested food moves to the colon and symptoms of bloating, cramping, gas, and diarrhea ensue, termed *the intermediate phase*.

A patient who experiences the late phase of dumping syndrome will experience symptoms within 1 to 3 hours of eating. Late phase is caused by reactive hypoglycemia, which arises from an excess release of insulin in response to a high intestinal concentration of carbohydrate and rapid absorption of glucose into the blood. This produces symptoms of sweating, shakiness, weakness, and confusion.

Treatment and Nutrition Intervention

Nutrition intervention is a mainstay of treatment, the postgastrectomy diet or antidumping diet (Box 10.7).[6] In addition, functional lactose intolerance tends to be a common problem after surgery. Treatment may also include drugs to slow gastric emptying, somatostatin and its synthetic analog orectide, and acarbose, an α-glycoside hydrolase inhibitor, which interferes with carbohydrate absorption.

BOX 10.7 Postgastrectomy Dietary Recommendations

1. Eat small, frequent meals.
2. Avoid large amounts of liquids with meals; consume fluids 1 to 2 hours before or after meals.
3. Avoid extremes in food temperature.
4. Avoid activity and lie down for 1 hour after meals.

1. Eat 50% to 60% of calories from complex carbohydrates, less than 15% of kilocalories from simple sugars.
2. Eat 20% of calories from protein with a protein-rich source at all meals.
3. Eat about 30% from fat; use medium-chain triglyceride product and pancreatic enzymes, as needed for fat malabsorption.
4. Consume diet moderate in sodium, 3 g of sodium or less daily.
5. Avoid concentrated sweets.
6. Avoid foods containing lactose.

ADIME 10.3 ADIME At-A-Glance: Dumping Syndrome

Assessment

- Low BMI, UWL, anorexia/decrease in appetite and food intake
- Abdominal pain, nausea and vomiting, steatorrhea
- Laboratory: hgb, hct; B_{12}

Nutrition Diagnosis

- Unintended weight loss RT dumping syndrome post partial gastrectomy and subsequent malabsorption, AEB recent UWL of 7% $\times$ 1 month, steatorrhea

Intervention

- Protein 1.0 g/kg to 1.2 g/kg
- Restrict to $<$15% of kcals from simple sugars
- 30% fat; MCT and PER for fat malabsorption
- Small, frequent meals
- Avoid lactose
- Supplement of B_{12}, Fe, other nutrients as needed

Monitoring and Evaluation

- Body weight
- Laboratory values for specific nutrients
- Control of GI symptoms

DISEASES OF THE LOWER GASTROINTESTINAL TRACT

Diverticular Disease: Diverticulosis and Diverticulitis

Disease Process

Diverticular disease includes diverticulosis and diverticulitis, of which the latter is considered a complication of the former. Diverticulosis is the asymptomatic presence of small herniations of the colon, most often the sigmoid colon, which form pouches, and diverticulitis refers to inflammation and/or infection of these pouches. This can occur throughout the intestine, but is most common in the sigmoid colon.[13] Potentially life-threatening complications can occur in diverticulitis and include intestinal obstruction, bleeding, abscess, fistula, and perforation.[14]

Because of the significant differences in disease prevalence between more economically developed and less developed countries, the Western diet has long been implicated in the etiology, particularly a low-fiber diet leading to constipation and straining during defecation.[15] However, a large population-based study compared patients with irritable bowel syndrome, which significantly increases risk for diverticular disease, of the two major forms, diarrhea predominant and constipation predominant.[16] They reported that diarrhea-predominant irritable bowel syndrome was the strongest predictor of diverticular disease. In addition, a meta-analysis showed that lowering dietary fiber intake reduced constipation.[17] A more definitive study using colonoscopy data reported that both a high-fiber diet and increased bowel movement frequency were associated with a higher prevalence of diverticulosis.[18]

Treatment and Nutrition Intervention

If a person has had diverticulitis in the past, future flare-ups, if not too severe, can often be treated at home by means of rest, fasting at first and then a clear liquid diet, and antibiotics and/or anti-inflammatory medications, if needed. As the symptoms subside, usually within a few days, nutrition therapy consists of a soft, low-fiber diet and gradual return to a normal level of fiber.[6] Although the evidence does not support a protective effect of a high-fiber diet in the prevention of diverticulosis, limited evidence suggests that it may reduce the risk of diverticulitis and subsequent complications.[19] In addition, some studies show a benefit with the use of specific probiotics and prebiotics with or without anti-inflammatory agents.[20–22]

In hospitalized patients, severe diverticulitis warrants complete bowel rest and only small sips of water or ice chips (Box 10.8).[6,23] When appropriate, the diet is progressed to clear liquids, and oral nutrition supplementation may be indicated depending on the need for extended nothing by mouth (NPO) or clear liquid diet status in conjunction with poor nutritional status upon admission. For most patients, antibiotics and bowel rest alleviate symptoms within 2 to 5 days. After a clear liquid, patients progress to a bland or GI soft diet, with no nuts, seeds, or fibrous vegetables. The diet is low fiber for up to 1 month, after which the patient should consume a high-fiber diet (Table 10.1).

BOX 10.8 Dietary Recommendations for Diverticular Disease

During Acute Diverticulitis Requiring Hospitalization

1. NPO or clear liquid diet, if bowel rest is indicated depending on severity

Diverticulosis (After Diverticulitis Has Subsided)

1. Gradual increase in daily fiber intake to DRI level of 14 g/1,000 calories
2. Ensure adequate daily intake of fluid, concomitant with increase in dietary fiber
3. Addition of probiotic supplement may be beneficial, although studies not conclusive

TABLE 10.1. Fiber Content of Foods

Food	Amount	Fiber (g)
Bread: whole wheat	1 slice	2
Cereal, bran	½ cup	10
Cereal, cooked oatmeal	½ cup	2
Fruit: apple, banana, kiwi, pear	1 med.	2
Legumes: cooked baked beans, kidney beans, navy beans	½ cup	8
Legumes: garbanzo, lima beans, lentils, split peas	½ cup	5
Vegetables: cooked broccoli green beans, corn, winter squash raw carrots, peppers	½ cup	3

ADIME 10.4 ADIME At-A-Glance: Diverticular Disease

Assessment

- Decrease in appetite and food intake
- Abdominal pain, nausea and vomiting, fever
- Diet Hx (fiber intake)
- Laboratory: hgb, hct

Nutrition Diagnosis

- Food and nutrition knowledge deficit RT to new Dx, AEB diet Hx

Intervention

- Advance from NPO to low fiber
- After discharge, gradual fiber increase to DRI
- Adequate fluid intake of fluid
- Possible probiotic supplement

Monitoring and Evaluation

- Fiber intake
- Laboratory values for specific nutrients
- Control of GI symptoms

Irritable Bowel Syndrome

Disease Process

Irritable bowel syndrome (IBS) is one of the most common functional gastrointestinal disorders, affecting up to 15% of the international population.[24,25] The cause of IBS is unknown, but theories suggest that people with IBS have an exaggerated response to specific stimuli, which include intolerance or hypersensitivity to specific substances in foods, infection, and gut hormones. Research also suggests potential participation in the pathophysiology of mucosal immune activation and inflammation, and alterations in intestinal permeability, serotonin metabolism, and the intestinal microbiome.[26,27]

Symptoms vary and can include abdominal cramping and pain, bloating, flatulence, and alternating bouts of both constipation and diarrhea or only one of these, with Rome III subgroups consisting of IBS alternating diarrhea and constipation (IBS-A), IBS with constipation (IBS-C), IBS with diarrhea (IBS-D), mixed type (IBS-M), and unclassified (IBS-U).[28] Because the symptoms are somewhat nonspecific and variable, it is important to rule out other LGI diseases. The Rome III diagnostic criteria specify the presence of recurrent abdominal pain or discomfort lasting a minimum of 3 days per month within the previous 3 months and two or more of the following: improvement with defecation, onset associated with a change in frequency of stool, onset associated with a change in form (appearance) of stool.

Treatment and Nutrition Intervention

Treatment emphasizes diet and lifestyle changes and, when needed, medications. Lifestyle changes emphasize establishing regular eating patterns, regular bowel habits, possible dietary changes, and stress reduction and management (Box 10.9).[6] A significant number of IBS patients are lactose intolerant, and other common problematic foods include caffeine, alcohol, gas-forming vegetables, and wheat or yeast.[29] To determine whether specific foods are provoking flare-ups, an elimination and reintroduction approach can be helpful for some patients,

BOX 10.9 Recommendations for Irritable Bowel Syndrome

1. Normalize eating patterns, eat at a relaxed pace at consistent times, with small, frequent meals, and ensure adequacy of all nutrients
2. Adjust diet for food allergies and intolerances; common problem foods include wheat, yeast, and eggs
3. Reduced lactose (if lactose intolerant)
4. Low-FODMAP diet (avoid foods high in fructose, sorbitol, xylitol and mannitol, and gas-forming foods)
5. Use of prebiotics and probiotics
6. Progress slowly to a diet adequate in fiber (25 to 35 g/d)
7. Ensure adequate fluid intake of 2 to 3 quarts of water daily
8. Foods to avoid: alcohol, black pepper, caffeine, chili powder, cocoa/chocolate, coffee, colas, garlic, red pepper, spicy foods, sugars
9. Avoid high-fat intake
10. Supplement with B-complex vitamins, calcium, vitamin D, and riboflavin (if lactose is not tolerated)
11. Supplement of 1 Tbsp daily of a bulking agent, such as Metamucil, may be helpful; avoid bran supplements, as it may be irritating

as can adherence to a diet in low–fermentable oligo-, di-, and monosaccharides and polyols (FODMAPs), particularly in the presence of small intestinal bacterial overgrowth (SIBO) (Box 10.10).[6,30,31] However, the contribution of SIBO to IBS remains controversial,[28] and a review of the low-FODMAP diet in IBS cited "very limited evidence" of effectiveness and patient difficulty in adherence to the diet.[32] Another potential treatment is the use of probiotics using species *Lactobacillus*, *Bifidobacterium*, *Escherichia*, and *Streptococcus* of various strains, with some studies reporting beneficial effects.[33,34]

The American College of Gastroenterology reviewed the various treatments in the management of IBS, with a comprehensive evaluation of studies and grading the quality of the evidence using GRADE (Grading of Recommendations Assessment, Development, and Evaluation). The quality of the evidence was assessed as very low, low, medium, and high

BOX 10.10 Low FODMAP Diet Recommendations

Foods High in FODMAPs: Limit or Avoid				
Fructans	Fructose	Galactans	Lactose	Polyols
Fruits: persimmon, watermelon *Grains*: rye and wheat products in high amounts *Vegetables*: artichokes, asparagus, beets, broccoli, brussels sprouts, cabbage, eggplant, fennel, garlic, leek, okra, onions, shallots *Other*: pistachios and products containing chicory, inulin	*Fruits*: apple, mango, pear, watermelon *Sweeteners*: agave, corn syrup, fructose, high-fructose corn syrup, honey	*Legumes*: baked beans, chickpeas, kidney beans, lentils, soybeans	*Cheeses*: cottage cheese, cream cheese, ricotta, and other soft unripened cheeses *Milk*: cow's, goat's, and sheep's milk and products from milk, such as ice cream and yogurt	*Fruits*: apple, apricot, avocado, blackberries, cherries, nectarine, peach, pear, plum, watermelon *Sweeteners*: Isomalt, maltitol, mannitol, sorbitol, xylitol *Vegetables*: cauliflower, corn, green bell pepper, mushrooms

Foods Low in FODMAPs: Appropriate for Diet

Fruits	Dairy	Grains	Vegetables	Miscellaneous
Banana, blueberries, boysenberries, cantaloupe, cranberries, grapes, grapefruit, honeydew, kiwi, lemon, lime, orange, passion fruit, raspberries, rhubarb, strawberries, tangerines	*Cheese*: brie, camembert, hard cheeses *Ice cream*: gelato, sorbet *Milk*: lactose-free milk, oat, rice, and soy milk (and tofu) *Yogurt*: lactose-free products	Arrowroot, corn products (polenta), gluten-free products, millet, oats, psyllium, quinoa, rice, spelled, tapioca	Alfalfa and bean sprouts, bamboo shoots, bok choy, carrot, celery, endive, ginger, green beans, lettuce, olives, parsnip, potato, pumpkin, red bell pepper, spinach, squash, sweet potato, tomato, turnip, yam, zucchini	*Sweeteners*: any artificial sweetener not ending in "ol," glucose, sucrose (table sugar)

and strength of the recommendation as weak or strong.[28] None of the typical nutrition and lifestyle recommendations for IBS patients was graded above "moderate" for quality of evidence, and all were graded as "weak" for strength of the recommendation (Table 10.2). However, given the wide range of symptoms in most IBS patients, it may be helpful to the individual IBS patient to employ these changes. Basic recommendations should include eating small, frequent meals at regular and consistent times, ensuring adequate fluid intake, and avoiding any foods that appear to cause problems. In addition to an elimination diet to find problem foods, a person with IBS can keep a food diary to record food and beverage intake and see if flare-ups are associated with certain foods.[6]

Medications typically focus on the specific symptom, such as antidiarrheal, anticholinergic, and antispasmodic drugs; antidepressants (tricyclic antidepressant or a selective serotonin reuptake inhibitor [SSRI]); and antibiotics (rifaximin [Xifaxan]), in a diagnosis of SIBO. In addition, there are two drugs developed specifically for IBS: alosetron (Lotronex) and lubiprostone (Amitiza).[35]

TABLE 10.2. American College of Gastroenterology Evidence and Recommendation Grading for IBS Management

Intervention	Quality of Evidence	Recommendation
Specialized diets	Very low	Weak
Fiber	Moderate	Weak
Psyllium (not bran)	Moderate	Weak
Prebiotics/synbiotics	Very low	Weak
Probiotics	Low	Weak
Peppermint oil	Moderate	Weak

Data from Ford AC, Moayyedi P, Lacy BE, et al. American College of Gastroenterology Monograph on the management of irritable bowel syndrome and chronic idiopathic constipation. *Am J Gastroenterol* 2014;109:S2–S26.

ADIME 10.5 ADIME At-A-Glance: Irritable Bowel Syndrome

Assessment

- Abdominal pain, nausea, diarrhea, constipation, abnormal stooling, xs flatulence
- Diet Hx (food intolerances, sensitivities), chronic laxative use, avoidance of specific foods
- Laboratory: specific nutrients, if diarrhea predominant IBS and/or avoidance of specific foods

Nutrition Diagnosis

- Altered GI function RT IBS Dx, AEB alternating diarrhea/constipation with subsequent avoidance of specific foods

Intervention

- Small, frequent meals; ensure adequacy of all nutrients
- Adjust diet for food allergies/intolerances; avoid lactose (if lactose intolerant [LI])
- Low-FODMAP diet
- Supplement prebiotics and probiotics
- Gradual increase to adequate in fiber, with adequate fluid
- Avoid high fat intake
- Supplement with B-complex vitamins, calcium, vitamin D, and riboflavin, if LI
- Possible supplement of 1 Tbsp daily of a bulking agent

Monitoring and Evaluation

- Meal pattern; Changes in stools (frequency, consistency)
- Fiber and fluid intake
- Laboratory values for specific nutrients
- Control of GI symptoms

Inflammatory Bowel Diseases

Disease Process

Inflammatory bowel disease (IBD) consists of two chronic diseases: Crohn disease (CD) and ulcerative colitis (UC), which both produce inflammation of the intestine. Both diseases tend to cause nutrient malabsorption, leading to malnutrition, and both can cause life-threatening complications[6] (Table 10.3). The diseases appear to represent heterogeneous disorders of potentially multiple etiologies with genetic and

TABLE 10.3. Differentiation Between Crohn Disease and Ulcerative Colitis

Parameter	UC	Crohn's
Typical age of onset	15–30	Same
Organ involved	Colon only	GIT anywhere
Tissues involved	Surface only	All layers
Distribution	Continuous	Segments
Cancer risk	Yes (10 years)	Probably
Rectal bleeding	Common	Occasional
Steatorrhea	No	Common
Diarrhea	Frequent	Frequent
Vomiting	Yes	Yes
Smoking	Lowers risk	Increases risk
Oral contraceptives	No effect on risk	Increases risk
Hormone replacement therapy	Increases risk	No effect on risk

environmental interactions, which cause the immunologic response that undergirds the disease processes.[36] Several aspects of the diseases are similar, but each also has its own pattern of attack and specific nutrient problems (Box 10.11). One significant difference between the two diseases is that surgery, which is often a necessity, can cure UC by removing the entire colon. In contrast, some patients with CD may require subsequent surgeries after the initial surgery, and the disease has no cure.[37]

Crohn Disease

CD is also known as regional enteritis, granulomatous ileitis, and ileocolitis. It can strike anywhere in the GI tract; however, it demonstrates a predilection for the terminal ileum. In contrast to UC, in which only the mucosa and submucosa are affected, all intestinal tissue layers may be affected.[38] Complications include obstruction, fissures, and fistulas, which increase the risk for mortality. The nutritional problems in

BOX 10.11 Nutrition Problems in Inflammatory Bowel Disease

Nutrient	UC	CD
Protein	Yes, because of inflammation, diarrhea, intake	Same
Fat	No	Yes, because of malabsorption
B_{12}	No	Yes, because of malabsorption, if ileal involvement
Vitamins A, D, E, and K	Yes, because of medications	Yes, because of malabsorption and medications
Fe	Yes, because of bleeding	Yes, because of bleeding and malabsorption, if duodenal involvement
Cu, Zn, Se	Yes, because of diarrhea	Yes, because of malabsorption and diarrhea

CD are potentially more severe compared with UC, because the small intestine is usually involved (Box 10.11).

Another nutritional concern is the potential for severe diarrhea, often steatorrhea from fat malabsorption, in cases of ileal involvement. In addition to direct nutrient malabsorption, people with CD experience pain and other GI symptoms that adversely affect appetite and worsen after eating, the latter of which may cause a fear of eating, further reducing nutrient and intake and worsening malnutrition.

Treatment and Nutrition Intervention

Treatment for CD depends on phase of the disease and, if during an exacerbation or "flare," its severity. Medications used in CD target specific problems; for example, during disease exacerbation, drugs target the inflammation, pain, and diarrhea, and may cause nutrition-related problems[39] (Box 10.12). In disease exacerbation that is not severe, patients can be treated on an outpatient basis, but if severe, hospitalization is necessary along with parenteral nutrition

BOX 10.12 Nutrition Implications of Medications Used in Inflammatory Bowel Disease

Drug Class	Drugs	Potential Nutrition Problems
5-Aminosalicylic acid derivative agents	Mesalamine rectal, mesalamine, sulfasalazine, balsalazide	Nausea, vomiting, acid reflux, diarrhea, folate depletion
Corticosteroids	Prednisone, methylprednisolone, budesonide, hydrocortisone, prednisolone	Fluid retention, increase in appetite, increase in blood glucose, nausea, weight gain; may need to reduce sodium; increase protein, potassium and calcium
Immunosuppressive agents	Mercaptopurine, methotrexate, tacrolimus	Anorexia, nausea, vomiting, mouth sores
Monoclonal antibodies	Infliximab, adalimumab, certolizumab pegol	Abdominal pain, nausea, vomiting, irritation of mouth or tongue
Alpha 4 integrin inhibitors	Natalizumab, vedolizumab	Diarrhea, stomach pain
Antibiotics	Metronidazole, ciprofloxacin	Anorexia, nausea, vomiting
Antidiarrheal agents	Loperamide, diphenoxylate–atropine	Anorexia, bloating, constipation, stomach pain with nausea and vomiting
Bile acid sequestrants	Cholestyramine, colestipol	Acid reflux, constipation, nausea, vomiting, stomach pain
Anticholinergic agents	Dicyclomine, hyoscyamine, propantheline	Dry mouth, nausea

(PN), although small monomeric/elemental enteral feedings may be tolerated (Box 10.13). A meta-analysis reported that exclusive enteral nutrition (EN) may be effective in some patients for induction of remission,[40] although compliance may be difficult.[41] Other nutrition intervention strategies include a lactose-free diet, which is usually a problem for patients with CD, supplementation with n-3 fatty acids, prebiotics and probiotics, low-FODMAP diet, and elimination–reintroduction diet, although data are conflicting and limited[41,42] (Box 10.13).

Patients should be encouraged to consume a nutrient-dense diet, with particular attention to specific nutrients in periods of remission in order to prevent nutrient deficiencies when a

BOX 10.13 Dietary Recommendations for Inflammatory Bowel Disease

In Acute Exacerbation, Depending on Severity:

1. Enteral feedings (that include glutamine, short-chain fatty acids) or parenteral nutrition, if severe
2. Progress to low-fat, low-fiber, high-protein, high-kilocalorie (if weight loss), small, frequent meals as tolerated
3. Avoid nuts, seeds, legumes, coarse grains
4. Avoid lactose, wheat, and gluten, if not tolerated
5. Vitamin/mineral supplements: vitamins D and B_{12}, folate; minerals iron, zinc, calcium, magnesium
6. If taking corticosteroids, limit sodium intake
7. If fat malabsorption (common with Crohn's), consider use of medium-chain triglycerides
8. Maintain good hydration

In Remission:

1. Eat a nutrient-dense diet, with adequate protein and energy
2. Gradually increase dietary fiber to recommended level; fruits and vegetables may be protective
3. Avoid foods high in oxalate (Box 10.16)
4. Avoid lactose, wheat, and gluten, if not tolerated
5. Increase foods high in antioxidants
6. Consider supplementation with n-3 fatty acids and glutamine
7. Consider use of probiotics/probiotic mixtures as indicated and prebiotics

disease exacerbation occurs with the nutrient malabsorption that may attend it.[42] Nutrients of concern include protein; fat-soluble vitamins; vitamins C, B_6, and B_{12} and folate; and the minerals iron, zinc, copper, calcium, potassium, and magnesium.

Ulcerative Colitis

Disease Process

Although symptoms are similar to CD, UC typically strikes the sigmoid segment of the colon, with extensive involvement of the rectum. It often spreads further up throughout the colon so that the entire organ may be affected, but it never involves the small intestine. Complications in UC are as severe as those for CD, including toxic colitis in which the organ begins to dilate. The dilation can happen in hours or days, and when severe, it is termed *toxic megacolon*, which can lead to perforation. Rectal bleeding is a common problem that often causes iron-deficiency anemia. Other nutritionally relevant problems include protein losses, electrolyte disturbances, dehydration, anorexia, and weight loss. In contrast to CD, most of the nutritional problems are not directly caused by malabsorption (Box 10.11). The diagnosis is made on the basis of a sigmoidoscopy, and this test also indicates the UC severity.

Treatment and Nutrition Intervention

Treatment for UC is similar to that for CD, with the goals of countering the inflammation, alleviating symptoms, and correcting dehydration and nutrient deficiencies.[2] And as with CD, when the disease is in remission, a high-protein, nutrient-dense diet is the best approach to stave off nutritional problems between exacerbations (Box 10.13). If the disease is not severe and is confined to the rectum, mesalazine suppository or budesonide rectal foam is used. In the case of left-sided colonic disease, mesalazine suppository and oral aminosalicylate enemas, suppositories, and foams containing budesonide or mesalamine are useful. When severe, oral medications are indicated (Box 10.12).[43]

ADIME 10.6 ADIME At-A-Glance: Inflammatory Bowel Disease

Assessment

- UWL, decreased appetite and intake
- Abdominal pain, nausea, diarrhea (UC), steatorrhea (Crohn's)
- Diet Hx, avoidance of specific foods
- Laboratory: hgb/hct, serum proteins, specific nutrients

Nutrition Diagnosis

- Inadequate oral intake R/T abdominal pain from UC, AEB UWL of 7% × 2 months and diet Hx
- Impaired nutrient utilization R/T malabsorption (Crohn's), AEB steatorrhea, 7% UWL × 2

Intervention

Acute:

- Enteral feedings (glutamine, short-chain fatty acids) or parenteral nutrition, if severe
- Progress to low-fat, low-fiber, high-protein, high-kilocalorie (if weight loss), small, frequent meals AT
- Avoid nuts, seeds, legumes, coarse grains; lactose, wheat, and gluten, if not tolerated
- Supplement of vitamins D and B_{12}, folate, Fe, Zn, Ca, Mg
- Limit sodium, if corticosteroids
- If Crohn's, consider use of MCT

Monitoring and Evaluation

- Weight
- Diarrhea, steatorrhea
- PO intake (esp protein)
- Laboratory values for specific nutrients
- Control of GI symptoms

Celiac Disease

Disease Process

Celiac disease, also known as nontropical sprue, gluten-induced sprue, gluten-induced enteropathy, and gluten-sensitive enteropathy, is caused by an inappropriate T-cell-mediated immune response to various compounds of specific grain proteins in genetically sensitive individuals, which causes inflammation and damage to mucosal cells in the proximal small intestine.[44] In wheat, the compound is gliadin, one of two protein components of the main protein gluten, with similar compounds in other grains including hordein in barley and secalin in rye.[45]

In addition to genetics, risk factors include Down syndrome, type 1 diabetes, chronic arthritis in childhood, and other autoimmune diseases.[44,46] Patient's disease presentation varies widely particularly at different ages with signs and symptoms from gastrointestinal, neurologic, hormonal, and skin disorders. Gastrointestinal symptoms can include abdominal bloating, pain, diarrhea, constipation, and children with IBS are four times more likely to have celiac disease.[47] The disease is characterized by malabsorption of nutrients with numerous nutritional problems including weight loss, anemia, bone disease, and growth deficits in children.

Antibody testing using immunoglobulin A anti-tissue transglutaminase antibody (IgA TTG) is the recommended first test for celiac disease, but the diagnostic standard for confirmation is upper endoscopy with at least six duodenal biopsies.[48]

Treatment and Nutrition Intervention

The treatment for celiac disease is the lifelong elimination of gliadin/gluten from the diet, which must be done as soon as possible to prevent extensive damage to the intestine.[48] Some patients with either a more severe or long-standing case may not respond to dietary intervention, and corticosteroids become necessary. As with IBD, damage of the intestinal tissue may necessitate the removal of the affected sections of the small intestine. And as with CD, this poses nutritional concerns because of the small intestine's role in nutrient digestion and absorption. In contrast to CD, however, removal of the toxin from the diet precludes further need for surgery. If a sufficient amount of small intestine is removed, this can cause short bowel syndrome (SBS).

Because of potentially long-standing nutrient malabsorption, it is important to identify and correct any nutrient deficiencies (Box 10.14), with special focus on vitamin D,

BOX 10.14 Dietary Recommendations in Celiac Disease

Initial Diagnosis

1. Correct any nutritional deficiencies (special attention to folate, vitamin D, calcium, iron).
2. Protein intake should be 1 to 2 g/kg body weight for adults.
3. Energy intake should be increased in cases of weight loss, or in growth deficits in children.
4. Reduce dietary fiber initially, and increase gradually as tolerated.
5. Avoid lactose and determine whether intolerance persists.
6. If fat malabsorption is present, the use of medium chain triglycerides is helpful.

Patient Education: Foods to Avoid

Breads, Cereals, and Grains

- Gluten, wheat, whole wheat flour, enriched flour, soft wheat flour, high-gluten flour, high-protein flour; all flour containing wheat, rye, or barley, bran, graham, wheat germ, malt, kasha, bulgur, spelt, kamut, triticale, couscous, farina, seitan, semolina, durum, durum flour, groats, millet, whole wheat berries, and wheat starch
- Commercially prepared mixes for biscuits, cornbread, muffins, pancakes, and waffles
- Pasta, regular noodles, spaghetti, macaroni, and most packaged rice dishes
- Bread crumbs, cracker meal, pretzels, and matzo
- Gelatinized starch, which may contain wheat protein

Milk/Dairy

- Malted milk, Ovaltine; chocolate milk with cereal additive
- Some sour cream, some yogurt, some nondairy creamers
- Products containing lactose, if lactose tolerance is present

Meat/Fish/Poultry

- Meats prepared with wheat, rye, or barley (bologna, chili, hot dogs, luncheon meats, and sandwich spreads)
- Creamed meats, breaded or bread-containing products (i.e., croquettes, Swiss steak, and meat loaf)
- Meats injected with hydrolyzed vegetable protein
- Tuna in vegetable broth, meat, or meat alternatives containing gluten stabilizers
- Eggs in sauces with gluten

(*continued*)

BOX 10.14 Dietary Recommendations in Celiac Disease (*continued*)

Fruits and Vegetables

- Breaded or creamed vegetables, or vegetables in sauce
- Some canned, baked beans
- Some commercially prepared vegetables and salads
- Thickened or prepared fruits, some pie fillings

Fats/Oils and Sweets

- Some commercially prepared salad dressings
- Some commercial candies, chocolate-coated nuts
- Commercial cakes, cookies, pies, and doughnuts made with wheat, rye, or barley
- Prepared dessert mixes including cookies and cakes
- Puddings thickened with wheat flour
- Ice cream or sherbet with gluten stabilizers; ice cream containing cookies, crumbs, or cheesecake; ice cream cones

Alcohol

- Ale, beer, gin, whiskies, vodka distilled from grain

Miscellaneous

- Herbal teas with malted barley or other grains with gluten (see Bread/Cereal/Grain list)
- Most canned soups, cream soups and soup mixes, bouillon
- Some curry powder, dry seasoning mixes, gravy extracts, meat sauces, catsup, mustard, horseradish, soy sauce, chip dips, chewing gum, distilled white vinegar, cereal extract, cereal beverages (Postum), root beer, yeast extract, malt syrup, malt vinegar, and commercial infant dinners with flour thickeners
- Caramel color and MSG may not be tolerated.

folate, iron, and calcium.[6] Additionally, protein should be increased to 1.0 to 2.0 g/kg body weight, with additional energy in cases of weight loss and growth deficits in children. If fat malabsorption is present, medium-chain triglycerides are also helpful. Lactose intolerance is likely to be a problem because of inflammation of mucosal tissue upon diagnosis, and it is important to avoid lactose long term, if intolerance persists after recovery.

The patient must avoid all sources of gluten in the diet, with the most obvious being foods that contain wheat, rye, and barley. At one time, oats were also eliminated from the diet, and while this is no longer the case, commercial oat products may be contaminated with wheat in processing. For this reason, it may be useful after the initial diagnosis to avoid oats and gradually introduce into the diet observing for signs of intolerance. In addition to obvious foods containing wheat, rye, or barley, the patient must also learn to read food labels for ingredients made from parts of one of the grains including cereal, starch, flour, thickening agents, emulsifiers, stabilizers, hydrolyzed vegetable proteins, caramel coloring, and monosodium glutamate (Box 10.14).[6]

ADIME 10.7 ADIME At-A-Glance: Celiac Disease

Assessment

- UWL, decreased appetite and intake
- Abdominal pain, nausea, diarrhea, steatorrhea
- Diet Hx, avoidance of specific foods
- Laboratory: anti-TTG antibodies, IgA, IgG, serum proteins, hgb/hct, specific nutrients

Nutrition Diagnosis

- Impaired nutrient utilization R/T malabsorption (Celiac), AEB steatorrhea, 7% UWL × 2 months

Intervention

- Protein 1.0 to 2.0 g/kg; energy for repletion/regain of lost weight
- Correct deficiencies (esp folate, vitamin D, Ca, Fe)
- Gradually increase fiber AT after initial reduction
- Avoid lactose, if LI
- MCT if fat malabsorption
- Instruction on gluten-free diet

Monitoring and Evaluation

- Weight
- Diarrhea, steatorrhea
- PO intake (esp protein)
- Laboratory values for specific nutrients
- Control of GI symptoms

Intestinal Surgery: Ostomy, Short Bowel Syndrome, Intestinal Transplant

Disease Process

Several gastrointestinal diseases, and intestinal cancer, may necessitate intestinal surgery that involves removal of sections of intestine. In the case of the colon, the entire organ may be removed with minimal long-term effects on nutrient absorption. However, many nutritional problems may arise depending on how much small intestine is lost: Loss of 50% or more of the small intestine produces nutrient malabsorption and places a patient at risk for SBS, and more than 75% of the small intestine is associated with a high mortality rate.[49,50]

The remaining bowel can adapt to recover intestinal function, and determinants of intestinal adaptability include type and location of the resection, patient age and nutritional status, and content of the diet.

After intestinal surgery to remove sections of the intestine, it may be necessary to create a stoma for waste elimination. In a colostomy, part of the colon, the rectum, and anus are removed, and the remaining segment of colon is brought out through the abdominal wall to form the stoma. An ileostomy involves a colectomy, removal of the entire colon, the rectum, and anus, and bringing the ileum through the opening. Ileostomy causes more problems because of the digestive and absorptive role of this portion of the small intestine.[51] In addition to nutritional problems, diet can influence various aspects of bowel regularity and stool consistency.

Ileostomy: Treatment and Nutrition Recommendations

An ileostomy produces a watery stool, making postsurgical adjustment more of a challenge than with colostomy. Also, ileostomy often causes fat malabsorption because bile is not reabsorbed, resulting in malabsorption of fat-soluble vitamins, which necessitates supplementation (Box 10.15).[6] Deficiency of vitamin B_{12} is also common, as absorption of

BOX 10.15 Dietary Recommendations for Ileostomy

1. A clear liquid diet follows surgery
2. Progress to a bland, low-fiber diet with extra kilocalories and protein (1.5 g/kg/d)
3. Continue with low-fiber diet for about 4 weeks; include sources of pectin such as oatmeal and applesauce
4. Choose a vitamin/mineral supplement with vitamins C and B_{12}, folate, calcium, magnesium, and iron
5. Maintain good hydration status and supplement with sodium and potassium, as needed, especially in hot weather
6. Avoid eating before bedtime
7. If gassiness is a problem, avoid cruciferous vegetables, legumes, and other potential gas-forming fruits and vegetables and FODMAPs (Box 10.10)
8. Follow additional recommendations for specific foods, as needed, for colostomy (Box 10.17)

BOX 10.16 Foods High in Oxalate

Beets	Rhubarb	Tea
Celery	Soy	Vitamin C supplements
Chocolate/cocoa	Spinach	Whole wheat
Nuts	Strawberries	
Peanut butter	Sweet potatoes	

the vitamin occurs in the terminal ileum. The risk for both kidney and gallstones increases with steatorrhea, and so it is important to monitor for and counter the development of these conditions and be prudent to avoid foods high in oxalate (Box 10.16). Ileostomy also causes excessive fluid losses, along with electrolytes, making dehydration a special concern. Obstruction is a possible complication, so thorough mastication of foods is important.

ADIME 10.8 ADIME At-A-Glance: Ileostomy

Assessment

- UWL, decreased appetite and intake
- Abdominal pain, nausea, diarrhea, steatorrhea
- Diet Hx, avoidance of specific foods
- Laboratory: serum proteins, hgb/hct, specific nutrients (esp B12)

Nutrition Diagnosis

- Altered GI function RT ileostomy, AEB diarrhea
- Impaired nutrient utilization (B_{12}) RT malabsorption from ileostomy, AEB low serum B_{12} level

Intervention

- Clear liquid diet post-surgery
- Progress to a bland, low-fiber diet, high kcal and protein (1.5 g/kg)
- Low fiber × 4 weeks with sources of pectin
- Supplement of vitamins C and B_{12}, folate, Ca, Mg, Fe
- Adequate fluids, possible Na and K supplement PRN, esp in hot weather
- Avoid eating before bedtime
- Low-FODMAP diet, if flatulence problem
- Low-oxalate diet

Monitoring and Evaluation

- Weight
- Diarrhea, steatorrhea
- PO intake (esp protein)
- Laboratory values for specific nutrients
- Control of GI symptoms

Colostomy: Treatment and Nutrition Recommendations

With a colostomy, the stool consistency is close to normal or normal, depending on how much of the colon was removed. If the colostomy is on the right side, the stool will be mushy, whereas a left-sided colostomy produces a firm stool. Odor is a significant problem for the person with a colostomy, and attention to specific foods that cause more of a problem is important. Because potential odor-causing foods are nutrient dense, it is better to focus on other approaches, such as deodorizers. Many of the same diet recommendations for ileostomy apply to colostomy, although the possible nutritional problems are more likely with ileostomy (Box 10.17).[6]

BOX 10.17 Dietary Recommendations for Colostomy

1. A clear liquid diet follows surgery, and an oral diet for most patients within 2 days
2. Progress to a low-fiber diet with extra kilocalories and protein (1.5 g/kg/d) and adequate vitamins and minerals
3. After approximately 2 weeks, gradually increase fiber intake
4. The following foods should be avoided only if they consistently cause undesirable effects, *as they may cause obstructions:*

   Bamboo shoots, bean sprouts, celery, citrus fruit membranes, coconut, coleslaw, corn, fruits with skins and seeds, green beans, lettuce, mushrooms, nuts, peas/pea pods, popcorn, potato skins, raw carrots, raw/dried fruit, relishes, seeds, spinach, tough meats, and vegetables.

May cause odor or gas

Antibiotics, asparagus, beer, broccoli, brussels sprouts, cabbage family vegetables, carbonated beverages, cauliflower, corn, cucumbers, deep fried foods, dried beans/peas, eggs, fish, melons, milk, mustard, nuts, onions, pastries, pickles, radishes, some vitamin/mineral supplements, spicy foods, strong-flavored cheeses, and turnips

May contribute to diarrhea

Beans, beer/wine, broccoli, coffee, fresh fruits/vegetables and juices, green leafy vegetables (esp spinach), highly spiced foods, licorice, and prune juice

1. Avoid high-oxalate foods (Box 10.16)
2. Foods such as applesauce, bananas, boiled milk, cheese, milk, peanut butter, rice, and tapioca may reduce diarrhea (reducing fluid intake does not reduce diarrhea, and it may cause dehydration)
3. Consume 1 to 2 quarts of fluid daily, between meals, with adequate or increased sodium

Dietary/Behavior Modifications

- Establish regular meal times
- Eat slowly and chew thoroughly with mouth closed
- Avoid chewing gum or drinking from straws to prevent excess gas
- Use cranberry juice, yogurt, buttermilk, and fresh parsley and spinach (as tolerated, in limited amounts) as natural deodorizers
- Use products such as Bean-O to reduce gas
- If a food has been eliminated from the diet because of diarrhea, constipation, odor, or gas, retest tolerance after 2 to 3 weeks

Short Bowel Syndrome

Disease Process

With removal of 50% or more of the small intestine in a resection, SBS is a prime concern, especially if the terminal ileum and ileocecal valve were removed.[49] A strict definition relative to length of intestine removed is not useful, since intestinal length varies widely as does ability to adapt, although gastroenterologists have proposed an SBS definition: "a condition resulting from surgical resection, congenital defect, or disease-associated loss of absorption, characterized by the inability to maintain protein-energy, fluid, electrolyte, or micronutrient balances when on a normal diet."[52] For diagnostic purposes, however, less than 200 cm of remaining small intestine is generally considered SBS.

The most significant nutritional problems associated with SBS arise from malabsorption (Box 10.18). Although the

BOX 10.18 Nutritionally Relevant Problems in Short Bowel Syndrome

Deficit or Problem	Result
Bile acid	Fat malabsorption, bacterial overgrowth
Absorptive surface	Malabsorption of nutrients
Fluid reabsorption	Dehydration
Increased motility, short GIT	Dumping syndrome, diarrhea
Loss of ileocecal valve	Bacterial overgrowth (B_{12} deficiency)
Oversecretion of gastric acid	Damage to duodenum, pancreatic enzyme activity altered
Pancreatic enzyme activity	Maldigestion, malabsorption
Fat malabsorption	Steatorrhea, increased risk for kidney stones, gallstones, fat-soluble vitamin deficiency, bone disease

survival rate declines as more of the intestine is removed, if the ileum and ileocecal valve remain intact, even an 80% resection can prove to be tolerated.[53] Resections of the jejunum initially cause significant malabsorption, because most nutrients are digested and absorbed within the first 40 inches of the small bowel. However, after the adaptation period, the ileum takes over this function, as the remaining intestine grows in length, diameter, and thickness.

Because of its importance in long-term survival, and the fact that it is the only controllable variable, enhancing the intestine's ability to adapt is the focus of treatment. Nutrition is the key to recovery and enhancing the intestine's adaptive ability. The reason is that many of the typical symptoms a patient with SBS will experience are nutritionally relevant: diarrhea, steatorrhea, weight loss, muscle wasting, bone disease, and malabsorption of several nutrients. SIBO is another nutritionally relevant problem that appears to be common in SBS.[54]

The occurrence of SIBO may positively affect energy extraction from carbohydrates; however, it presents several deleterious nutritional consequences. The bacterial overgrowth can cause inflammation and atrophic changes that produce nutrient malabsorption. In addition, the excess microbes deconjugate bile acids, causing fat malabsorption, and compete for B_{12}, exacerbating the potential for deficiency of the vitamin. Other gastrointestinal symptoms resulting from SIBO also aggravate diarrhea, which can adversely affect food intake, and may increase the risk of intestinal failure–associated liver disease (IFALD), a serious complication that can cause cholestasis, steatosis, and fibrosis, leading to cirrhosis.[55]

Treatment and Nutrition Intervention

Treatment and nutrition intervention focuses on managing symptoms, enhancing intestinal adaptation, and maintaining adequate nutritional and hydration status (Box 10.19).[6] A major problem for most SBS patients is voluminous diarrhea, which, if not controlled, can adversely affect nutritional status and bowel recovery. Although diet alone cannot control the

BOX 10.19 Dietary Recommendations for Short Bowel Syndrome

Phase 1: Immediately Following Intestinal Resection Surgery

1. Parental nutrition (PN) is required. The extent of the resection and overall health of the subject will determine the duration of PN.
2. Enteral nutrition (EN) may be useful, and should begin as soon as possible after surgery

Phase 2: Initiation of Oral Feedings

1. Fat: If colon is present, diet should be <30% (MCT may be useful); without colon, 30% to 40% of calories.
2. Carbohydrate: If colon is present, diet should be 50% to 60%; without colon, 40% to 50% of calories; both must restrict simple sugars.
3. Protein: 20% to 30% of calories, emphasis on high biologic value sources.
4. As oral diet tolerance improves:
   - 5 to 10 g/d soluble fiber, if stool output is >3 L/d
   - Avoid high-oxalate foods (Box 10.16), not in patients with end jejunostomy/ileostomy
   - Vitamin/mineral supplements that include calcium, magnesium, zinc, iron, manganese, vitamin C, selenium, potassium, folic acid, B_{12} and B-complex vitamins, and water miscible forms of vitamins A, D, E, and K
   - Salt: increase in patients with end jejunostomy/ileostomy
   - Fluids: oral rehydration solution may be needed; total fluid may need to be restricted
   - If supplemental MCT oil is used, divide it into doses of 1 Tbsp with meals
   - Modified FODMAP restriction, avoid fructose, high fructose corn syrup, sugar alcohols such as sorbitol, and limit lactose only if intolerant

Diet and Behavior Modifications

- Smaller, more frequent meals: 4 to 6 meals/d
- Consume fluids between meals in small amounts

diarrhea, careful food selection and fluid intake can help reduce fecal output and optimize nutrient absorption.[56]

Medications are useful in managing the symptoms of diarrhea, steatorrhea, and SIBO, such as those that slow gastric emptying and intestinal motility and reduce gastric secretion, which can help to increase nutrient digestion and absorption. However, it is important to note that reduced absorptive surface area and accelerated transit time typically cause drug malabsorption.

Feeding progresses are a stepwise process in three phases that will vary with the patient and their specific resection, and it may take years.[57] The first phase is within 1 to 3 months after surgery, characterized by voluminous diarrhea, fluid losses, and significantly limited absorption. For the majority of patients, PN is the first method of feeding.[56–58] If the patient has become nutritionally compromised because of the disease state that necessitated the surgery, PN support is vital in providing adequate energy for repletion. As soon as possible, EN should start, as this stimulates adaptation of the bowel remnant.

In the second phase, 4 to 12 months, nutrient absorption begins to improve, and the patient begins to regain weight. Depending on the extent of the resection, PN may need to continue from 3 weeks to 6 months and may be done at home after discharge. In the final phase, which lasts 13 to 24 months, bowel adaptation results in a return to more normalized nutrient absorption. The timing of the different dietary changes is variable but may take months or even years before a patient can resume a regular diet, and some patients cannot be weaned off PN.

Once oral intake has begun, key dietary points include consuming smaller, more frequent meals, avoiding all forms of simple sugars, and paying careful attention in chewing foods extremely well. Although widely recommended and used, studies on the efficacy of compounds, such as glutamine, somatropin, a recombinant human growth hormone, and glucagons, in promoting intestinal adaptation are limited.[56–58] A recently approved drug, Teduglutide, an analog of naturally occurring glucagon-like peptide-2 (GLP-2), has shown some effectiveness in SBS patients on PN.[58] Bowel rehabilitation programs have claimed some success in weaning SBS patients off PN sooner, although more long-term outcome data are needed.[51]

ADIME 10.9 ADIME At-A-Glance: Short Bowel Syndrome (and Intestinal Transplant)

Assessment

- Current PO intake or nutrition support regimen
- Length and location of remaining functional bowel
- GI symptoms including vomiting, diarrhea
- Ostomy output and hydration status
- Lab values
- Baseline vitamin levels (vitamins A, D, E, B_1, B_2, B_6, B_{12}, and C, and folic acid) and mineral levels (chromium, copper, manganese, selenium, and zinc)[4]

Nutrition Diagnosis

- TPN dependent because of malabsorption RT short gut syndrome or intestinal dysmotility
- Complications with TPN RT liver cholestasis, central vein thrombosis, line sepsis, or severe dehydration

Intervention

- Short term:
  - POD 1 to 2: initiate PN
  - POD 3 to 7: initiate enteral feedings and taper PN as tube feedings increase
  - 2 weeks: begin clear liquids and advance as tolerated to regular diet, taper enteral feedings as oral intake increases
- Long term:
  - Small, frequent meals with supplements and ORS
  - Low fiber with complex carbohydrates
  - Limit lactose and concentrated sweets, low oxalate
  - Limit fat with chylous ascites

Monitoring and Evaluation

- PO intake and tolerance using food journals
- Weight, protein status
- I & Os (ostomy output, hydration)
- Electrolyte balance
- Labs:
  - Monthly: zinc
  - Every 6 months: vitamins D, B_{12}, and B_6, iron studies, lipid panel
  - Every year: vitamins A and C, selenium, copper, manganese, chromium[6]

Intestinal Transplantation

—*Thomas Pietrowsky, MS, RD, and Maria Segovia, MD*

Intestinal transplantation is an option for patients with intestinal failure who suffer severe complications because of total parenteral nutrition (TPN) dependence. Intestinal failure is defined as the loss of absorptive capacity of the small bowel as result of severe GI disease or surgically induced short gut syndrome.[59] The total number of intestine transplants performed annually in the United States increased to 139 in 2014.[60] Both transplant outcomes and patient survival rates over 1, 3, and 5 years have improved over the past decade.[59]

Indications for and Types of Intestinal Transplant

Patients with intestinal failure are eligible for intestine transplant if they meet any of the following criteria according to the Centers for Medicare and Medicaid Services (CMS):

- Imminent or evident liver failure of TPN-induced liver injury.
- Thrombosis of at least two central veins
- Two or more episodes of line sepsis per year that require hospitalization
- Single episode of line-related fungemia, septic shock, or acute respiratory distress
- Recurrent episodes of severe dehydration despite intravenous fluid supplementation[59]

Types of intestinal transplants are as follows:

- Isolated intestine: intestinal failure without liver disease
- Combined liver/intestine: intestinal failure with TPN-associated liver failure
- Multivisceral: includes the stomach, pancreas, and intestine with or without the liver. Indicated in patients with massive gastrointestinal polyposis, traumatic loss of abdominal viscera, extensive abdominal desmoid tumors, locally aggressive nonmetastasizing neoplasms, generalized hollow visceral myopathy/neuropathy, and complete thrombosis of the splanchnic arterial or portal venous systems.[61]

Nutrition Before Intestine Transplant

When evaluating patients for intestine transplant, a thorough nutritional assessment should be performed. The evaluation should assess medical history and current diagnoses, diet history including oral intake and nutritional support, amount and location of remaining functional bowel, GI symptoms, anthropometrics including weight history, laboratory values, ostomy output, and appropriateness of the current diet order or TPN regimen. Collaboration with home infusion providers is important when assessing labs and changes with home TPN prescriptions. Living environment should also be considered, including persons in the household and who will perform shopping and meal preparation.

Once a patient is deemed a candidate for intestine transplant, there are several nutritional goals to consider. Maintaining adequate hydration is vital to help preserve renal function, and additional intravenous hydration may be needed to replace fluid losses. Preserving kidney function prior to transplant is especially important since some posttransplant medications, including tacrolimus, can have potentially nephrotoxic effects.[62] Hepatic function should be preserved by adjusting parenteral lipids and dextrose as needed to help avoid hepatic steatosis. Since patients can experience significant weight loss of 20% or more of their pretransplant weight in the postoperative period, optimization of nutritional status is vital for improving outcomes after transplant.[63] Measuring pertinent serum vitamin and trace element levels and correcting deficiencies are also recommended in the pretransplant phase.[62]

Posttransplant Nutrition—Short Term

Nutritional goals in the early posttransplant period are similar to other major surgeries (Box 10.19). Adequate nutrition is critical to help promote weight gain, decrease risk of infection, and improve wound healing. The ultimate nutritional goal posttransplant is to reach nutritional autonomy in which the patient can maintain weight, electrolyte balance, and adequate hydration.

The transition to an oral diet can occur rather quickly after transplant. PN can usually be started 24 to 48 hours after surgery. Calorie intake should be increased as tolerated to 30 to 35 kcal/kg. Recommended protein requirements are 1.5 to 2.0 g/kg. PN can be weaned as enteral nutrition is initiated and increased, and some centers will place feeding tubes at the time of transplant. Surgical complications, episodes of rejection, or infections may delay PN weaning.[64]

Enteral nutrition should be initiated as soon as possible after surgery to help maintain gut integrity. Enteral feedings can generally be initiated 3 to 7 days post transplant once allograft motility is established.[62] Routes of administration can vary among transplant centers. Feedings should be started at full strength and advanced slowly (5 to 10 mL/h) every 12 to 24 hours to goal rate. Polymeric formulas are usually tolerated well. Formulas that are lower in potassium but maintain a high protein content may be beneficial because of the risk of hyperkalemia from some immunosuppression medications,[62] and lower fat formulas may be used if chylous ascites develops.

Although the rate of diet advancement is individualized, an oral diet can usually be initiated within 2 weeks after transplant. A clear liquid diet should be started and advanced as tolerated to a regular diet. Patients should be started on a low-fiber diet consisting of small, frequent meals. Lactose should also be limited in patients who show signs of lactose intolerance. Concentrated sweets should be restricted if patients experience diarrhea or hyperglycemia. Fats can contribute a significant source of calories and generally should not be restricted unless there is a medical indication, such as chylous ascites. Oral rehydration solutions should also be added once diet is initiated to help avoid dehydration.

Posttransplant Nutrition—Long Term

Tolerance to diet can vary, and some patients may have difficulty tolerating lactose and concentrated sweets long term. Food journals are useful for assessing oral intake and any GI symptoms with eating. Nutrition therapy should emphasize maintaining weight and protein status, adequate hydration, and electrolyte balance. Suggested nutritional labs for monitoring long term include the following:

- Monthly: zinc
- Every 6 months: vitamin D, vitamin B_{12}, vitamin B_6, iron studies, lipid panel
- Every 12 months: vitamin A, vitamin C, selenium, copper, manganese, chromium[64]

As oral intake improves over time, intestine transplant patients can be at a higher risk of becoming overweight or obese. Therefore, education and reinforcement of healthy eating guidelines are prudent. Conversely, many patients can have eating issues because of anxiety from GI symptoms they experienced before transplant. Psychologists can be valuable members of the transplant team, especially in helping intestine transplant patients return to a regular diet.

Although intestine transplant is still a relatively new medical procedure, in concert with intensive nutritional therapy, many patients with intestinal failure can discontinue TPN and experience an improved quality of life.

References

1. Booth CL, Thompson KS. Barrett's esophagus: A review of diagnostic criteria, clinical surveillance practices and new developments. *J Gastrointest Oncol* 2012;3(3):232–242.
2. Hyun JJ, Bak Y-T. Clinical significance of hiatal hernia. *Gut Liver* 2011;5(3):267–277.
3. Enns R, Kazemi P, Chung W, et al. Eosinophilic esophagitis: Clinical features, endoscopic findings and response to treatment. *Can J Gastroenterol* 2010;24(9):547–551.
4. UpToDate. Patient information: Achalasia (Beyond the Basics). Available at: http://www.uptodate.com/contents/achalasia-beyond-the-basics. Accessed December 30, 2015.
5. Ito T, Jensen RT. Association of long-term proton pump inhibitor therapy with bone fractures and effects on absorption of calcium, vitamin B12, iron, and magnesium. *Curr Gastroenterol Rep* 2010;12(6):448–457.

6. Academy of Nutrition and Dietetics. *Nutrition Care Manual.* Available at: https://www.nutritioncaremanual.org. Accessed December 29, 2015.
7. Wu WKK, Cho CH. The pharmacological actions of nicotine on the gastrointestinal tract. *J Pharmacol Sci* 2004;94(4):348–358.
8. WebMD. Digestive Disorders Health Center. What is *H. pylori*? Available at: http://www.webmd.com/digestive-disorders/h-pylori-helicobacter-pylori. Accessed December 29, 2015.
9. Peura DA. *Helicobacter pylori* and ulcerogenesis. *Am J Med* 1996;100(5A):19S–25S.
10. Goldstein JL, Cryer B. Gastrointestinal injury associated with NSAID use: A case study and review of risk factors and preventative strategies. *Drug Healthc Patient Saf* 2015;7:31–41.
11. Centers for Disease Control and Prevention. *Helicobacter pylori* and peptic ulcer disease. Available at: http://www.cdc.gov/ulcer/history.htm. Accessed December 29, 2015.
12. Medscape. Dumping Syndrome. Available at: http://emedicine.medscape.com/article/173594-overview. Accessed December 31, 2015.
13. Peery AF, Sandler RF. Diverticular disease: Reconsidering conventional wisdom. *Clin Gastroenterol Hepatol* 2013;11(12):1532–1537.
14. Tursi A, Papagrigordiadis S. Review article: The current and evolving treatment of colonic diverticular disease. *Aliment Pharmacol Ther* 2009;30:532–546.
15. Painter NS, Burkitt DP. Diverticular disease of the colon: A deficiency disease of western civilization. *BMJ* 1971;2:450–454.
16. Jung HK, Choung RS, Locke GR, et al. Diarrhea-predominant irritable bowel syndrome is associated with diverticular disease: A population-based study. *Am J Gastroenterol* 2010;105(3):652–661.
17. Ho K-S, Tan CYM, Mohd Daud MA, et al. Stopping or reducing dietary fiber intake reduces constipation and its associated symptoms. *World J Gastroenterol* 2012;18(33):4593–4596.
18. Peery AF, Barrett PR, Park D, et al. A high-fiber diet does not protect against asymptomatic diverticulosis. *Gastroenterology* 2012;142:266–272.
19. Crowe FL, Appleby PN, Allen NE, et al. Diet and risk of diverticular disease in Oxford cohort of European Prospective Investigation into Cancer and Nutrition (EPIC): Prospective study of British vegetarians and non-vegetarians. *BMJ* 2011;343:d4131.
20. Tursi A, Brandimarte G, Elisei W, et al. Randomised clinical trial: Mesalazine and/or probiotics in maintaining remission of

symptomatic uncomplicated diverticular disease—A double-blind, randomised, placebo-controlled study. *Aliment Pharmacol Ther* 2013;38:741–751.

21. Annibale B, Maconi G, Lahner E, et al. Efficacy of *Lactobacillus paracasei* sub. paracasei F19 on abdominal symptoms in patients with symptomatic uncomplicated diverticular disease: A pilot study. *Minerva Gastroenterol Dietol* 2011;57:13–22.
22. Lahner E, Esposito G, Zullo A, et al. High-fiber diet and *Lactobacillus paracasei* B21060 in symptomatic uncomplicated diverticular disease. *World J Gastroenterol* 2012;18:5918–5924.
23. Escott-Stump S. *Nutrition and Diagnosis-Related Care*. 8th ed. Philadelphia, PA: Wolters Kluwer; 2015:442–444.
24. Lovell RM, Ford AC. Global prevalence of, and risk factors for, irritable bowel syndrome: A meta-analysis. *Clin Gastroenterol Hepatol* 2012;10:712–721.
25. Quigley EM, Abdel-Hamid H, Barbara G, et al. A global perspective on irritable bowel syndrome: A consensus statement of the World Gastroenterology Organisation Summit Task Force on irritable bowel syndrome. *J Clin Gastroenterol* 2012;46:356–366.
26. Barbaro M, Di Sabatino A, Cremon C, et al. Interferon-γ is increased in the gut of patients with irritable bowel syndrome and modulates serotonin metabolism. *Am J Physiol Gastrointest Liver Physiol* 2016;310(6):G439–G447. doi:10.1152/ajpgi.00368.2015.
27. Lacy BE. The science, evidence, and practice of dietary interventions in irritable bowel syndrome. *Clin Gastroenterol Hepatol* 2015;13(11):1899–1906.
28. Ford AC, Moayyedi P, Lacy BE, et al. American College of Gastroenterology Monograph on the management of irritable bowel syndrome and chronic idiopathic constipation. *Am J Gastroenterol* 2014;109:S2–S26.
29. Böhn L, Störsrud A, Liljebo T, et al. Diet low in FODMAPs reduces symptoms of irritable bowel syndrome as well as traditional dietary advice: A randomized controlled trial. *Gastroenterology* 2015;149(6):1399–1407.
30. Molina-Infante J, Serra J, Fernandez-Bañares F, et al. The low-FODMAP diet for irritable bowel syndrome: Lights and shadows. *Gastroenterol Hepatol* 2016;39(2):55–65. doi:10.1016/j.gastrohep.2015.07.009.
31. International Foundation for Function Gastrointestinal Disorders. The Low FODMAP Diet Approach: What are FODMAPs? Available at: http://www.aboutibs.org/site/treatment

/low-fodmap-diet/what-are-fodmaps. The Low FODMAP Diet Approach: Measuring FODMAPs in Foods. Available at: http://www.aboutibs.org/site/treatment/low-fodmap-diet/measuring. Accessed January 22, 2016.

32. Does a low FODMAP diet help IBS? *Drug Ther Bull* 2015;53(8):93–96. doi:10.1136/dtb.2015.8.0346.
33. Charbonneau D, Gibb RD, Quigley EM. Fecal excretion of *Bifidobacterium infantis* 35624 and changes in fecal microbiota after eight weeks of oral supplementation with encapsulated probiotic. *Gut Microbes* 2013;4:201–211.
34. Guglielmetti S, Mora D, Gschwender M, et al. Randomised clinical trial: *Bifidobacterium bifidum* MIMBb75 significantly alleviates irritable bowel syndrome and improves quality of life—A double-blind, placebo-controlled study. *Aliment Pharmacol Ther* 2011;33:1123–1132.
35. Mayo Clinic. Irritable Bowel Syndrome: Treatment and Drugs. Available at: http://www.mayoclinic.org/diseases-conditions/irritable-bowel-syndrome/basics/treatment/con-20024578. Accessed January 22, 2016.
36. Tsianos EV, Katsanos KH, Tsianos VE. Role of genetics in the diagnosis and prognosis of Crohn's disease. *World J Gastroenterol* 2012;18(2):105–118.
37. Cottone M, Orlando A, Viscido A, et al. Prevention of postsurgical relapse and recurrence in Crohn's disease. *Aliment Pharmacol Ther* 2003;17(s2):38–42.
38. Hanauer SB. Inflammatory bowel disease: Epidemiology, pathogenesis, and therapeutic opportunities. *Inflamm Bowel Dis* 2006;12:S3–S9.
39. Medscape. Crohn Disease. Management: Pharmacotherapy. Available at: http://emedicine.medscape.com/article/172940-overview#showall. Accessed February 1, 2016.
40. Zachos M, Tondeur M, Griffiths AM. Enteral nutritional therapy for induction of remission in Crohn's disease. *Cochrane Database Syst Rev* 2007:CD000542.
41. Yamamoto T, Nakahigashi M, Saniabadi AR. Review article: Diet and inflammatory bowel disease—Epidemiology and treatment. *Aliment Pharmacol Ther* 2009;30:99–112.
42. Donnellan C, Yann LH, Lal S. Nutritional management of Crohn's disease. *Therap Adv Gastroenterol* 2013;6(3):231–242.
43. Medscape. Ulcerative Colitis. Management. Available at: http://emedicine.medscape.com/article/183084-overview#a1. Accessed February 2, 2016.

44. Farrell RJ, Kelly CP. Celiac sprue. *N Engl J Med* 2002;346:180–188.
45. Murray JA. The widening spectrum of celiac disease. *Am J Clin Nutr* 1999;69:354–365.
46. Reilly NR, Fasano A, Green PHR. Presentation of celiac disease. *Gastrointest Endosc Clin N Am* 2012;10(22):613–621.
47. Cristofori F, Fontana C, Magistà A, et al. Increased prevalence of celiac disease among pediatric patients with irritable bowel syndrome. *JAMA Pediatr* 2014;168(6):555–560.
48. Rubio-Tapia A, Hill ID, Kelly CP, et al. ACG clinical guidelines: Diagnosis and management of celiac disease. *Am J Gastroenterol* 2013;108(5):656–676.
49. Matarese LE, O'Keefe SJD, Kandil HM, et al. Short bowel syndrome: Clinical guidelines for nutrition management. *Nutr Clin Pract* 2005;20(5):493–502.
50. Vanderhoof JA, Langnas AN. Short-bowel syndrome in children and adults. *Gastroenterology* 1997;113:1767–1778.
51. Fessler TA. A dietary challenge: Maximizing bowel adaptation in short bowel syndrome. *Today's Dietitian* 2007;9(1):40.
52. O'Keefe SJ, Buchman AL, Fishbein TM, et al. Short bowel syndrome and intestinal failure: Consensus definitions and overview. *Clin Gastroenterol Hepatol* 2006;4:6–10.
53. Dieleman LA, Heizer WD. Nutritional issues in inflammatory bowel disease. *Gastroenterol Clin North Am* 1998;27(2):435–435.
54. DiBaise JK, Young RJ, Vanderhoof JA. Enteric microbial flora, bacterial overgrowth and short bowel syndrome. *Clin Gastroenterol Hepatol* 2006;4:11–20.
55. Raphael BP, Duggan C. Prevention and treatment of intestinal failure-associated liver disease in children. *Semin Liver Dis* 2012;32(4):341–347.
56. Escott-Stump S. *Nutrition and Diagnosis-Related Care*. 8th ed. Philadelphia, PA: Wolters Kluwer; 2015:475.
57. Parrish CS, DiBaise JK. Short bowel syndrome in adults—Part 2: Nutrition therapy for short bowel syndrome in the adult patient. *Pract Gastroenterol* 2014:40–51.
58. Medscape. Short-Bowel Syndrome Treatment & Management. Available at: http://emedicine.medscape.com/article/193391-treatment#d9. Accessed February 3, 2016.
59. Centers for Medicare and Medicaid Services. Decision Memo for Intestinal and Multivisceral Transplantation. Available at: https://www.cms.gov/medicare-coverage-database/details/nca-decision-memo.aspx?NCAId=42&NcaName=Intestinal+

and+Multivisceral+Transplantation&NCDId=280&ncd-ver=2&IsPopup=y&bc=AAAAAAAACAAAAA%3D%3D&. Accessed January 29, 2016.

60. Smith JM, Skeans MA, Horslen SP, et al. Intestine. *Am J Transplant* 2016;16:99–114. doi:10.1111/ajt.13669.
61. Abu-Elmagd KM. Intestinal transplantation: Indications and patient selection. In: Langnas AN, Goulet R, Quigley EM, eds. *Intestinal Failure: Diagnosis, Management and Transplantation*. Malden, MA: Blackwell Publishing; 2008:245–253.
62. Matarese LE. Nutrition interventions before and after adult intestinal transplantation: The Pittsburgh experience. *Pract Gastroenterol* 2010;89:11–26.
63. Sharkey L, Kratzing C, Rutter C, et al. Nutritional status after intestinal and multivisceral transplant. *Gut* 2014;63:A267. doi:10.1136/gutjnl-2014-307263.573.
64. Burch T. Nutritional management for intestinal and multivisceral transplant. Lecture presented at: Transplant Institute Lecture Series at Henry Ford Hospital; December 2, 2015; Detroit, MI.

NOTES

Notes

Notes

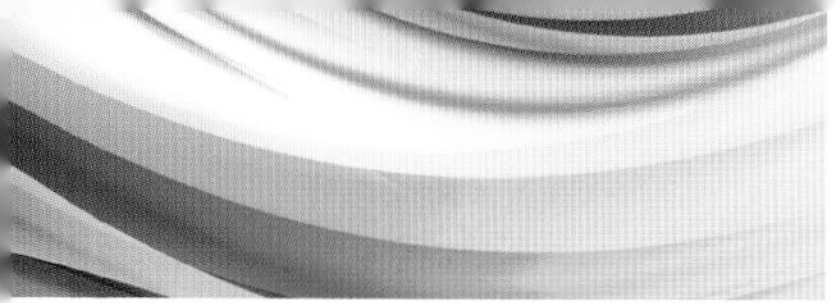

CHAPTER

Hepatobiliary Disease 11

The liver, pancreas, and gall bladder have been referred to as the "accessory organs" because of their participation in digestion. Given the crucial role the liver, in particular, plays in nutrient absorption, metabolism, synthesis, and storage, diseases affecting this organ can profoundly and adversely affect nutritional status. The pancreas, a dual organ of both endocrine and exocrine function, critically participates in digestion and also in blood glucose regulation. Problems with this organ affect both of these functions. The gall bladder's role is limited, with minimal potential effect on nutritional status. However, the presence of gallstones, which affects up to 20% of Americans, 33% of whom will develop acute cholecystitis, may necessitate nutrition intervention.[1]

LIVER DISEASE

Several conditions can cause inflammation or damage to the liver and adversely affect organ function, including exposure to toxins or hepatotoxic drugs, infection, physical injury, genetic abnormality resulting in accumulation of minerals, or an autoimmune response. Because of the organ's role in the metabolism of most nutrients, liver diseases have significant potential to negatively affect nutritional status, and these include hepatitis, hepatic steatosis (fatty liver), and cirrhosis, with excessive alcohol intake being a common trigger for all.

In advanced liver disease, malnutrition is the most common complication occurring in up to 90% of hospitalized patients, and it is even more common in alcohol-induced liver disease.[2]

The pathophysiologic processes underlying the various forms of liver disease, such as inflammation and lipid infiltration, can lead to irreversible diffuse fibrosis of hepatic tissue known as cirrhosis, or end-stage liver disease (ESLD). Prior to this advanced stage, the liver has extensive regenerative ability and reserve capacity, posing a challenge for diagnosis, as significant function must be lost before disease is clinically evident.

Liver function tests (LFTs) provide information on the presence and extent of liver disease[3] (Box 11.1). LFTs indicate the functional status of the liver, as with the synthesis of proteins such as serum albumin and prothrombin, and indication of liver injury, as with various enzymes. These enzymes include aspartate aminotransferase (AST) and alanine aminotransferase (ALT). Although not specific for liver disease, other enzymes that indicate biliary tract obstruction, whether in the liver or in the bile channels outside the liver, include alkaline phosphatase (ALP) and gamma-glutamyl transpeptidase (GGT).

Hepatitis

Disease Process

Hepatitis is inflammation of the liver induced by the presence of a toxin, such as alcohol, medications and some dietary supplements, environmental toxins, or viral infection[4] (Box 11.2). The viral forms of hepatitis include viruses A, B, C, D, and E, with D only arising in patients with hepatitis B virus (HBV), as it requires a helper function of HBV for replication.[5] Both hepatitis A virus (HAV) and hepatitis E virus (HEV) are spread by contact with infected persons or consumption of infected foods, generally from the fecal–oral route. The other forms are transmitted parenterally through contaminated blood and body fluids. Patients with HAV generally recover within

BOX 11.1 Liver Function Abnormalities in Liver Disease

Function	Test	Derangement
Bile synthesis	Bilirubin (serum, urine, fecal); direct (conjugated) and indirect (unconjugated)	Bilirubin not excreted in feces (clay-colored); indirect bilirubin high in liver disease and direct bilirubin high in biliary tract disease
Carbohydrate metabolism	Oral glucose tolerance test, blood glucose	Normal until advanced disease; low in acute disease; high in chronic disease
Lipid metabolism	Triglyceride, lipoproteins/ cholesterol, ketones	All low in severe disease
Protein metabolism	**Urea:** BUN, NH_3	BUN low, NH_3 high in advanced disease
	Plasma proteins: albumin, transferrin, amino acid ratios (BCAA vs. AAA), A1AT	Low protein levels BCAA: AAA ratio skewed toward higher AAA
	Prothrombin time (PT)	PT increased
	Enzymes: ALT, AST, GGT, ALP	High

3 to 6 months, and rarely develop chronic liver disease.[6] In contrast, chronic liver disease develops in up to 6% of adults and 90% of infants infected with HBV and 85% of hepatitis C virus (HCV) patients.[5]

Acute hepatitis proceeds through three stages: prodromal, icteric, and posticteric. The prodromal phase is generally of

BOX 11.2 Dietary Supplements Associated with Hepatitis

Comfrey
Chaparral
Germander
Green tea extract
Jin Bu Huan
Kava
Ma Huang
Saw Palmetto
Skullcap
Yohimbe

Bodybuilding and weight loss supplements of all types are the most likely to cause liver damage (most are proprietary formulations).

2 weeks in duration after exposure and ends with the onset of jaundice (icteric). If infection is the cause, the patient can transmit the virus during this time. Symptoms may include nausea, anorexia, low-grade fever, and hepatomegaly. In the icteric phase, which can last up to 1 month, up to 85% of patients will be jaundiced, although it is less likely to occur in children and even less likely in infants.[7] In this stage, symptoms include clay-colored stools, dark urine, and abdominal pain in 40% of patients.

Patients with HBV and HCV are often asymptomatic, and in the case of type C, symptoms arise only after extensive hepatic damage. In the recovery phase, after jaundice, the liver is still enlarged, but function begins to return. Patients with HBV and HCV may develop chronic liver disease after recovery, and although uncommon in HAV, relapsing hepatitis A may occur and is more common in the elderly.

Treatment and Nutrition Intervention

In acute hepatitis, the goals are to promote liver regeneration and prevent further injury, if a toxin is the cause. The nutritional therapy components include an adequate diet, repletion of energy reserves (anorexia and gastrointestinal symptoms often result in weight loss), higher protein (1.0 to 1.2 g/kg body weight), adequate carbohydrate to spare protein for tissue synthesis[8] (Box 11.3). Small, frequent meals facilitate provision of adequate energy and nutrient intake and may be needed because of anorexia, gastrointestinal symptoms, and early satiety. If disease progresses to chronic liver disease and cirrhosis, more problems with eating and nutrient restrictions can make consuming adequate food and fluids more difficult.

ADIME 11.1 ADIME At-A-Glance: Hepatitis

Assessment

- Low BMI, UWL, anorexia/early satiety, decrease in appetite and food intake
- Abdominal pain, fatigue, nausea and vomiting
- Ascites, edema, jaundice
- CT scans, abdominal ultrasound, ERCP, cholangiogram
- Viral antibodies, LFTs, electrolytes, glucose, hepatic proteins, vitamins/minerals

Nutrition Diagnosis

- Inadequate oral intake RT decreased appetite from abdominal pain, AEB recent UWL of 5% × 2 weeks, and PO intake of <50%

Intervention

- Provision of higher energy/protein diet (30 to 35 kcal/kg, 1.0 to 1.2 g/kg)
- Progress as tolerated to small, frequent feedings
- Provision of supplement of B-complex, vitamins C and K, zinc, as needed
- Adequate fluids

Monitoring and Evaluation

- Body weight, dry weight
- PO intake (food, fluid)
- Laboratory values
- Control of GI symptoms

BOX 11.3 Nutrition Intervention for Hepatitis

Higher energy (30 to 35 kcal/kg body weight)
Higher protein (1.0 to 1.2 g/kg body weight)
Carbohydrate (50% to 55% energy)
B-complex, vitamins C and K, zinc
Adequate fluids
Progress as tolerated to small, frequent feedings

Nonalcoholic Fatty Liver Disease and Nonalcoholic Steatohepatitis

Disease Process

Fatty liver consists of an accumulation of lipids in hepatic tissue because of an imbalance between endogenous synthesis, reduced oxidation, or delivery to the organ and removal via very-low-density lipoprotein (VLDL). It can arise as an early and reversible stage of liver disease from alcohol abuse, but when this is not the cause, it is nonalcoholic fatty liver disease (NAFLD). In up to a third of patients with NAFLD, inflammation and liver cell death lead to nonalcoholic steatohepatitis (NASH).[9]

Although the condition is reversible, it may progress to chronic and irreversible damage. NAFLD is also an independent risk factor for the development of type 2 diabetes.[10] Several toxins and conditions can cause NAFLD, including drugs; environmental toxins; specific diseases such as diabetes, obesity, insulin resistance (IR), and dyslipidemia; surgical procedures such as jejunal ileal bypass; and long-term parenteral nutrition.

Treatment and Nutrition Intervention

If related to toxins, eliminating the underlying cause is the most important treatment component. Dietary treatment is similar to that for hepatitis.[8] Supplementation with vitamin E and α-lipoic acid may improve disease markers in NAFLD,[11] and coffee, tea, and caffeine appear to be protective against the development of fibrosis.[12,13]

ADIME 11.2 ADIME At-A-Glance: Nonalcoholic Fatty Liver Disease

Assessment

- Low BMI, UWL, decrease in appetite and food intake, or high BMI/waist circumference (diabetes, insulin resistance, dyslipidemia)
- Hepatotoxic drugs or alcohol, diabetes, obesity, insulin resistance, dyslipidemia, jejunal ileal bypass, long-term TPN
- Abdominal pain, fatigue, nausea and vomiting
- Ascites, edema, jaundice
- CT scans, abdominal ultrasound, ERCP, cholangiogram
- LFTs, electrolytes, glucose, hepatic proteins, vitamins/minerals

Nutrition Diagnosis

- Inadequate oral intake RT decreased appetite from abdominal pain, AEB recent UWL of 5% × 2 weeks, and PO intake of <50%

Intervention

- Provision of higher energy/protein diet (30 to 35 kcal/kg, 1.0 to 1.2 g/kg); restricted energy, if high BMI
- Progress as tolerated to small, frequent feedings
- Provision of supplement of B-complex, vitamins C and K, zinc, as needed
- Adequate fluids
- If diabetes/insulin resistance, CHO management for glycemic control
- Possible benefit of supplementation: vitamin E and α-lipoic acid
- Coffee, tea, and caffeine may help prevent fibrosis

Monitoring and Evaluation

- Body weight, dry weight
- PO intake (food, fluid)
- Laboratory values
- Control of GI symptoms

Cirrhosis

Disease Process

Cirrhosis is a chronic degenerative disease, in which hepatic tissue becomes fibrous, with impairment of liver function and leading ultimately to liver failure. It is the final stage of many forms of chronic liver disease. With progression to ESLD, the fibrosis becomes increasingly extensive, with fewer remaining functional hepatocytes. In the United States, the most common cause is HCV, with alcoholic liver disease being the next leading cause.[14] Potential complications include malnutrition, esophageal varices, ascites, edema, fat malabsorption, portal hypertension, IR, and hepatic encephalopathy (HE).

Of these complications, IR develops in 60% of cirrhosis patients and leads to diabetes in 20%. If acute variceal hemorrhage occurs, risk for mortality is 15% to 55% within 6 weeks of diagnosis.[15,16] One of the most serious complications is HE, which affects 50% to 80% of patients with cirrhosis.[17] HE is a spectrum of neuropsychiatric abnormalities, which occurs in four stages, leading to coma (hepatic coma), and is a major concern, as the stage four mortality rate approaches 80%. A preliminary stage "0" subclinical, which had been termed *subclinical HE*, is now recognized as minimal hepatic encephalopathy (MHE). In MHE, no changes in behavior or personality can be identified, but there is impaired psychomotor testing, with minimal changes in memory, concentration, intellectual function, and coordination.

When HE arises from cirrhosis, common precipitating factors include electrolyte abnormalities, specific medications, infection, and gastrointestinal bleeding. Somatic protein depletion has been shown to increase the risk for HE.[18] Although the exact cause of HE is not known, it involves the shunting of portal blood from systemic to collateral circulation. One theory relates to the altered ratio of aromatic amino acids (AAAs), phenylalanine, tyrosine, and tryptophan, to branched-chain amino acids (BCAAs), leucine, isoleucine, and valine. Although ammonia is not the primary causative agent in HE, its levels are always elevated with impending HE and are therefore involved in some way.

Treatment and Nutrition Intervention

Aspects of both treatment and nutrition intervention focus on the goals of maintenance of adequate nutrition, prevention tissue catabolism, and the control of complications[8] (Box 11.4).

BOX 11.4 Nutrition Intervention for Cirrhosis and Hepatic Encephalopathy

Cirrhosis

Protein

1.2 to 1.5 g/kg (70 to 100 g), as tolerated

Source: lower AAA (meats) in favor of more BCAA (vegetable, dairy)

Fat

If steatorrhea, MCT and omega-3 fats may be helpful, as will small, frequent meals

Sodium

Restrict 2 to 3 g, if edema, ascites; possible fluid restricted, if ascites (1.0 to 1.5 L/d); may depend on use of diuretic

Texture

If esophageal varices, use soft, low fiber

Energy

Indirect calorimetry is best to determine energy (may vary as to 25% to 70% above resting energy needs); based on dry weight

General

High kcal, CHO (prevent hypoglycemia, but if diabetes is present, CHO management)

Small, frequent meals

Vitamin supplement (B-complex, folic acid)

Fat-soluble vitamins

No alcohol

Avoid raw shellfish

Hepatic Encephalopathy

Chronic: as above, and oral BCAA supplement may be beneficial

Acute: NPO for 24 hours, provide IV glucose; use of enteral feeding, if unable to progress to oral intake; possible benefit of BCAA and L-acetylcarnitine supplement

Dietary restrictions in the control of complications may need to be liberalized to promote optimal intake and prevent or reverse malnutrition, which develops in as many as 90% of patients, and is more prevalent in patients with alcoholic cirrhosis.[2,19] Sodium restriction of 2,000 mg may be needed for controlling edema and ascites, and fluid restriction if hyponatremia is present.[8,20] Since cirrhosis adversely affects immunity, patients with cirrhosis should avoid raw shellfish, which can contain *Vibrio vulnificus*, a virulent bacterium that causes serious infection. In addition, infection can increase the rate of protein catabolism.[2]

The diet should include adequate energy of up to 75% higher than calculated needs, and energy determinations must be based on dry weight. In the presence of diabetes, IR, and hyperglycemia, management of carbohydrate intake is also important. Fat malabsorption with steatorrhea is common, and omega-3 fatty acids and medium-chain triglyceride (MCT) may be useful, along with dividing meals into small, frequent feedings. However, MCT can cause diarrhea and acidosis, so its use should be carefully monitored.[20] The diet should include high-quality protein of 1.0 g to 1.5 g/kg body weight, and dietary sources of BCAA (dairy, eggs, and vegetable) rather than AAA (meats) may be helpful. Oral BCAA supplementation may also be useful in improving protein status and preventing malnutrition, as well as improving abnormal glucose tolerance.[2,21] A systematic review reported that oral BCAA supplementation, but not intravenous, significantly improved manifestations of HE.[22]

Vitamin and mineral supplementation is important, consisting of vitamin C; folate; B-complex; water-soluble forms of vitamins A, D, E, and K; and calcium, potassium, magnesium, and zinc. Supplementation of vitamins A and D, however, must not be excessive so as to avoid hepatotoxicity. As with preventing progression in reversible forms of liver disease, coffee intake also appears to have the same effect in cirrhosis, with one study reporting significant benefits at four cups or more cups daily leading its authors to state, *Are we ready to write a prescription for coffee? Most likely, "yes." There is sufficient evidence to provide biological plausibility for coffee as an antifibrotic.*[23]

Treatment of the onset of HE includes administration of lactulose, a synthetic disaccharide that reduced ammonia in the gut, and antibiotics such as rifaximin to reduce bacterial production of ammonia and toxins.[22] Microbial alterations in the gut arise in tandem with decompensated cirrhosis, which is characterized by the disease complications including HE.[24] For this reason, prebiotics and probiotics may be clinically useful, and lactulose is sometimes classified as a prebiotic, although further research is needed to demonstrate supplement efficacy without adverse effects.[25,26] However, patients should be encouraged to follow a dietary intake of both fiber and probiotic foods.[20]

Nutrition intervention depends on the stage of HE, with acute HE requiring nothing by mouth (NPO) status for 24 hours and administration of IV dextrose.[20] If a patient cannot resume oral intake, enteral nutrition is warranted beginning with protein at 0.5 g/kg body weight and increased to 1.0 to 1.5 g/kg. The efficacy of BCAA in acute HE remains controversial, with more evidence pointing to benefits in chronic HE cirrhosis patients.[17,27] One study reported benefits of BCAA supplemented with L-acetylcarnitine in patients with cirrhotic hepatic coma.[28] For cirrhosis patients with MHE, prevention of hypoglycemia is important, and, if needed, gradual administration over several days beginning at 15 to 20 kcal/kg progressing to 35 to 40 kcal/kg.[21,24] In addition, prevention of malnutrition is important, and adequate protein intake is key in this regard, with most MHE and chronic HE patients being able to tolerate a daily intake of more than 60 to 80 g of protein per day.[17]

ADIME 11.3 ADIME At-A-Glance: Cirrhosis and Hepatic Encephalopathy

Assessment

- Low BMI, UWL, anorexia/early satiety, decrease in appetite and food intake
- Abdominal pain, fatigue, nausea and vomiting, steatorrhea
- Ascites, edema, jaundice, GI bleeding (esp esophageal varices)
- Alcohol, hepatotoxic drugs, diabetes, obesity, insulin resistance, dyslipidemia, jejunal ileal bypass, long-term TPN
- CT scans, abdominal ultrasound, ERCP, cholangiogram
- LFTs (esp ammonia), electrolytes, glucose, hepatic proteins, hgb/hct, chol, vitamins/minerals

(*continued*)

ADIME 11.3 ADIME At-A-Glance: Cirrhosis and Hepatic Encephalopathy (*continued*)

Nutrition Diagnosis

- Inadequate oral intake RT decreased appetite from abdominal pain, AEB recent UWL of 5% × 2 weeks, and PO intake of <50%

Intervention

- Provision of higher-protein diet (1.2 to 1.5 g/kg, as tolerated); BCAA protein sources vs. AAA
- Oral BCAA supplementation, if protein not tolerated
- If steatorrhea, MCT and omega-3 fats
- CHO to prevent hypoglycemia; if diabetes, CHO management
- Small, frequent feedings
- Restrict Na 2 to 3 g, if edema, ascites; possible fluid restricted if ascites (1.0 to 1.5 L/d), depending on use of diuretic
- If esophageal varices, soft, low fiber
- Provision of supplement of B-complex, fat-soluble vitamins
- Avoidance of raw shellfish, alcohol
- Adequate fluids

Monitoring and Evaluation

- Body weight, dry weight
- PO intake (food, fluid)
- Laboratory values
- Control of GI symptoms and other symptoms
- Prevention of neurologic symptoms (HE)

GALLBLADDER DISEASE

Disease Process

The presence of gallstones is cholelithiasis, and problems with the organ generally stem from this common condition, affecting up to 25 million in the United States.[29] Relatively static conditions give rise to biliary sludge, which is thought to promote the crystals to form and later become gall stones.[30] Constituents of the stones include bilirubin, cholesterol, calcium salts, lipid, protein, and other materials. Although the majority of people with gallstones are asymptomatic, serious complications include cholecystitis (inflammation of the organ), pancreatitis, and cancers of the gallbladder and liver.

Risk factors for the development of gallstones include being female, obese, Mexican American, Native American, the use of estrogen and oral contraceptives, and long-term total parenteral nutrition. In addition, several diseases and conditions increase the risk, including diabetes, metabolic syndrome, intestinal diseases causing ileal dysfunction such as Crohn disease, cystic fibrosis, sickle cell disease, bariatric surgery, and rapid weight loss.[30,31] Genetic susceptibility confers considerable risk of a fivefold higher rate. Epidemiologic studies have implicated low-fiber diets high in energy and refined carbohydrates. In contrast, higher intakes of vitamin C, coffee, and calcium appear to be protective.[30]

The disease becomes symptomatic with either stone impaction in the cystic duct or inflammation. The former causes either epigastric or right upper quadrant (RUQ) pain of varying intensity with nausea and vomiting, often after a high-fat meal. Inflammation causes similar but more severe symptoms, sometime accompanied by fever and leukocytosis, often requiring hospitalization.

Treatment and Nutrition Intervention

Nutrition recommendations for patients with chronic cholecystitis include following a diet low in fat with adequate fiber and vitamin C, and reduced energy, if weight loss is indicated.[32] In acute cholecystitis requiring hospitalization, nutrition intervention includes NPO status with progression to a low-fat diet. With gallbladder removal, cholecystectomy, patients should follow a low fat for several months until hepatic compensation develops, with gradual progression to normal levels.

PANCREATIC DISEASE

Disease of the pancreas can significantly impact nutritional status, given the dual role of the organ, that is, exocrine and endocrine. Dysfunction related to the former role will affect digestion and absorption of nutrients, potentially resulting in malnutrition, whereas dysfunctions of the latter cause diabetes mellitus. Because of the direct malabsorption that occurs with failure of the exocrine pancreas, nutritional assessment and intervention are critical in preventing malnutrition.

Acute Pancreatitis

Disease Process

Acute pancreatitis (AP) is a sudden inflammation of the pancreas resulting in 210,000 hospitalizations annually in the United States.[33] AP can lead to chronic pancreatitis (CP) and is linked to pancreatic cancer, with a fourfold higher cancer risk for patients over the age of 70 compared with those aged 41 to 50.[34] Symptoms are similar for AP and CP and include pain of varying intensity in the upper abdomen radiating to the back, nausea, vomiting, and steatorrhea. In AP, serum levels of pancreatic enzymes, lipase and amylase, are elevated; however, in CP, they may be close to normal because of atrophy of the pancreatic parenchyma, leading to fibrosis in advanced disease.[35]

The most common cause of AP is the presence of gallstones in the common bile duct, accounting for 45% of cases, followed by alcohol abuse, which accounts for 35% and can result in pancreatitis within hours of or up to 2 days after heavy ingestion.[36] Additional causes of AP include genetic predisposition and obstruction of the pancreatic duct, which can arise from narrowing of the duct or pancreatic cancer, hypercalcemia, hypertriglyceridemia, abdominal trauma or surgery, various medications and microbes (Box 11.5), and cigarette smoking.[37]

Treatment and Nutrition Intervention

Medical nutrition therapy for AP depends on the severity of the patient's condition (Box 11.6).[8,38,39] In mild cases, a low-fat oral diet can begin immediately in the absence of nausea and vomiting, and once pain has subsided.[40] In moderate AP hospitalized patients, NPO status on admission can progress

BOX 11.5 Medications and Microbes Causing Acute Pancreatitis

Medications	Microbes
Azathioprine	Mumps
Thiazide	Coxsackie B virus
Valproic acid	Cytomegalovirus (CMV)
Dideoxyinosine	Candida
Sulfasalazine	HIV
Trimethoprim–sulfamethoxazole	*Salmonella*
Pentamidine	Shig*ella*
Tetracycline	*E. coli*
	Legionella
	Leptospirosis

BOX 11.6 Dietary Recommendations for Acute Pancreatitis

Feeding Progression

Initial status: NPO
Mild: can advance to small, frequent oral low-fat feedings; MCT if steatorrhea; pancreatic enzyme replacement with each meal
Mild to moderate: nasogastric or nasojejunal feedings; formula containing peptides and MCT
If unable to feed enterally: parenteral nutrition

General

If inflammation extensive, protein and energy needs higher
If alcohol abuse, supplement thiamin (100 mg), folate (1 mg), general multivitamin
Abstinence from alcohol

to an oral diet when bowel function returns, usually within a few days for most patients, without the need for a clear liquid diet. In severe cases, nasogastric or nasojejunal delivery of enteral is the preferred nutrition therapy, which will help prevent infectious complications. Enteral formulas containing peptides and MCT have been shown to be effective.[38] If enteral feeding is not possible, or if nutrient needs cannot be achieved by this method, parenteral nutrition is warranted.

If inflammation is extensive, protein and energy needs are high because of catabolism. Patients with fat malabsorption should receive fat-soluble vitamin supplementation. Alcohol should be avoided by all patients, and in those with a history of alcohol abuse, daily supplemental thiamin (100 mg), folate (1 mg), and general multivitamin are indicated.[8]

In patients with steatorrhea, pancreatic enzymes with each oral feeding will promote nutrient absorption.

ADIME 11.4 ADIME At-A-Glance: Acute Pancreatitis

Assessment

- Low BMI, UWL, decrease in appetite and food intake
- Abdominal pain, nausea and vomiting, steatorrhea
- Hypovolemia
- Alcohol abuse
- Laboratory: amylase, lipase, CRP, glucose, electrolytes, lipids

Nutrition Diagnosis

- Inadequate oral intake RT decreased appetite from abdominal pain, AEB recent UWL of 5% × 2 weeks, and PO intake of <50%

Intervention

- Progress from NPO status: if mild, small, frequent oral low-fat feedings; MCT if steatorrhea; pancreatic enzyme replacement with each meal
- Mild to moderate: NGT or nasojejunal formula containing peptides and MCT
- If unable to feed enterally: parenteral nutrition
- In extensive inflammation, protein and energy needs higher
- If alcohol abuse, supplement thiamin (100 mg), folate (1 mg), general multivitamin
- Supplement of fat-soluble vitamins, B_{12}
- Abstinence from alcohol, caffeine (GI stimulant), smoking

Monitoring and Evaluation

- Body weight, dry weight
- PO intake (food, fluid)
- Laboratory values
- Control of GI symptoms and other symptoms

Chronic Pancreatitis

Disease Process

CP involves inflammation, which after resolution results in irreversible fibrosis and calcification of pancreatic tissue.[41] Some CP patients will have episodes of AP, and as the disease progresses, acinar cells are destroyed and nutrient malabsorption occurs, causing steatorrhea, which can lead to malnutrition. Beta cells may also be destroyed with disease progression, producing diabetes in 33% of patients.[42] Symptoms are similar to those of AP with severe abdominal pain, which subsides over time as the disease worsens; however, some patients have no pain.[33]

The most common cause of CP is heavy alcohol ingestion over several years, which accounts for 90% of cases.[36] As with alcohol, other causes are similar to those of AP and include genetic pancreatic diseases (cystic fibrosis is the most common), gallbladder disease, hypercalcemia, hypertriglyceridemia, hyperparathyroidism, organ trauma, certain medications, and autoimmune diseases. CP can also occur after an episode of AP in which the pancreatic duct is damaged, causing inflammation of the organ and the development of scar tissue.

Treatment and Nutrition Intervention

Abstinence from alcohol and tobacco is an important aspect of intervention to remove the underlying disease cause, in the case of alcoholic CP, and to prevent further damage to the pancreas, as both appear to have both direct and indirect toxic effects on the organ.[33] In CP, eating may exacerbate the chronic abdominal pain, which can reduce food intake and leads to further weight loss, which mainly arises from nutrient malabsorption, particularly fat.[8,43] In addition, limited evidence suggests that resting energy expenditure is 30% to 50% higher in CP patients.[44] For all of these reasons, nutrient deficiencies and protein energy malnutrition are common, particularly in alcoholic CP. Goals for nutritional intervention include repletion of nutritional status and reduction of malabsorption. Pancreatic replacement enzymes are important therapeutic agents to achieve these goals.

Recommendations for dietary fat intake vary, from a low-fat diet[33,42] to moderate[43] to as high as the patient can tolerate[8] (Box 11.7). In addition, MCT may be helpful if steatorrhea cannot be controlled. For most patients, protein should be 1.0 to 1.5 g/kg body weight.[43] However, protein needs may be as high as 2.0 g/kg in a severely compromised patient who has had significant weight loss. Small, frequent meals (four to eight) are better tolerated and may promote higher absorption, particularly of dietary fat. Supplementation with fat-soluble vitamins and vitamin B_{12} and possibly other micronutrients is often warranted because of chronic nutrient malabsorption in general and fat in particular. Some patients may require enteral nutrition, if they are unable to consume adequate energy through dietary intake. This may include nocturnal feedings, depending on the patient's nutritional status and tolerance.[43]

BOX 11.7 Dietary Recommendations for Chronic Pancreatitis

Protein: 1.0 g/kg body weight, up to 2.0 g/kg for repletion
Small, frequent meals (4 to 8)
Pancreatic enzyme replacements with each meal
Fat variable, based on tolerance; MCT, if steatorrhea severe
Adequate diet or supplement: calcium, magnesium, fat-soluble vitamins, B-complex vitamins, vitamin C, zinc
Abstinence from alcohol

ADIME 11.5 ADIME At-A-Glance: Chronic Pancreatitis

Assessment

- Low BMI, UWL, decrease in appetite and food intake
- Abdominal pain, nausea and vomiting, steatorrhea
- Hypovolemia
- Alcohol abuse
- Laboratory: amylase, lipase, CRP, glucose, electrolytes, lipids

Nutrition Diagnosis

- Impaired nutrient utilization RT to Dx and nonadherence to PER with meals, AEB steatorrhea and recent UWL of 5% × 2 weeks

ADIME 11.5 ADIME At-A-Glance: Chronic Pancreatitis (*continued*)

Intervention

- Small, frequent meals (4 to 8)
- Pancreatic enzyme replacements with each meal
- Fat variable, based on tolerance; MCT, if steatorrhea severe
- Adequate diet or supplement: calcium, magnesium, fat-soluble vitamins, B-complex vitamins, vitamin C, zinc
- Abstinence from alcohol, smoking

Monitoring and Evaluation

- Body weight
- PO intake
- Laboratory values
- Control of GI symptoms and other symptoms

Pancreaticoduodenectomy (Whipple Procedure)

Procedure and Nutrition Intervention

Pancreatic cancer accounts for 3% of all cancer cases in the United States and 7% of cancer mortality.[45] The disease may necessitate a pancreaticoduodenectomy, or Whipple procedure (WP), which involves removal of the head of pancreas, distal bile duct, gall bladder, duodenum, first few centimeters of jejunum, approximately 50% of the distal stomach, and pylorus.[46] Numerous nutrition problems typically arise, including gastroparesis, dumping syndrome, diabetes, malabsorption, lactose intolerance, weight loss, and malnutrition.[47] Specific nutrient deficiencies that can develop include vitamins A, D, E, K, and B_{12}, and minerals iron, calcium, zinc, copper, and selenium.

Nutrition intervention targets all of the potential nutrition problems.[47] The specific dietary measures include small, frequent meals (five to six), limited fluid at meals (up to 5 oz) and drinking fluids up to 40 minutes after a meal, avoidance of simple sugars and sugar alcohols, inclusion of protein at every meal, and limiting fat to less than 30% of total calories. In addition, if lactose intolerance occurs, the patient should be instructed to avoid lactose and use specialized products in which lactose has been prehydrolyzed. The patient should also be encouraged to eat slowly and chew all foods thoroughly. A vitamin and mineral supplement is also an important part of nutrition intervention with close monitoring for weight loss and possible malnutrition.

References

1. Medscape. Cholecystitis. Available at: http://emedicine.medscape.com/article/171886-overview#a6. Accessed February 19, 2015.
2. Cheung K, Lee SS, Raman M. Prevalence and mechanisms of malnutrition in patients with advanced liver disease, and nutrition management strategies. *Clin Gastroenterol Hepatol* 2012;10(2):117–125.
3. Lab Tests Online. Available at: https://labtestsonline.org/nderstanding/conditions/liver-disease/start/1. Accessed February 20, 2016.
4. Farrell GC. Liver disease caused by drugs, anesthetics, and toxins. In: Feldman M, Friedman LS, Sleisenger MH, eds. *Sleisenger and Fordtran's Gastrointestinal and Liver Disease: Pathophysiology, Diagnosis, Management*. Philadelphia, PA: Saunders; 2002:1403–1447.
5. Centers for Disease Control and Prevention. Viral Hepatitis. Available at: http://www.cdc.gov/hepatitis/. Accessed February 20, 2016.
6. Lai M, Chopra S. Hepatitis A Overview. In: *UptoDate*. Available at: http://www.uptodate.com/contents/hepatitis-a-beyond-the-basics. Accessed February 20, 2016.
7. Medscape. Hepatitis A Clinical Presentation. Available at: http://emedicine.medscape.com/article/177484-clinical. Accessed February 22, 2016.
8. Academy of Nutrition and Dietetics. *Nutrition Care Manual*. https://www.nutritioncaremanual.org. Accessed February 23, 2016.
9. MedicineNet.com. Fatty Liver. Available at: http://www.edicinenet.com/fatty_liver/page4.htm. Accessed February 23, 2016.
10. Sung KC, Wild SH, Byrne CD. Resolution of fatty liver and risk of incident diabetes. *J Clin Endocrinol Metab* 2013;98(9):3637–3643.
11. Basu PP, Shah NJ, Aloysius NM, et al. Effect of vitamin E and alpha lipoic acid in nonalcoholic fatty liver disease: A randomized, placebo-controlled, open-label, prospective clinical trial (VAIN trial). *Open J Gastroenterol* 2014;4:199–207.

12. Molloy JW, Calcagno CJ, Williams CD, et al. Association of coffee and caffeine consumption with fatty liver disease, nonalcoholic steatohepatitis, and degree of hepatic fibrosis. *Hepatology* 2012;55:429–436.
13. Khalaf N, White D, Kanwal F, et al. Coffee and caffeine are associated with decreased risk of advanced hepatic fibrosis among patients with hepatitis C. *Clin Gastroenterol Hepatol* 2015;13(8):1521–1531.
14. National Institute of Diabetes & Digestive & Kidney Diseases. Cirrhosis. Available at: http://www.niddk.nih.gov/health-information/health-topics/liver-disease/cirrhosis/Pages/facts.aspx. Accessed March 11, 2016.
15. Cabrera L, Tandon P, Abraldes JG. An update on the management of acute esophageal variceal bleeding. *Gastroenterol Hepatol* 2016. doi:10.1016/j.gastrohep.2015.11.012.
16. Bambha K, Kim WR, Pedersen R, et al. Predictors of early re-bleeding and mortality after acute variceal haemorrhage in patients with cirrhosis. *Gut* 2008;57(6):814–820.
17. Cleveland Clinic. Hepatic Encephalopathy. Available at: http://www.clevelandclinicmeded.com/medicalpubs/diseasemanagement/hepatology/hepatic-encephalopathy/. Accessed March 11, 2016.
18. Merli M, Giusto M, Lucidi C. Muscle depletion increases the risk of overt and minimal hepatic encephalopathy: Results of a prospective study. Metab Brain Dis 2013;28:281–284.
19. Teiusanu A, Andrei M, Arbanas T, et al. Nutritional status in cirrhotic patients. *Maedica* 2012;7(4):284–289.
20. Escott-Stump S. *Nutrition Diagnosis-Related Care*. 8th ed. Philadelphia, PA: Wolters Kluwer; 2015:502–507.
21. Tajiri K, Shimizu Y. Branched-chain amino acids in liver diseases. *World J Gastroenterol* 2013;19(43):7620–7629.
22. Gluud LL, Dam G, Borre M, et al. Lactulose, rifaximin or branched chain amino acids for hepatic encephalopathy: What is the evidence? Metab Brain Dis 2013;28(2):221–225.
23. Dranoff JA, Feld JJ, Lavoie EG, et al. How does coffee prevent liver fibrosis? Biological plausibility for recent epidemiological observations. *Hepatology* 2014;60(2):464–467.
24. Amodio P, Canesso F, Montagnese S. Dietary management of hepatic encephalopathy revisited. *Curr Opin Clin Nutr Metab Care* 2014;17(5):448–452.
25. Bémeur C, Butterworth RF. Nutrition in the management of cirrhosis and its neurological complications. *J Clin Exp Hepatol* 2014;4:141–150.

26. Amodio P, Bemeur C, Butterworth R, et al. The nutritional management of hepatic encephalopathy in patients with cirrhosis: International Society for Hepatic Encephalopathy and Nitrogen Metabolism Consensus. *Hepatology* 2013;58(1):325–336.
27. Als-Nielsen B, Koretz RL, Kjaergard LL, et al. Branched-chain amino acids for hepatic encephalopathy. *Cochrane Database Syst Rev* 2003;2:CD001939.
28. Malaguarnera M, Risino C, Cammalleri L, et al. Branched chain amino acids supplemented with L-acetylcarnitine versus BCAA treatment in hepatic coma: A randomized and controlled double blind study. *Eur J Gastroenterol Hepatol* 2009;21(7):762–770.
29. Stinton LM, Shaffer EA. Epidemiology of gallbladder disease: Cholelithiasis and cancer. *Gut Liver* 2012:6(2):172–187.
30. Njeze GE. Gallstones. *Niger J Surg* 2013;19(2):49–55.
31. National Institute of Diabetes & Digestive & Kidney Diseases. Gallstones. Available at: http://www.niddk.nih.gov/health-information/health-topics/digestive-diseases/gallstones/Pages/facts.aspx. Accessed March 14, 2016.
32. Escott-Stump S. *Nutrition Diagnosis-Related Care*. 8th ed. Philadelphia, PA: Wolters Kluwer; 2015:535–536.
33. National Institute of Diabetes & Digestive & Kidney Diseases. Pancreatitis. Available at: http://www.niddk.nih.gov/health-information/health-topics/liver-disease/pancreatitis/Pages/facts.aspx. Accessed March 14, 2016.
34. Munigala S, Kanwal F, Xian H, et al. Increased risk of pancreatic adenocarcinoma after acute pancreatitis. *Clin Gastroenterol Hepatol* 2014;12(7):1143–1150.
35. Medscape. Chronic Pancreatitis Workup. Available at: http://emedicine.medscape.com/article/181554-workup. Accessed March 15, 2016.
36. Cleveland Clinic. Pancreatitis. Available at: http://my.clevelandclinic.org/health/diseases_conditions/hic_Pancreatitis/dd_overview. Accessed March 14, 2016.
37. Barreto SG. How does cigarette smoking cause acute pancreatitis? *Pancreatology* 2016;16(2):157–163. doi:10.1016/j.pan.2015.09.002.
38. Mirtallo J, Forbes A, McClave S, et al. International consensus guidelines for nutrition therapy in pancreatitis. *JPEN J Parenter Enteral Nutr* 2012;36(3):284–291.
39. Anand N, Park JH, Wu BU. Modern management of acute pancreatitis. *Gastroenterol Clin North Am* 2012;41:1–8.

40. Tenner S, Baillie J, DeWitt J, et al. American College of Gastroenterology Guideline: Management of acute pancreatitis. *Am J Gastroenterol* 2013;108(9):1400–1415.
41. Johns Hopkins Medicine. Gastroenterology and Hepatology. FAQs About Chronic Pancreatitis. Available at: http://www.hopkinsmedicine.org/gastroenterology_hepatology/diseases_conditions/faqs/chronic_pancreatitis.html. Accessed March 15, 2016.
42. Medscape. Chronic Pancreatitis. Available at: http://emedicine.medscape.com/article/181554-overview. Accessed March 15, 2016.
43. Rasmussen HH, Irtun O, Olesen SS, et al. Nutrition in chronic pancreatitis. *World J Gastroenterol* 2013;19(42):7267–7275.
44. Hébuterne X, Hastier P, Péroux JL, et al. Resting energy expenditure in patients with alcoholic chronic pancreatitis. *Dig Dis Sci* 1996;41:533–539.
45. American Cancer Society. What are the key statistics about pancreatic cancer? Available at: http://www.cancer.org/cancer/pancreaticcancer/detailedguide/pancreatic-cancer-key-statistics. Accessed March 17, 2016.
46. Mayo Clinic. Whipple Procedure. Available at: http://www.mayoclinic.org/tests-procedures/whipple-procedure/basics/definition/prc-20021393. Accessed March 17, 2016.
47. Marcason W. What is the Whipple procedure and what is the appropriate nutrition therapy for it? *J Acad Nutr Diet* 2015;115(1):168.

Notes

NOTES

Notes

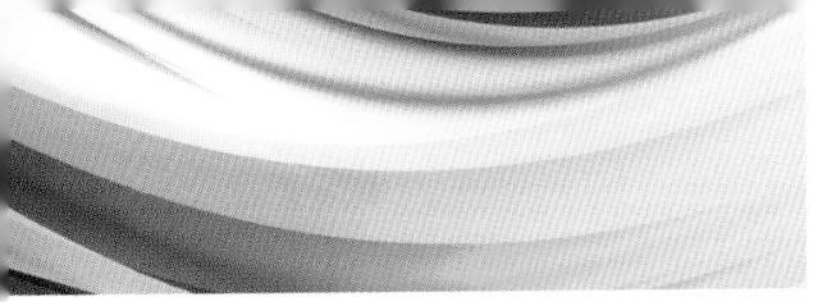

CHAPTER

12 Kidney Disease

Tilakavati Karupaiah, PhD, APD, AN

Acute kidney injury in hospitalized patients and patients with progressive chronic kidney disease account for the majority of kidney cases requiring nutrition intervention. Prevalence in the United States for end-stage kidney disease (ESKD) is 2,034 per million and continues to rise by approximately 21,000 cases per year.[1] High-risk groups include African Americans, Native Americans, and Asians, with rates of 3.7, 1.4, and 1.5 times greater compared with that of whites, respectively.

ACUTE KIDNEY INJURY

Acute kidney injury (AKI) represents an abrupt reduction in glomerular filtration rate (GFR), resulting in the reduced ability of the kidney to excrete metabolic wastes with dysregulation of fluid, electrolyte, and acid–base homeostasis.[2] It often results from an illness, surgery, or severe trauma, but can also be caused by a rapidly progressive, intrinsic renal disease.[1] AKI is reversible in many cases if diagnosed and treated early; however, there is a significantly increased long-term risk of chronic kidney disease and ESKD for many AKI survivors even after initial recovery of kidney function. AKI is now increasingly recognized as a risk factor for the development of chronic kidney disease. Severe AKI occurs in

>5% of critically ill patients and is associated with mortality rates of 40% to 70%.[2]

Disease Process

AKI is suspected when there is a rapid rise in serum creatinine (SCr) associated with oliguria.[3] The causes of AKI are varied and can be divided into three general categories:

- As an adaptive response to severe volume depletion and hypotension, with the kidney's structure and function intact (prerenal)
- In response to inflammatory, ischemic, or cytotoxic insults, which affects both kidney structure and function (intrinsic renal)
- When the passage of urine is blocked (postrenal)[3]

The majority of AKI cases arise from prerenal causes and are multifactorial, particularly in the critically ill setting.[2] A listing of the causes of AKI in each category can be found in Table 12.1.

The basis for the clinical diagnosis of AKI is based on changes in SCr and/or urine output as surrogates for changes in GFR. A system for the classification of the increasing severity of AKI has been established by an International Work Group of the Kidney Disease: Improving Global Outcomes (KDIGO) initiative, and is referred to by the acronym RIFLE (Table 12.2).[2,5] The three severity grades (risk, injury, and failure) are based on the magnitude of increase in SCr and/or the duration of oliguria. The two outcome stages (loss of kidney function and ESKD) are defined by the duration of loss of kidney function. Although the RIFLE classification system provides an important tool for staging the severity of AKI for conducting epidemiologic studies and in the design of clinical trials, the National Kidney Foundation–Kidney Disease Outcomes Quality Initiative (NKF-KDOQI) does not recommend use of this system in the diagnosis and clinical management of AKI patients in acute care settings in the United States.[4]

TABLE 12.1. Causes of Acute Kidney Injury

AKI Category	Causes

Prerenal (decreased blood flow)	• Hypotension from any cause
	• Congestive heart failure
	• Systemic vasodilation (e.g., sepsis, neurogenic shock)
	• Volume depletion
	  • Renal loss from diuretic overuse, osmotic diuresis (e.g., diabetic ketoacidosis)
	  • Extrarenal loss from vomiting, diarrhea, burns, excessive sweating, blood loss
	• Hypercalcemia

Intrinsic renal	• Ischemia
	  • Sepsis or direct infections
	  • Atheroembolism or thromboembolism
	  • Thrombotic microangiopathy
	  • Systemic necrotizing vasculitides
	  • Hypoperfusion from systemic hypotension
	• Toxins
	  • Endogenous (e.g., hemolysis, rhabdomyolysis, tumor lysis syndrome, myeloma)
	  • Exogenous (drugs, radiographic contrast agents, bacteria, fungi, viruses)
	• Acute glomerular or tubulointerstitial nephritis
	• Tumor
	• Stones
	• Scar tissue formation
	• Tissue inflammation

Postrenal (obstruction)	• Stones • Tumor • Prostate hypertrophy • Neurogenic bladder • Bladder, prostate, or cervical cancer

Data from (i) Gilbert SJ, Weiner DE. *National Kidney Foundation's Primer on Kidney Diseases*. 6th ed. Philadelphia, PA: Elsevier Saunders; 2014 and (ii) Mahboob R, Shad F, Smith MC. Acute kidney injury: A guide to diagnosis and management. *Am Fam Physician* 2012;86(7):631–639.

TABLE 12.2. RIFLE Classification for Categorizing Acute Kidney Injury Severity

Class	Serum Creatinine Criteria[a]	Urine Output Criteria
Risk	Increased to >1.5 times baseline	<0.5 mL/kg/hr for >6 hr
Injury	Increased to >2.0 times baseline	<0.5 mL/kg/hr for >12 hr
Failure	Increased to >3.0 times baseline, or an increase of ≥0.5 mg/dL to a value of ≥4 mg/dL	<0.3 mL/kg/hr for >12 hr or anuria for >12 hr
Loss	Need for KRT >4 wk	
End-stage kidney disease	Need for KRT >3 mo	

[a]Increase in serum creatinine should be both abrupt (within 1–7 d) and sustained (>24 hr).

Data from Mahboob R, Shad F, Smith MC. Acute kidney injury: A guide to diagnosis and management. *Am Fam Physician* 2012;86(7):631–639.

Treatment and Nutrition Intervention

The AKI patient typically presents with metabolic derangements resulting from both the uremic burden and inflammatory processes. Therefore, metabolic acidosis, hyperkalemia, and protein catabolism need to be assessed. Stress hyperglycemia with peripheral insulin resistance is a distinctive clinical feature of critical illness. Short-term dialysis may be necessary to treat AKI, with the goal of preventing renal damage and returning the kidneys to baseline function. Medications may include the following:

- IV sodium chloride to correct dehydration
- Diuretics, such as furosemide, to correct fluid overload
- Bicarbonate to correct severe acidosis

- Potassium-exchange resins to bind potassium in the gut to correct hyperkalemia
- Insulin to correct hyperglycemia

Specific nutritional goals are based on whether or not dialysis is planned to reduce the uremic burden, and the presence of multiple organ complications. Careful daily monitoring of the metabolic status of the AKI patient is necessary, and nutritional goals should be determined based on these findings. Table 12.3 lists the nutritional recommendations and monitoring parameters for patients with AKI.

ADIME 12.1 ADIME At-A-Glance: Acute Kidney Injury

Assessment

- Ht, wt, BMI, wt changes, dry wt, SBW
- Labs: blood pressure, serum creatinine, BUN, GFR, albumin, electrolytes, calcium, phosphorus, inflammatory markers (CRP), acid–base balance (pH, CO_2, chloride), I&Os
- Food history/logs, vitamin/mineral/supplement use, appetite status
- NFPE: presence of edema, muscle wasting, subcutaneous fat loss

Nutrition Diagnosis

- Inadequate protein energy intake RT AKI (stress hypermetabolism/catabolism), initiation of CRRT, and decreased ability to consume sufficient protein/energy AEB unintentional weight loss of 1.8% in 1 week, intake $<25\% \times 3$ days, and new NPO status

Intervention

- Initiate enteral nutrition Nepro at 20 mL/hr via NG tube and increase by 10 mL/hr every 8 hours to goal rate of 45 mL/hr to provide 1,944 kcal, 87 g protein, 785 mL free water
- Request metabolic cart study

Monitoring and Evaluation

- Goal rate for EN reached by day 2
- Reassess energy needs based on metabolic cart study

TABLE 12.3. Nutrition Intervention and Monitoring in Acute Kidney Injury

Nutrient Rationale	Recommended Amounts: ASPEN	Recommended Amounts: KDIGO	Monitor
Protein • Avoid net negative nitrogen balance associated with hypercatabolism • Sufficient to reduce serum urea and improve urinary output • Sufficient to maintain somatic and visceral protein status • Replace protein losses from KRT • Correct hyperkalemia	1.2–2.0 g/kg/d On hemodialysis or CRRT: additional 0.2 g/kg/d up to 2.5 g/kg/d	Not on dialysis: 0.8–1.0 g/kg/d On HD or PD: 1.0–1.5 g/kg/d On CRRT: up to 1.7 g/kg/d	BUN Serum creatinine Serum chloride Urine output GI tolerance
Energy • Sufficient to spare protein for synthesis • Sufficient to prevent tissue protein catabolism • Titrate for stress-induced hyperglycemia	25–30 kcal/kg/d (use usual body weight for normal weight patients; use ideal body weight for obese or critically ill) Indirect calorimetry is preferred.	20–30 kcal/kg/d in patients with any stage of AKI Indirect calorimetry is preferred.	Blood glucose Insulin dose

Electrolytes		
• Sodium—restriction during oliguric phase • Potassium—hyperkalemia from tissue catabolism; control to prevent cardiac arrhythmias	Sodium—20–40 mEq/d (2–3 g) during oliguric phase Potassium—30–50 mEq/d during oliguric phase Phosphorous—limit as needed Restriction not required on dialysis	Blood levels of sodium, potassium, and phosphorous
Fluid		
• Control in early oliguric phase • Net intake must balance output. • Maintain normal blood pressure	500 mL + previous days output Restriction not required on dialysis	I/O charts Weight change Blood pressure IVs Parenteral or enteral fluid volumes

ASPEN, American Society for Parenteral and Enteral Nutrition; CRRT, continuous renal replacement therapy.

Data from (i) Kidney Disease: Improving Global Outcomes (KDIGO) Acute Kidney Injury Work Group. KDIGO Clinical Practice Guideline for Acute Kidney Injury. *Kidney Int Suppl* 2012;2:1–138, (ii) Palevsky PM, Liu KD, Brophy PD, et al. KDOQI US commentary on the 2012 KDIGO Clinical Practice Guideline for Acute Kidney Injury. *Am J Kidney Dis* 2013;61(5):649–672, (iii) McClave SA, Taylor BE, Martindale RG, et al. Guidelines for the provision and assessment of nutrition support therapy in the adult critically ill patient: Society of Critical Care Medicine (SCCM) and America Society for Parenteral and Enteral Nutrition (ASPEN). *JPEN J Parenter Enteral Nutr* 2016;40(2):159–211, (iv) Fiaccadori E, Maggiore U, Giacosa R, et al. Enteral nutrition in patients with acute renal failure. *Kidney Int* 2004;65(3):999–1008, and (v) Davies AR, Morrison SS, Bailey MJ, et al. A multicenter, randomized controlled trial comparing early nasojejunal with nasogastric nutrition in critical illness. *Crit Care Med* 2012;40(8):2342–2348.

CHRONIC KIDNEY DISEASE

Chronic kidney disease (CKD) represents a gradual and progressive loss of kidney function, which is irreversible. The GFR, which is a measure of kidney function, decreases proportionately from stages 1 to 5 CKD in tandem with acidosis, anemia, bone disorders, and uremic symptoms (Box 12.1).[3] The progression in GFR decline (termed *renal insufficiency*) is inversely proportional to SCr levels.[3] Initially, as renal tissue loses function, there are few signs or symptoms because the remaining tissue increases its performance (renal adaptation). At a GFR that has fallen to 50% of normal, up to 75% of renal tissue function may already be lost.[5] The principle causes leading to CKD are diabetic nephropathy and hypertension, which together account for up to two-thirds of all cases.[1] The nutritional management of CKD patients differs based on the stage of the disease and dialysis status.

CKD: Nondialysis

Disease Process

In the nondialysis (ND) stage of CKD, also referred to as CKD ND, preservation of kidney function for as long as possible becomes the main goal.[6] Early renal insufficiency is characterized by increasing blood urea nitrogen (BUN) and SCr concentrations and decreasing creatinine clearance.[3] As the GFR declines, the progressive loss of functioning nephrons impairs a range of physiologic functions in the CKD patient relative to acid–base balance, potassium and phosphate excretion, vitamin D metabolism, increased renin production, impaired erythropoietin production, and retention of protein metabolites.[3]

The development of the uremic syndrome quantitatively and qualitatively characterizes the deterioration of cardiovascular, neurologic, hematologic, immunologic, and other systems.[3] Increased catabolism leads to malnutrition and acidosis, which further increases the uremic burden. By stages 4 and 5 CKD, full blown uremia is a complex clinical picture comprising fatigue, anorexia, weight loss, itching, muscle cramps, pericarditis, and sensory and cognitive disturbances.[3,7]

BOX 12.1 Definition and Classification of Chronic Kidney Disease

Definition of CKD Based on the NKF-KDOQI Guidelines[a]:

1. Kidney damage for ≥3 months, with or without decreased kidney function. Kidney damage is defined as pathologic abnormalities or markers of damage, including abnormalities in blood, in urine test, or on diagnostic imaging studies.
2. Decreased kidney function measured by GFR <60 mL/min/1.73 m^2 for ≥3 months, with or without kidney damage

Stage	Description	GFR[b]	Symptoms	Action
Pre-CKD	At increased risk	>90 with CKD risk factors		• Screening for CKD • CKD risk reduction
1	Kidney damage with normal or increased GFR	≥90	Albuminuria, proteinuria, hematuria	• Diagnosis and treatment • Treatment of comorbid conditions • Slowing progression • CVD risk reduction
2	Kidney damage with mild decrease in GFR	60–89	Albuminuria, proteinuria, hematuria	• Estimating progression

(*continued*)

BOX 12.1 Definition and Classification of Chronic Kidney Disease (*continued*)

Stage	Description	GFR[b]	Symptoms	Action
3[a]	Moderate decrease in GFR	30–59	Early to chronic renal insufficiency	• Evaluating and treating complications • Start nutrition intervention
4	Severe decrease in GFR	15–29	Chronic renal insufficiency, late renal insufficiency, pre-ESKD	• Preparation for KRT • Nutrition counseling
5	Kidney failure	<15	Renal failure, uremia, ESKD	KRT if uremia is present

[a]KDIGO guidelines established in 2012 further divide stage 3 CKD into the following categories, with concurrence from NKF-KDOQI:

- 3a (GFR 45–59): mild to moderate decrease in GFR or early renal insufficiency.
- 3b (GFR 30–44): moderate to severe decrease in GFR or chronic renal insufficiency.

[b]Glomerular filtration rate (mL/min/1.72 m^2).

CVD, cardiovascular disease.

Data from National Kidney Foundation KDOQI. Clinical Practice Guidelines for chronic kidney disease: Evaluation, classification, and stratification. *AM J Kidney Dis* 2002;39(Suppl 1):S1–S266.

Treatment and Nutrition Intervention

Laboratory values should be monitored at least monthly and reviewed with the patient to determine any necessary therapeutic interventions (Table 12.4). Some values may

TABLE 12.4. Commonly Monitored Laboratory Values in Kidney Disease

Test	Normal Chronic Kidney Disease Range
Albumin	WNL for laboratory >4.0 is ideal
Blood urea nitrogen	7–20 mg/dL; 60–80 mg/dL (dialysis) Based on well-dialyzed patient with good intake
Calcium–phosphorus product	<55 mg/dL
Corrected calcium[a]	<10.2 mg/dL 8.4–9.5 mg/dL is ideal
Chloride	WNL
CO_2, total	>22
Cholesterol	WNL
Creatinine	0.8–1.4 mg/dL; 2–15 mg/dL
Ferritin	>100 mg/mL
Glucose	WNL
Hematocrit	33%–36% (dialysis)
Hemoglobin	11–12 g/dL
Phosphorus	3.5–5.5 (dialysis); 2.7–4.6 (nondialysis 3–4 stage)
Potassium	3.5–5.5
Parathyroid hormone, intact	150–300 pg/mL (stage 5); 70–110 (stage 4); 35–70 (stage 3)
Sodium	WNL

[a]Ca = total calcium mg/dL + 0.8 [4 – serum albumin g/dL].

WNL, within normal limits.

Data from (i) National Kidney Foundation KDOQI. Clinical Practice Guidelines for chronic kidney disease: Evaluation, classification, and stratification. *AM J Kidney Dis* 2002;39(Suppl 1):S1–S266 and (ii) National Kidney Foundation KDOQI. *Clinical Practice Guidelines for Bone Metabolism and Disease in Chronic Kidney Disease*. New York: National Kidney Foundation; 2004.

be monitored more frequently, such as hemoglobin, hematocrit, calcium, and phosphorus. These lab values can be affected by medications or acute medical conditions, and in both cases, more frequent monitoring will significantly improve patient outcomes. Some biochemical parameters, such as lipid profile, are tested less frequently, generally on a quarterly basis.

Primary goals in the treatment of CKD include the preservation of kidney function and maintaining adequate nutritional status, thus delaying the need for dialysis as long as possible. The NKF has issued national guidelines, KDOQI, which provide evidence-based clinical practice guidelines for all stages of CKD.[2] These guidelines strongly recommend nutrition evaluation and monitoring as early as stage 2 or 3. To prevent further decline of kidney function, the cornerstone of treatment is intensive control of diabetes and hypertension, if present. Nutritional intervention can help to control uremic symptoms such as anorexia, diarrhea, and vomiting that frequently accompany the decline in GFR (Table 12.5). Preventing malnutrition in the predialysis patient is of critical importance to overall patient outcome.[3] In planning diets for patients, the rationale for multiple nutrient recommendations must be considered and adjusted to patient needs accordingly:

- **Energy and protein** calculations are typically based on standard body weight (SBW) or actual body weight and provide for maintenance only. Calorie provision should be adequate to prevent protein catabolism for gluconeogenesis. Activity level and stress factor should be taken into account when planning for caloric and protein requirements. High biologic value (HBV) protein should provide at least 50% of the total protein consumed.[8]
- **Potassium** may be liberalized if potassium-depleting diuretics are in use. Restrictions are implemented only with hyperkalemia. Once a potassium restriction is needed, diabetic patients should use caution in selecting items for the treatment of hypoglycemic reactions (Table 12.6).

TABLE 12.5. KDOQI Nutrition Guidelines for CKD ND (Stages 1–4 CKD)

Nutrients	Stages 1–4 CKD
Protein (g/kg/d)	0.8 (with GFR >25)
	0.6–0.75 (with GFR <25)
Energy (kcal/kg/d)	35 < 60 years
	30–35 ≥ 60 years
Phosphorus (mg/d)	Based on laboratory values
	Restrict to 800–1,000 mg/d in stages 3–4 CKD when serum phosphorus is elevated and/or when plasma levels of intact PTH are elevated above target range of the CKD stage
Sodium (g/d)	2–4; based on labs and blood pressure
Potassium (g/d)	Adjust per laboratory values
Calcium (mg/d)	1,200; maintain serum calcium WNL
Fluid (mL/d)	Unrestricted with normal urine output. May need restriction with CHF

WNL, within normal limits; CHF, congestive heart failure.
Data from National Kidney Foundation KDOQI. Clinical Practice Guidelines for chronic kidney disease: Evaluation, classification, and stratification. *AM J Kidney Dis* 2002;39(Suppl 1):S1–S266.

TABLE 12.6. Low Potassium Hypoglycemic Interventions (15 g CHO)

Food Item	Portion Size
Regular gelatin	½ cup
Honey	1 Tbsp
Regular soda or apple juice	½ cup
Sherbet or sorbet	½ cup
Glucose	1 tube
Glucose tablets	3

Data from Council on Renal Nutrition of the National Kidney Foundation. In: McCann L, ed. *Pocket Guide to Nutrition Assessment of the Patient with Chronic Kidney Disease*. 5th ed. New York: National Kidney Foundation; 2015.

- **Very-low-sodium** diets are generally not palatable enough to sustain adequate calorie and protein intake for most patients. Initiation of dialysis should be considered when the dietary restrictions are such that palatability of the diet prevents adequate intake.[9]
- Controlling **phosphorus** intake will automatically limit calcium intake, since many high-phosphorus foods are also rich in calcium. Early control of phosphorus intake will help control the serum phosphorus and parathyroid hormone (PTH) levels. The phosphorus level is also controlled with the addition of phosphate-binding medications. These medications, taken with each meal and snack, bind phosphorus in the gastrointestinal (GI) tract and reduce the amount of phosphorus absorbed into the blood. Educate patient to read food labels to identify phosphorus sources.
- Elemental **calcium** intake from both the diet and medications should be limited to 2,000 mg daily. Patients should read labels to avoid products that are fortified with calcium.
- **Fluid** needs to be limited in predialysis patients only when congestive heart failure appears imminent (stages 4 to 5). Fluid restrictions for patients on diuretics may cause progression of renal failure because of volume depletion.

ADIME 12.2 ADIME At-A-Glance: Chronic Kidney Disease

Assessment

- Ht, wt, BMI, wt changes, dry wt, SBW
- Labs: blood pressure, serum creatinine, BUN, GFR, electrolytes, calcium, phosphorus microalbuminuria, inflammatory markers (CRP), Hgb, Hct, iron
- Food history/logs, vitamin/mineral/supplement use, appetite status
- NFPE: presence of edema, muscle wasting, subcutaneous fat loss

Nutrition Diagnosis

- Excessive sodium intake RT intake of foods high in sodium × 7 days AEB elevated blood pressure, reported intake of sodium of >4 g/d, and 3+ pitting edema in hands and feet

ADIME 12.2 ADIME At-A-Glance: Chronic Kidney Disease (*continued*)

Intervention

- Nutrition prescription: add 2 g sodium restriction
- Review sodium-containing foods
- Review label reading and meal planning

Monitoring and Evaluation

- Improvements in blood pressure and edema
- Food intake logs to show decreased sodium intake and appropriate food choices; have patient submit logs for 1 week

CKD: Dialysis

Initiation of dialysis as a kidney replacement therapy (KRT) option starts at stage 5 CKD when GFR falls to <15 mL/min/1.72 m^2, although initiation at higher levels of kidney function may be necessary for some patients.[7] KDOQI refers to dialysis-dependent CKD as CKD 5D.

The two main types are hemodialysis (HD) and peritoneal dialysis (PD). In HD, blood from an artery circulates through a mechanical dialyzer, where it is filtered and returned to the body via the parallel vein. HD is an intermittent therapy that takes place 3 times per week, with sessions lasting 3 to 5 hours. HD is typically performed at a dialysis center; however, at-home dialysis treatments are becoming more popular. In PD, the patient's own peritoneum serves as the filtration membrane. The dialysis solution (dialysate) is placed into the peritoneal cavity, periodically drained, and replaced with a fresh solution via a catheter (the process is called an exchange). To allow for removal of waste products from the blood, a hyperosmolar dextrose dialysate is used, which results in some dextrose being absorbed by the patient during the process. The daily amount of dextrose absorbed depends on the concentration of dextrose used for each exchange and on the number of exchanges (Box 12.2). Currently, three concentrations of PD dialysate are available: 1.5%, 2.5%, and 4.25%. The dextrose and kilocalorie absorption should be taken into consideration when developing a diet plan for peritoneal

BOX 12.2 Simple Estimation of Dextrose Kilocalories Absorbed from Peritoneal Dialysis

- Continuous cycling peritoneal dialysis (CCPD)[a] allows **40%** dextrose absorption.
- Continuous ambulatory peritoneal dialysis (CAPD) allows **60%** dextrose absorption.
- Each gram of dextrose = 3.4 kcal

Dialysate Dextrose Concentration	Grams of Dextrose/L	kcal/L from Dextrose	kcal/L with CCPD (40%)	kcal/L with CAPD (60%)
1.5%	15 g	51 kcal	21 kcal	31 kcal
2.5%	25 g	85 kcal	34 kcal	51 kcal
4.25%	42.5 g	144.5 kcal	57.8 kcal	86.7 kcal

Example: A CAPD patient uses 4 L of 1.5% dialysate and 4 L of 4.25% dialysate daily.
4 L of 1.5% = 124 kcal (31 kcal/L × 4 L)
4 L of 4.25% = 346 kcal (86.7 kcal/L × 4 L)
Total kcal absorbed from dextrose = **470**

[a]CCPD is an automated form of peritoneal dialysis and may also be referred to as APD.

Data from Council on Renal Nutrition of the National Kidney Foundation. In: McCann L, ed. *Pocket Guide to Nutrition Assessment of the Patient with Chronic Kidney Disease*. 5th ed. New York: National Kidney Foundation; 2015.

patients. It is important to monitor patients with diabetes closely for glucose control. In both HD and PD, the diet is more liberalized compared with that in the predialysis state.

Treatment and Nutrition Intervention

Laboratory values monitored in CKD can be found in Table 12.4. A listing of nutrient needs for dialyzed patients can be found in Table 12.7, with additional considerations for specific nutrients as follows:

- **Energy and protein** needs should be based on SBW or adjusted edema-free body weight (aBW_{ef}).[8]

TABLE 12.7. Daily Nutrient Needs for Dialyzed Patients

	Hemodialysis	Peritoneal Dialysis
Protein (g/kg)	1.2 stable	1.2–1.3
At least 50% HBV	1.2–1.3 acutely ill or PEW	
Energy (kcal/kg)	35 for age <60 years	35 for age <60 years Include dextrose kcals absorbed from PD
	30–35 for age ≥60 years	30–35 for age ≥60 years Include dextrose kcals absorbed from PD
Potassium (g/d)	2–3	3–4
	Adjust per serum levels	Adjust per serum levels; typically unrestricted
Sodium (g/d)	2–3	2–4
Phosphorus (mg/d)	800–1,000	800–1,000
	Or 10–17 mg/kg/d	Or 10–17 mg/kg/d
Calcium (mg/d)	≤1,000; maintain serum calcium WNL	800; maintain serum calcium WNL
Fluid (mL/d)	750–1,000 plus urine output in 24 hr	1,000–2,000 depending on urine output, cardiac status, blood pressure; adjust to maintain fluid balance

WNL, within normal limits.

Data from (i) Kidney Disease: Improving Global Outcomes (KDIGO) CKD Work Group. KDIGO 2012 Clinical Practice Guideline for the evaluation and management of chronic kidney disease. *Kidney Int Suppl* 2013;3:1–150, (ii) National Kidney Foundation KDOQI. Clinical Practice Guidelines for chronic kidney disease: Evaluation, classification, and stratification. *AM J Kidney Dis* 2002;39(Suppl 1):S1–S266, and (iii) National Kidney Foundation KDOQI. *Clinical Practice Guidelines for Bone Metabolism and Disease in Chronic Kidney Disease.* New York: National Kidney Foundation; 2004.

$$aBW_{ef} = BW_{ef} + [(SBW - BW_{ef}) \times 0.25],$$

where BW_{ef} is actual edema-free body weight and SBW is the standard body weight (NHANES II data)

Goals should be adjusted for stress, illness, and infections as needed. Protein recommendations for dialysis are higher because of losses through the artificial kidney membrane and blood loss in HD, and through the peritoneal membrane in PD. PD patients in particular face a high risk of protein malnutrition, partly because of greater losses of amino acids and proteins (8 to 10 g/d) in the dialysate through the daily exchanges. Appetite suppression, as a direct effect of dialysate dextrose calories as well as from uremia, may contribute to suboptimal food intake. HBV protein should account for at least 50% of the protein allowance.[8] Total calories for PD patients should be adjusted for the calories absorbed from the dialysate to control potential obesity, hyperlipidemia, and hyperglycemia (in patients with diabetes).

- **Potassium** restriction is only necessary if the patient is hyperkalemic. Potassium allowance is liberalized in PD because of frequent dialysis exchanges that consistently remove potassium; potassium supplementation may be needed at times to maintain serum levels in the normal range. HD patients may have increased potassium needs when potassium-depleting diuretics are used or increased losses are related to the etiology of the renal failure, as in polycystic kidney disease or high residual kidney function. For diabetic patients requiring the standard potassium restriction, care should be taken in selecting interventions for hypoglycemic reactions (Table 12.6).
- **Sodium** intake is limited to help control volume expansion, thirst, and edema. High dietary intake and inadequate sodium removal during HD result in excess fluid intake and hypertension. Chronic extracellular volume overload is associated with higher cardiovascular morbidity and mortality. The PD diet is more liberal in sodium because of greater losses to the dialysate.

- **Phosphorus** intake is limited to maintain serum phosphorus levels in goal range and reduce stimulation of PTH secretion.[9] The phosphorus level is also controlled with the inclusion of phosphate-binding medications. These medications, taken with meals and snacks, bind phosphorus in the GI tract and reduce the amount of phosphorus absorbed into the blood. Educate patient to read food labels to identify phosphorus sources.
- Elemental **calcium** intake should be limited to 2,000 mg daily from oral intake and medication.[9] Calcium-based phosphate binders and calcium-fortified foods that are widespread in the food supply must be given close attention in meeting this dietary limitation. Renal osteodystrophy is common in both dialysis groups and typically in the form of *osteomalacia* (bone demineralization), *osteitis fibrosa cystica,* which is caused by elevated PTH, and *metastatic calcification* of joints and soft tissue. Limiting calcium and phosphorous, and treatment with calcitriol and phosphate binders plays a large role in improving these skeletal disorders. Monitoring of serum phosphorous and calcium levels should be more frequent when patients are on calcitriol therapy. Calcitriol should be discontinued in the presence of elevated calcium-phosphorous product, especially with severe hyperparathyroidism.
- **Fluid** limitations are dictated by the amount of urine output and interdialytic weight gains. Goal fluid gains between HD treatments should not exceed 5% of the estimated dry weight. Patients should be free of shortness of breath, edema (peripheral, facial, and ascites), and significant elevation in blood pressure prior to treatment. Fluid intake is more liberal in PD.
- **Vitamin** requirements can follow the recommended dietary allowance (RDA). Nutrition supplements designed specifically for dialysis patients can be useful because these products offer the best nutrient profile with limited fluid for a dialysis patient; however, many patients can also tolerate the standard or basic supplements. Intake

of vitamins and minerals may be decreased because of the restriction of foods containing potassium, which limits fruit and vegetable intake. Water-soluble vitamins are also lost through dialysis. Peripheral neuropathy and hyperoxalemia, particularly in HD, are associated with high-dose pyridoxine and vitamin C supplementation. Vitamin A supplementation leads to retention and toxicity. Megavitamin therapy should be discouraged.

Malnutrition and Dialysis

Malnutrition is common in dialysis patients and can be either protein only (in PD) or protein energy malnutrition (in HD). Presence of malnutrition aggravates comorbidities, leading to poor prognosis. Causative factors are reduced dietary intake, poor appetite, increased uremia, metabolic acidosis, increased catabolism, and the dialysis procedure itself. Adherence to low- or very-low-protein diets from the predialysis period inadvertently sets up the suboptimal nutrient milieu contributive to malnutrition in KRT.[11]

Inflammation can be present in dialysis patients, which may lead to cachexia and muscle wasting. This severe form of malnutrition, identified as protein energy wasting (PEW), is persistent, as inflammation, uremia, and hypercatabolism lead to depletion of muscle and fat stores.[12] PEW is associated with reduced strength, poor physical activity, poor quality of life, and higher risk of death. The International Society of Renal Nutrition and Metabolism (ISRNM) has provided guidelines for PEW diagnosis (Box 12.3).

The following corrective interventions may be implemented when providing medical nutrition therapy (MNT) for a malnourished dialysis patient:

- The average protein consumption in ESKD patients is low (less than 1 g/kg/d in ~50% of subjects) along with an equivalent caloric deficit. Thus, nutritional intervention should start early for patients whose spontaneous intake is <30 kcal/kg/d and <1.0 g/kg/d of protein.[13]

BOX 12.3 The ISRNM Criteria for PEW Diagnosis

1. Serum chemistry: low serum levels of albumin, transthyretin, or total cholesterol
2. Body mass: unintentional weight loss over time, decreased BMI or total body fat percentage
3. Muscle mass: decreased muscle mass over time, mid arm muscle circumference, or creatinine appearance
4. Dietary intake: unintentional decreased protein (DPI) or decreased energy intake (DEI)

Note: Diagnosis of PEW requires 3 out of 4 main components.
BMI, body mass index.
Data from Fouque D, Kalantar-Zadeh K, Kopple J, et al. A proposed nomenclature and diagnostic criteria for protein-energy wasting in acute and chronic kidney disease. *Kidney Int* 2008;73:391–398.

- In patients reporting poor appetite, consider diet liberalization and food preferences in meal planning. Intake of foods higher in potassium, sodium, and phosphorus in limited amounts can help the patient increase total calories and protein. Intake of protein-rich food or oral supplements (snacks or light meals) is effective in mitigating the catabolism associated with HD and to increase total protein intake.[14]
- If intake remains inadequate, use of appetite stimulants, liquid supplements, protein, and calorie modulars, as well as more aggressive interventions (tube feeding or parenteral nutrition), should be considered.
- Oral nutrition supplementation (ONS) is recommended as the first step of nutritional support for ESKD patients with suboptimal dietary intake.[13,15] ONS can add up to 10 kcal/kg and 0.3 to 0.4 g of protein/kg daily to spontaneous intake, helping the patient to achieve nutritional targets. Nutrition supplements designed specifically for kidney disease patients can be useful. These supplements have nutrient profiles that fit either low or high protein

requirements, are calorically dense, and can help meet fluid, phosphorus, potassium, and sodium limitations. Many protein modular products in the form of powders, bars, and cookies are available as options for improving protein deficits.

- Intradialytic parenteral nutrition (IDPN) is now proposed as an intensive treatment option to address PEW by the ISRNM.[13] IDPN is the administration of nutrients (usually a mixture of amino acids, dextrose, and lipid emulsions) during each dialysis session, through the extracorporeal circulation lines. IDPN is recommended only if the patient has a spontaneous intake of at least 20 kcal/kg/d and 0.8 to 0.9 g/kg/d of proteins.[13,16] Safe IDPN administration in each dialysis session involves the delivery of not more than 1 L of fluids, 1000 kcal, and 50 g of amino acids.[16]

Pregnancy and Dialysis

Pregnancy in women with ESKD is rare and carries very high rates of neonatal complications, including miscarriage, stillbirths, prematurity, and small-for-gestational-age births.[3] Many nephrologists prescribe long and frequent HD for pregnant women with ESKD, which is necessary to maintain fluid balance, control blood pressure, and reduce uremic toxins of both the mother and the growing fetus.[3] However, the current evidence base is too weak to determine or recommend an optimal session duration.[6] HD sessions offered 6 times per week improve pregnancy-related outcomes.[6] A Canadian dialysis cohort study reported live birth rates of 48% in woman dialyzed ≤20 hr/wk, 75% in women dialyzed for 30 hr/wk, and 85% in women dialyzed for >36 hr/wk.[17] Using this Canadian study evidence, an ungraded statement was made that live birth rates increase with increasing time per HD session.[6]

The nutritional management of the pregnant patient should be on an empirical basis with the following considerations[6]:

- Pregnant patients are likely to be dialyzed daily (BUN is maintained below a range of 50 to 60), allowing for more diet liberalization in all areas.

- Daily protein intake should increase by an additional 20 g above standard dialysis calculations, and energy intake should increase by 100 to 300 kcal.
- Trace elements should be monitored to determine whether supplementation is needed.
- Monitoring of the maternal and infant weight gain is important, and post-dialysis weight should be used for reference.
- Close monitoring of interdialytic weight gain will determine signs and symptoms of fluid overload, and if excessive, fluid removal is necessary.
- Worsening anemia in the pregnant patient requires synthetic erythropoietin, iron, and folate supplementation to support increased blood volume.

Medications in CKD: Nondialysis and Dialysis

The CKD medications are functionally diverse, targeting the symptoms of kidney functions that are declining in stages 3 to 4 CKD patients, and are absent in dialysis patients (Table 12.8). Phosphate binders, intravenous iron, and PTH-suppressing medications will have dose titration based on the laboratory results.[8] Dose titration is generally addressed monthly in a chronic dialysis patient. Aside from these CKD-specific medications, comorbidity presence of diabetes, hyperlipidemia, and/or hypertension will also add to the medication list of CKD patients. All patients should be monitored for common side effects of medications that may contribute to GI intolerance as well as drug–nutrient interactions.[10]

Posttransplant Considerations

Kidney transplantation is the preferred KRT option of CKD patients. KDOQI guidelines refer to non–dialysis-dependent CKD of any stage (1 to 5), with a kidney transplant as CKD–T.[6]

In the immediate postoperative period, protein needs are increased to offset postsurgical hypercatabolism and to enhance wound healing.[10] In this period, fluid restriction may be needed in a patient with significant fluid overload,

TABLE 12.8. Common Medications in CKD

Category	Medication	Comments
Phosphate binders		• All binders must be taken with each meal and snack
• Calcium-based	• Phoslo, Calphron, Eliphos (calcium acetate); Tums, Os-cal, Caltrate (calcium carbonate)	• Monitor for hypercalcemia
• Calcium-free, aluminum-free	• Renvela (sevelamer carbonate), Renagel (sevelamer), Fosrenol (lanthanum carbonate)	• Dose is titrated based on serum phosphorus level and diet intake. • Renagel may exacerbate metabolic acidosis and should be monitored during use.
• Iron-based	• Auryxia (ferric citrate) • Velphoro (sucroferric oxyhydroxide)	• May cause dark stools
• Aluminum-based	• Aluminum hydroxide	• Use of aluminum should be limited to <14 days because of risk of aluminum toxicity.
Potassium binder	• Veltassa (patiromer)	• Binds many oral medications, reducing their effectiveness; other oral meds must be administered at least 6 hr before or 6 hr after Veltassa • Binds to magnesium, so monitor for hypomagnesemia

Vitamin supplements		
Renal-specific formulas	• Dialyvite, Nephrocaps, Nephro-Vite, Rena-Vite • NephPlex, RenaPlex	• Taken daily, usually in the evening to accommodate dialysis treatment days when fluid is removed • Use to replace water-soluble vitamin losses
Iron supplements		
• Oral iron	• Ferrous sulfate, ferrous gluconate, ferrous fumarate	• Oral iron should not be taken with binders.
• IV iron	• Venofer (iron sucrose), Ferrlecit (sodium ferric gluconate complex in sucrose), Infed (iron dextran)	• IV iron is administered during hemodialysis treatments.
Vitamin D		
• Oral vitamin D • Oral and IV vitamin D • IV vitamin D • Oral calcimimetic agent	• Rocaltrol (calcitriol)[a] • Hectorol (doxercalciferol), Zemplar (paricalcitol)[a] • Calcijex (calcitriol)[a] • Sensipar (cinacalcet)[a]	• Oral agents are to be taken consistently as ordered. • IV forms are administered during hemodialysis. • Calcium levels should be monitored closely with use of Rocaltrol and Sensipar.

[a]All agents used to manage PTH levels.

Data from (i) National Kidney Foundation KDOQI. Clinical Practice Guidelines for chronic kidney disease: Evaluation, classification, and stratification. *AM J Kidney Dis* 2002;39(Suppl 1):S1–S266, (ii) Veltassa. Available at: http://www.relypsa.com/our-medicine/veltassa/. Accessed April 3, 2016, (iii) RxLis: The internet drug index. Available at: http://www.rxlist.com. Accessed April 3, 2016, and (iv) Phosphate binders. Available at: http://emedicine.medscape.com/article/241185-medication#3. Accessed April 3, 2016.

but in long-term maintenance, fluid is generally unrestricted. In the stable chronic posttransplant period, most patients should follow the general nutrition guidelines for any healthy individual. Table 12.9 lists the nutrient recommendations for posttransplant patients. Immunosuppressive treatment to prevent kidney allograft rejection is a lifelong strategy and the cornerstone of successful transplantation; however, associated comorbidities such as hyperlipidemia, diabetes mellitus, hypertension, obesity, and osteoporosis may necessitate the need for nutrition intervention.[3]

TABLE 12.9. Daily Nutrient Needs for Kidney Transplant Patients

Nutrients	Acute Posttransplant	Long-Term Maintenance
Protein (g/kg)	1.2–2.0	0.8–1.0
Energy (kcal/kg)	30–35	25–35; maintain healthy body weight
Potassium (g)	2–4; maintain serum levels WNL	Individualize based on serum level, graft function, and immunosuppressant therapy
Sodium (g)	2–4; based on blood pressure and fluid balance	2–4; based on blood pressure, immunosuppressant effect on fluid balance
Phosphorus	RDA; individualize based on serum levels	RDA; individualize based on serum levels
Fluid	Limit if edema or volume overload is present	Unrestricted, unless overloaded

WNL, within normal limits.

Data from Council on Renal Nutrition of the National Kidney Foundation. In: McCann L, ed. *Pocket Guide to Nutrition Assessment of the Patient with Chronic Kidney Disease*. 5th ed. New York: National Kidney Foundation; 2015.

REFERENCES

1. United States Renal Data System. *2015 USRDS Annual Data Report: Epidemiology of Kidney Disease in the United States*. Bethesda, MD: National Institutes of Health, National Institute of Diabetes and Digestive and Kidney Diseases; 2015.
2. Kidney Disease: Improving Global Outcomes (KDIGO) Acute Kidney Injury Work Group. KDIGO Clinical Practice Guideline for Acute Kidney Injury. *Kidney Int Suppl* 2012;2:1–138.
3. Gilbert SJ, Weiner DE. *National Kidney Foundation's Primer on Kidney Diseases*. 6th ed. Philadelphia, PA: Elsevier Saunders; 2014.
4. Palevsky PM, Liu KD, Brophy PD, et al. KDOQI US commentary on the 2012 KDIGO Clinical Practice Guideline for Acute Kidney Injury. *Am J Kidney Dis* 2013;61(5):649–672.
5. McMillan JI. Chronic Kidney Disease. Merck Manual Professional Version. Available at: http://www.merckmanuals.com/professional/genitourinary-disorders/chronic-kidney-disease/chronic-kidney-disease. Accessed March 31, 2016.
6. National Kidney Foundation. KDOQI Clinical Practice Guideline for hemodialysis adequacy: 2015 update. *Am J Kidney Dis* 2015;66(5):884–930.
7. Kidney Disease: Improving Global Outcomes (KDIGO) CKD Work Group. KDIGO 2012 Clinical Practice Guideline for the evaluation and management of chronic kidney disease. *Kidney Int Suppl* 2013;3:1–150.
8. National Kidney Foundation KDOQI. Clinical Practice Guidelines for chronic kidney disease: Evaluation, classification, and stratification. *AM J Kidney Dis* 2002;39(Suppl 1):S1–S266.
9. National Kidney Foundation KDOQI. *Clinical Practice Guidelines for Bone Metabolism and Disease in Chronic Kidney Disease*. New York: National Kidney Foundation; 2004.
10. Council on Renal Nutrition of the National Kidney Foundation. In: McCann L, ed. *Pocket Guide to Nutrition Assessment of the Patient with Chronic Kidney Disease*. 5th ed. New York: National Kidney Foundation; 2015.
11. Kovesdy CP, Kopple JD, Kalantar-Zadeh K. Management of protein-energy wasting in non-dialysis-dependent chronic kidney disease: Reconciling low protein intake with nutritional therapy. *Am J Clin Nutr* 2013;97:1163–1177.

12. Fouque D, Kalantar-Zadeh K, Kopple J, et al. A proposed nomenclature and diagnostic criteria for protein-energy wasting in acute and chronic kidney disease. *Kidney Int* 2008;73:391–398.
13. Ikizler TA, Cano NJ, Franch H, et al. Prevention and treatment of protein energy wasting in chronic kidney disease patients: A consensus statement by the International Society of Renal Nutrition and Metabolism. *Kidney Int* 2013;84:1096–1107.
14. Kalantar-Zadeh K, Ikizler TA. Let them eat during dialysis: An overlooked opportunity to improve outcomes in maintenance hemodialysis patients. *J Ren Nutr* 2013;3:157–163.
15. Kalantar-Zadeh K, Cano NJ, Budde K, et al. Diets and enteral supplements for improving outcomes in chronic kidney disease. *Nat Rev Nephrol* 2011;7:369–384.
16. Sabatino A, Regolisti G, Antonucci E, et al. Intradialytic parenteral nutrition in end stage renal disease: Practical aspects, indications and limits. *J Nephrol* 2014;27:377–383.
17. Luders C, Castro MC, Titan SM, et al. Obstetric outcome in pregnant women on long-term dialysis: A case series. *Am J Kidney Dis* 2010;56:77–85.

Notes

Notes

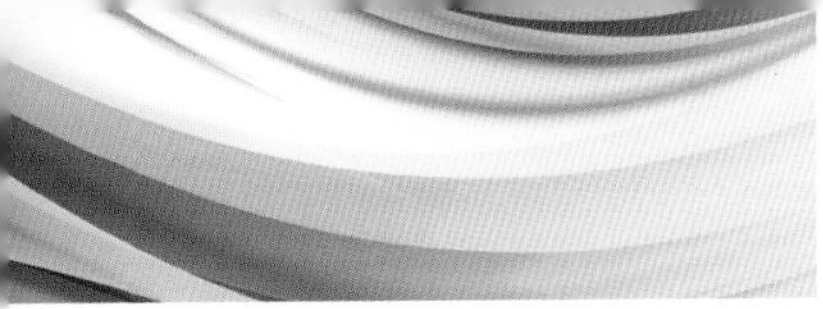

CHAPTER 13

Pulmonary Disease

Chronic lower respiratory disease is the third leading cause of death in the United States.[1] Currently, more than 35 million Americans are living with chronic lung diseases such as asthma, emphysema, or chronic bronchitis. Pulmonary diseases have a significant impact on nutritional status, and the clinician's role is crucial in nutrition assessment and patient education to prevent or correct malnutrition.

CHRONIC OBSTRUCTIVE PULMONARY DISEASE

Disease Process

Chronic obstructive pulmonary disease (COPD) is characterized by persistent airflow limitation that is usually progressive and associated with an enhanced chronic inflammatory response in the airways and lungs to noxious particles or gases.[2] COPD comprises chronic bronchitis (clinically defined) and emphysema (pathologically or radiologically defined). COPD patients typically have chronic bronchitis or emphysema, or a mixture of both.[3,4] Common causes of COPD include cigarette smoking, pipe smoking, and cigar smoking; passive exposure to cigarette smoking; occupational dust and chemicals; air pollution; and genetic factors. The nutritional interventions for emphysema and bronchitis are similar.

Chronic Bronchitis

Chronic bronchitis is characterized by a chronic, productive cough (occurring on most days for a minimum of 3 months, for 2 consecutive years), inflamed bronchial tubes, excess mucus production, and shortness of breath.[4] Patients with chronic bronchitis, often called "blue bloaters" because of cyanosis and edema in the extremities, usually present with right-sided cardiac failure and little to no weight loss.[5] Chronic bronchitis becomes chronic obstructive bronchitis if spirometric evidence of airflow obstruction develops, which happens in a minority of patients.[4]

Emphysema

Emphysema involves the destruction of lung parenchyma, leading to loss of elastic recoil and loss of alveolar septa and radial airway traction, which increases the tendency for airway collapse. Lung hyperinflation, airflow limitation, and air trapping follow.[4] These patients, often called "pink puffers" because of reddish complexion and hyperventilation, are typically thin and breathe with pursed lips. Wheezing, shortness of breath, and chronic mild cough are common. Nutritional depletion is significantly greater in patients with emphysema than in those who have chronic bronchitis.[5]

Treatment and Nutrition Intervention

COPD patients are at risk of weight loss and nutritional deficiencies because of a 15% to 25% increase in resting energy expenditure (REE) owing to difficulty breathing, a higher energy cost of daily activities, reduced caloric intake relative to need because of dyspnea, and the catabolic effect of inflammatory cytokines.[4] Additional factors that may influence energy requirements include chronic infections, chest physical therapy, and pulmonary rehabilitation exercise programs.[6] Medical nutrition therapy (MNT) should focus on prevention and treatment of weight loss and other comorbidities.[7]

Energy, Macronutrients, and Fluid

- Indirect calorimetry (IC), when available, is the preferred method of determining energy expenditure in COPD patients, especially during an exacerbation.[6] When using predictive equations to assess energy needs, increases for the presence of inflammation or physiologic stress and the level of physical activity must be included.

- A high-kilocalorie, high-protein diet is necessary to correct malnutrition in stable COPD patients. Start with 30 to 35 kcal/kg and 1.2 to 1.7 g protein/kg.[5] Body mass index (BMI) and weight change should be used to evaluate weight status.
- When utilizing nutrition support, overfeeding (providing more than 35 kcal/kg unless measured by IC) should be avoided, particularly in patients with hypercapnia. Energy intake should be kept at or below estimated needs to avoid excessive CO_2 production. The routine use of high-fat, low-carbohydrate diets for hypercapnic patients is not warranted.[5]
- Patients with stable COPD generally have normal fluid requirements. Fluid intake should be 1 mL/kcal in the absence of any mitigating circumstances such as vomiting, diarrhea, infection, or fever.[6]

Patient Education

- Gas-forming foods may cause discomfort for some patients because they bloat the abdomen and make breathing more difficult. Foods to avoid/use in moderation include onions, cauliflower, broccoli, melons, peas, corn, cucumbers, cabbage, brussels sprouts, turnips, raw apples, and beans—except green beans. Fried and greasy foods can also cause gas or bloating.
- Use medications that make breathing easier and/or clear airways about 1 hour before eating.
- If the patient is using oxygen, make sure it is worn during food procurement, preparation, and eating.
- Eat small, frequent meals and snacks to help compensate for shortness of breath and possible limited oxygen supply to gastrointestinal (GI) tract. Drink beverages at the end of the meal to avoid early satiety.[5]
- Consider food choices that are easy to chew, swallow, and digest, with nutrients easily absorbed.
- Provide strategies to increase the nutrient density of foods, such as adding the following to foods to increase caloric

and/or protein content: butter, margarine, whipped cream, half and half, cream cheese, sour cream, salad dressings, mayonnaise, honey, jam, sugar, granola, dried fruits, cottage or ricotta cheese, whole milk, powdered milk, ice cream, yogurt, eggs, nuts, seeds, wheat germ, peanut butter.
- Avoid excess sodium, as it may increase edema and make breathing more difficult. Provide patient with list of high-sodium foods.
- Encourage consumption of foods high in omega-3 fatty acids (salmon, haddock, mackerel, tuna, other fish sources).[6]
- Encourage consumption of a diet that meets the recommended dietary allowance (RDA) for antioxidant vitamins A, C, and E.[6]

ADIME 13.1 ADIME At-A-Glance: COPD

Assessment

- Ht, wt, BMI, unintentional wt loss
- Labs: Hgb, Hct, electrolytes, serum iron, arterial blood gases
- Appetite/interest in eating, fatigue, diminished ability to shop for food and prepare meals, SOB, food intake
- NFPE: barrel chest, digital clubbing, cyanosis, loss of fat/muscle, edema

Nutrition Diagnosis

- Unintentional weight loss RT generalized fatigue and decreased ability to walk and stand while preparing food AEB 6.5% wt loss in 30 days
- Inadequate mineral intake (iron) RT decreased intake AEB low serum iron, Hgb, and Hct levels

Intervention

- Small, frequent mini-meals and snacks using easy-to-prepare, nutrient-dense food choices
- Add oral supplements (Ensure) to increase caloric and nutrient intake
- Add iron supplement to daily multivitamin
- Consult physician regarding possible need for oxygen therapy during food preparation and eating
- Refer to social work for possible at-home meal delivery service

Monitoring and Evaluation

- Improvements in caloric intake
- Monitor weight changes

CYSTIC FIBROSIS

Disease Process

Cystic fibrosis (CF) is an autosomal recessive genetic disease of the mucus and sweat glands. CF is characterized by the secretion of thick, tenacious mucus that obstructs the ducts and glands of the respiratory tract, sweat and salivary glands, intestine, pancreas, liver, and reproductive tract. Complications include bronchitis, pneumonia, glucose intolerance, and malabsorption caused by decreased availability of digestive enzymes, decreased bicarbonate secretion, decreased bile acid reabsorption, and decreased nutrient absorption by intestinal microvilli.[6,8]

CF is caused by a defect in the cystic fibrosis transmembrane conductance regulator (CFTR) gene, which codes for a chloride transporter found on the surface of the epithelial cells that line the lungs and other organs. There are channels in these lining cells through which sodium and chloride ions can pass. Normally, the movement of ions brings water to the surface of the airway and keeps the mucus moist. The defective gene acts to block the chloride channels, which causes the mucus to dry out. It is difficult for a person to shift the thick mucus, which then becomes prone to infection by bacteria. This defect also accounts for the high levels of sodium and chloride that are present in the saliva, tears, and sweat of patients with CF.[9] In the digestive tract, the mucus blocks the movement of digestive enzymes into the duodenum, and if left untreated, this lack of pancreatic digestive enzymes can lead to malnutrition. Individuals with CF also have difficulties absorbing the fat-soluble vitamins A, D, E, and K.[6]

Treatment and Nutrition Intervention

The risk for malnutrition in CF patients is high because of increased nutrient needs, decreased intake, and malabsorption. The goals of nutritional care include controlling malabsorption with pancreatic enzyme replacement; providing adequate energy, protein, and other nutrients; and preventing nutritional deficiencies. There are three time periods during which special attention should be given to nutrition for CF patients[10]:

- Birth to 12 months of age
- First 12 months post diagnosis
- Pubertal growth period (girls aged 9 to 16 and boys aged 12 to 18)

Energy

Energy requirements for patients with CF vary widely, and many factors such as gender, age, basal metabolic rate (BMR), physical activity, severity of lung disease, and severity of malabsorption must all be considered when determining appropriate energy levels. Nutrition management guidelines are dependent on the disease progression, with calorie needs increasing as pulmonary and GI function decline.[10]

- For patients with CF who are growing normally without malabsorption, the total daily energy requirement is consistent with 100% to 110% of the estimated energy requirement (EER) from the DRIs for age and sex.[6] DRI EER information can be found in Table 3.9 of this book.
- Needs can increase to 120% to 150% of the EER, with increased activity and severity of disease (with some teenagers needing 3,000 to 4,000 kcal/d).
- Needs can be as high as 200% of EER, during episodes of acute respiratory tract infections or disease exacerbations.
- Nocturnal tube feedings may be used to prevent or treat growth failure or malnutrition (usually providing 30% to 50% of established nutritional needs).

Protein and Fluid

Protein needs are 150% to 200%, or higher, of standard protein needs compared with a healthy population, not to exceed 4 g/kg/d except for cases of severe malabsorption.[6,10] This may translate into 4 g/kg for infants, 3 g/kg for children, 2 g/kg for teens, and 1.5 g/kg for adults.[5–7] Patients with CF typically have normal fluid requirements, unless an underlying disease process requires a restriction such as heart or kidney failure.

Patient Education

- Encourage intake of omega-3 fatty acids to reduce inflammation.
- Vitamin/mineral supplementation should include a daily CF-specific vitamin, with dosing depending on age and laboratory fat-soluble vitamin levels. Vitamin K should also be given to all patients who are taking antibiotics secondary to depletion of beneficial GI flora.[10]
- Additional micronutrient supplementation may vary depending on laboratory values and dietary intake, but can include additional vitamin D, iron, and calcium.[6,10]
- Pancreatic enzyme capsules are taken by mouth with all meals and snacks that contain fat and/or protein. Enzymes work best for approximately 30 to 45 minutes. For infants and young children, capsules can be opened and the microspheres mixed with a soft, acidic food, such as applesauce. Avoid mixing enzymes with milk-based foods such as yogurt or pudding, or anything with pH >6.0 (the alkaline pH will destroy the enteric coating and inactivate the enzymes by exposing them to stomach acid).
- CF patients need sodium replacement[6,10]:
  - Infants: 1/8 tsp (12 mEq Na) salt per day from 0 to 6 months of age, not to exceed 4 mEq/kg/d
  - Increase to 1/4 tsp (25.2 mEq Na) daily for 6 to 12 months of age, not to exceed 4 mEq/kg/d
  - Greater than 1 year of age: very liberal salt diet especially in hot climates or with high activity

Cystic Fibrosis-Related Diabetes

Cystic fibrosis-related diabetes (CFRD) is a unique type of diabetes that is prevalent in the CF population. CFRD is unique because it has features of both type 1 and type 2 diabetes, including insulin insufficiency from pancreatic scarring, and insulin resistance.[11]

CF patients should be screened annually for CFRD starting at age 10 with a 2-hour oral glucose tolerance test. Insulin is currently the only medication that has proven effective in CFRD; oral agents are not indicated. Nutrition therapy incorporates carbohydrate counting so insulin can be adjusted at mealtimes, but dietary restrictions are kept to a minimum to avoid weight loss. Patients should be encouraged to balance regular meals and snacks, and insulin should be dosed accordingly.

ADIME 13.2 ADIME At-A-Glance: Cystic Fibrosis

Assessment

- Ht (length in children), wt, BMI, head circumference, mid-arm circumference, triceps skinfold, growth velocity
- Labs: serum vitamin A, D, E levels, PT/PTT, fasting plasma glucose; A1C (quarterly); fecal elastase levels (newly diagnosed patients), Hgb, Hct, zinc levels
- Appetite/oral intake, steatorrhea, abdominal pain, edema
- Eating behaviors in children
- Physical activity level (exercise)
- Pancreatic enzyme replacement therapy

Nutrition Diagnosis

- Inadequate oral intake RT increased nutrient needs owing to chronic lung disease and shortened meal times AEB decline in growth velocity and shortened meal time owing to typical childhood behaviors

Intervention

- Increase caloric intake by adding two snacks per day and additional calories to prepared foods with butter, milk, gravy, etc.
- Provide at least two servings per day of oral supplements of choice
- Educate family on importance of increasing calories and nutrients to support lung function and reverse decline in growth velocity
- Refer to psychologist for help with mealtime behaviors to maximize intake

Monitoring and Evaluation

- Improvements in growth
- Consider tube feeding if weight goals are not achieved

RESPIRATORY FAILURE

Disease Process

Respiratory failure (RF) is a life-threatening impairment of the gas-exchange functions of the lungs, either oxygenation or carbon dioxide elimination, or both. RF is defined as either hypoxemic (drop in blood oxygen levels) or hypercapnic (rise in arterial carbon dioxide levels). Hypoxemic RF (type I) is characterized by an arterial oxygen tension (Pa_{O_2}) of <60 mm Hg, with a normal or low carbon dioxide tension (Pa_{CO_2}). Type 1 is the most common form of RF, and some examples include cardiogenic or noncardiogenic pulmonary edema, pneumonia, and pulmonary hemorrhage. Hypercapnic RF (type II) is characterized by a Pa_{CO_2} of >50 mm Hg. Type II RF patients who are breathing room air often develop hypoxemia as well. Common causes of type II RF include drug overdose, neuromuscular disease, chest wall abnormalities, and severe airway disorders, such as asthma and COPD.[12,13]

RF can be either acute or chronic. Acute hypercapnic RF develops quickly, over minutes to hours, and usually results in a pH <7.3. Chronic RF develops over several days or longer, allowing time for renal compensation and an increase in bicarbonate concentration. Therefore, the pH is usually only slightly decreased.[12]

Arterial Blood Gases

The confirmation of the diagnosis of RF is based on arterial blood gas (ABG) analysis. ABG measurement is a blood test that is performed to determine the oxygen, carbon dioxide, and bicarbonate content, as well as the pH (acidity), of the blood. Its main use is in pulmonology, as many lung diseases feature poor gas exchange, but it is also used in nephrology and electrolyte disturbances. In pulmonology, the test is used to evaluate respiratory diseases and conditions that affect the lungs, to measure the effectiveness of ventilation and oxygen therapy, and to evaluate overall acid–base balance.[14,15] See Table 13.1 for ABG components.

TABLE 13.1. Arterial Blood Gases

Analyte	Normal Range	Interpretation
pH	7.35–7.45	<7.35 = acidosis >7.45 = alkalosis <6.8 or >7.8 is usually fatal.
Pa_{CO_2}	35–45 mm Hg	Partial pressure of carbon dioxide in arterial blood (reflects CO_2 concentration). A high Pa_{CO_2} (respiratory acidosis) indicates hypoventilation; a low Pa_{CO_2} (respiratory alkalosis) indicates hyperventilation.
Pa_{O_2}	70–100 mm Hg	Partial pressure of oxygen in arterial blood. On room air. Values below 60 may require immediate action and possibly mechanical ventilation.
Sa_{O_2}	94%–100%	Saturation of hemoglobin available for transporting oxygen in the arteries.
HCO_3	22–26 mEq/L	Bicarbonate-metabolic indicator of kidney's role in maintaining normal pH values. A low HCO_3 indicates metabolic acidosis; a high HCO_3 indicates metabolic alkalosis.
CO_2	19–24 mEq/L	Dissolved carbon dioxide in the blood.
Base excess	–2 to 2 mEq/L	Represents the amount of buffering anions in the blood, with HCO_3 being the largest. A negative-base excess (deficit) indicates metabolic acidosis. A positive-base excess indicates metabolic alkalosis or compensation to prolonged respiratory acidosis.

Data from (i) Grogono AW. Acid-base tutorial. Tulane University Departments of Anesthesiology. Available at: www.acid-base.com/index.php. Accessed February 20, 2016 and (ii) Pagana KD, Pagan TJ. *Mosby's Manual of Diagnostic and Laboratory Tests*. 5th ed. St. Louis, MO: Elsevier Mosby; 2014:109–118.

Acid–Base Balance

When the pulmonary system is compromised by diseases such as RF or COPD, the ability of the lungs to regulate acid–base balance can be affected. Acid–base balance within the body is required to provide an optimal environment for enzymatic and cellular activity. When normal physiology is altered, acid–base imbalances may result. These can be defined as either acidosis or alkalosis. When the acid–base disturbance results from a primary change in HCO_3^-, it is a metabolic disorder; when the primary disturbance alters blood $Paco_2$, it is a respiratory disorder. Compensation for these disturbances can be respiratory or metabolic in nature and is intended to minimize further pH changes.[14] Box 13.1 lists acid–base disturbances and the body's physiologic response.[8,14,15]

BOX 13.1 Acid–Base Disturbances

Respiratory Acidosis

- **Common causes:** asphyxia, respiratory depression (drugs, central nervous system trauma), pulmonary disease (pneumonia, COPD, respiratory underventilation)
- **Mechanism of compensation:** Kidneys will retain HCO_3 and excrete H^+ to increase pH.

	Uncompensated	Compensated
pH	<7.35	Normal
$Paco_2$	↑	↑
HCO_3	Normal	↑

Respiratory Alkalosis

- **Common causes:** hyperventilation (anxiety, pain, respiratory overventilation), pulmonary emboli
- **Mechanism of compensation:** Kidneys will excrete HCO_3 and retain H^+ to decrease pH.

	Uncompensated	Compensated
pH	>7.45	Normal
$Paco_2$	↓	↓
HCO_3	Normal	↓

(continued)

BOX 13.1 Acid–Base Disturbances (*continued*)

Metabolic Acidosis

- **Common causes:** diabetic ketoacidosis, shock, renal failure, intestinal fistula, diarrhea, starvation
- **Mechanism of compensation:** Respiratory rate increases, and so lungs "blow off" excess CO_2 to increase pH.

	Uncompensated	Compensated
pH	<7.35	Normal
$Paco_2$	Normal	↓
HCO_3	↓	↓

Metabolic Alkalosis

- **Common causes:** excessive vomiting, diuretics, hypercalcemia, antacid overdose
- **Mechanism of compensation:** Respiratory rate decreases to retain CO_2 and decrease pH.

	Uncompensated	Compensated
pH	>7.35	Normal
$Paco_2$	Normal	↑
HCO_3	↑	↑

Treatment and Nutrition Intervention

Mechanical ventilation is used when a patient's spontaneous ventilation is inadequate to maintain life. In addition, it is indicated as a measure to control ventilation in critically ill patients and as prophylaxis for impending collapse of other physiologic functions. Physiologic indications include respiratory or mechanical insufficiency and ineffective gas exchange.[16]

It is important for the dietitian working in intensive care to be familiar with ventilator modes and settings. This information is useful when conducting nutrition assessments and calculating nutritional requirements for RF patients on mechanical ventilation. Table 13.2 describes common ventilator modes.

TABLE 13.2. Ventilator Modes

Mode	Name	Description
ACV	Assist-control ventilation	Triggered by patient breaths, but if patient fails to trigger the threshold, a mechanically controlled breath is delivered.
CMV	Continuous mandatory ventilation	Ventilator delivers breaths at a set rate and volume or pressure, regardless of patient effort.
CPAP	Continuous positive airway pressure	Positive pressure applied during spontaneous breathing and maintained throughout the entire respiratory cycle, without ventilator assistance.
IMV	Intermittent mandatory ventilation	Combination of spontaneous and CMV—patient can breathe spontaneously between ventilator breaths that are delivered at a set rate and volume or pressure.
MMV	Mandatory minute ventilation	Patient breathes spontaneously, yet a minimum level of minute ventilation is ensured.
PEEP	Positive end-expiratory pressure	Positive pressure applied during machine breathing and maintained at end-expiration.
PSV	Pressure support ventilation	Provides a preset level of positive pressure during each inspiratory effort by the patient.
SIMV	Synchronized intermittent mandatory ventilation	Combines spontaneous and IMV. Intermittent ventilator breaths are synchronized to spontaneous breaths to reduce competition between the ventilator and the patient. If no inspiratory effort is sensed, the ventilator delivers a breath.

Energy and Protein

The use of predictive equations to estimate energy expenditure is a regular part of the nutrition assessment completed by a dietitian. However, in a critically ill patient with pulmonary disease, normal predictive equations may be of little value. The measurement of REE through IC has been shown to be more accurate than published formulas used to predict REE.[17] IC is the measurement of gas exchange used to indicate a patient's cellular metabolic activity. IC measures oxygen consumption and carbon dioxide production to calculate REE and the respiratory quotient. This information can be used to prevent over- and underfeeding of patients. Therefore, IC is the preferred method of determining energy expenditure in critically ill patients.

- If IC is not available, then start with 20 to 25 kcal/kg to avoid overfeeding (25 to 30 kcal/kg in ambulatory patients).
- Once initiated, monitor pulmonary status, body weight, and fluid balance closely to avoid overfeeding.
- Two predictive equations have been shown to be useful in the critical care setting for patients on mechanical ventilation.[7] The Penn State (2003b) and the Modified Penn State (2010) equations can be used and are found in Box 13.2.
- Protein should be provided at 1.2 to 1.5 g/kg/d.[5]

Respiratory Quotient

The respiratory quotient (RQ) measures the ratio of the volume of carbon dioxide (V_{CO_2}) produced to the volume of oxygen consumed (V_O). This is represented by the following equation:

$$RQ = V_{CO_2}/V_{O_2}$$

The RQ was once thought to be useful as a means to determine the source of substrate metabolism (fat, carbohydrate, or protein), although this assumption was never verified by research.[17] Stored CO_2 in the body can be mobilized with

BOX 13.2 Predictive Equations for Patients on Mechanical Ventilation

Penn State (2003b) equation: Use for nonobese or obese patients

$$\text{RMR} = \text{Mifflin}\ (0.96) + V_E\ (31) + T_{max}\ (167) - 6{,}212$$

Modified Penn State (2010) equation: Use for obese patients

$$\text{RMR} = \text{Mifflin}\ (0.71) + V_E\ (64) + T_{max}\ (85) - 3{,}085$$

Both equations above use the Mifflin–St. Jeor equation

Men: $\text{RMR} = (9.99 \times W) + (6.25 \times H) - (4.92 \times A) + 5$

Women: $\text{RMR} = (9.99 \times W) + (6.25 \times H) - (4.92 \times A) - 161$

RMR, resting metabolic rate; V_E, expired minute ventilation; T_{max}, maximum body temp in previous 24 hour in degree Celsius; W, weight in kg using actual BW; H, height in cm; A, age.

Data from Academy of Nutrition and Dietetics, Evidence Analysis Library. *Critical Illness: Critical Illness Guidelines: Determination of Resting Metabolic Rate.* 2012. Available at: http://www .eatrightpro.org/resources/research/evidence-based-resources/evidence-analysis-library. Accessed February 1, 2016.

hyperventilation, and would thus reflect an increase in CO_2 excretion but not necessarily production, which would have an erroneous effect on the measured RQ. A clinical benefit of the measured RQ is to validate an IC study. Measured values of RQ that fall outside the physiologic range of 0.67 to 1.3 can infer serious problems with test validity, and almost always represent human or machine calibration errors. In addition, the RQ may be used as a measure of tolerance to feeding. A significant rise in measured RQ, especially above 1.0 in response to enteral or parenteral feeding, may indicate mild respiratory compromise and the need for alteration in the nutrition support regimen. However, the application of the RQ as a marker of substrate use has limited clinical usefulness.[18]

BOX 13.3. Common Respiratory Abbreviations

ABG	Arterial blood gas
ARDS	Adult respiratory distress syndrome
BP	Blood pressure
CF	Cystic fibrosis
CO_2	Carbon dioxide
COPD	Chronic obstructive pulmonary disease
CPAP	Continuous positive airway pressure
CVP	Central venous pressure
CWP	Coal worker's pneumoconiosis
DOE	Dyspnea on exertion
ET	Endotracheal tube
FEV	Forced expiratory volume
FEV_1	Forced expiratory volume in 1 sec
FIO_2	Fraction of inspired oxygen
HCO_3	Bicarbonate
IF	Inspiratory force
$Paco_2$	Partial pressure of arterial carbon dioxide
Pao_2	Partial pressure of arterial oxygen
PEEP	Positive end-expiratory pressure
Sao_2	Saturation of arterial hemoglobin with oxygen
SOB	Shortness of breath
TLC	Total lung capacity
V_T	Tidal volume
VC	Vital capacity

References

1. Centers for Disease Control and Prevention. Leading Causes of Death. Available at: http://www.cdc.gov/nchs/fastats/leading causes-of-death.htm#. Accesses February 20, 2016.
2. Global Initiative for Chronic Obstructive Lung Disease (GOLD). Global strategy for the diagnosis, management, and prevention of chronic obstructive pulmonary disease. Updated 2014. Available at: http://www.goldcopd.org/uploads/users/files/GOLD_Report_2014_Jan23.pdf. Accessed February 20, 2016.
3. Centers for Disease Control and Prevention. What is COPD? Available at: http://www.cdc.gov/copd/index.html. Accessed February 20, 2016.

4. Wise RA. Chronic Obstructive Pulmonary Disease. Merck Manual Professional Version. Available at: http://www.merckmanuals.com/professional/pulmonary-disorders/chronic-obstructive-pulmonary-disease-and-related-disorders/chronic-obstructive-pulmonary-disease-(copd). Accessed February 20, 2016.
5. Escott-Stump S. *Nutrition and Diagnosis-Related Care*. 8th ed. Philadelphia, PA: Wolters Kluwer; 2015:315–318.
6. Academy of Nutrition and Dietetics. Nutrition Care Manual. https://www.nutritioncaremanual.org. Accessed February 21, 2016.
7. Academy of Nutrition and Dietetics, Evidence Analysis Library. *Critical Illness: Critical Illness Guidelines: Determination of Resting Metabolic Rate*. 2012. Available at: http://www.eatrightpro.org/resources/research/evidence-based-resources/evidence-analysis-library. Accessed February 1, 2016.
8. Mahan LK, Escott-Stump S, Raymond JL. *Krause's Food and the Nutrition Care Process*. 13th ed. St. Louis, MO: Elsevier Saunders; 2012:788–794.
9. Cystic fibrosis transmembrane conductance regulator, CFTR Online Mendelian Inheritance in Man (OMIM). John Hopkins University. Available at: http://omim.org/entry/602421. Accessed February 20, 2016.
10. Texas Children's Hospital. *Pediatric Nutrition Reference Guide*. 10th ed. Houston, TX: Texas Children's Hospital; 2013.
11. Cystic Fibrosis Foundation. Cystic Fibrosis-Related Diabetes. Available at: https://www.cff.org/Living-with-CF/Cystic-Fibrosis-Related-Diabetes/. Accessed February 20, 2016.
12. Kaynar AM. Respiratory failure. Available at: www.emedicine.com/med/topic2011.htm. Accessed February 20, 2016.
13. Hall JB, McShane PJ. Overview of Respiratory Failure. Merck Manual Professional Version. Available at: https://www.merckmanuals.com/professional/critical-care-medicine/respiratory-failure-and-mechanical-ventilation/overview-of-respiratory-failure. Accessed February 20, 2016.
14. Grogono AW. Acid-base tutorial. Tulane University Departments of Anesthesiology. Available at: www.acid-base.com/index.php. Accessed February 20, 2016.
15. Pagana KD, Pagan TJ. *Mosby's Manual of Diagnostic and Laboratory Tests*. 5th ed. St. Louis, MO: Elsevier Mosby; 2014:109–118.
16. Byrd RP. Mechanical ventilation. Available at: www.emedicine.com/med/topic3370.htm. Accessed February 20, 2016.

17. Siobal MS, Baltz JE. A Guide to the Nutritional Assessment and Treatment of the Critically Ill Patient. Produced by the American Association for Respiratory Care. 2013. Available at: https://c.aarc.org/education/nutrition_guide/nutrition_guide.pdf. Accessed February 20, 2016.
18. McClave SA, Lowen CC, Kleber MJ, et al. Clinical use of the respiratory quotient obtained from indirect calorimetry. *JPEN J Parenter Enteral Nutr* 2003;27(1):21–26.

NOTES

NOTES

Appendix A
Laboratory Assessment

Kelly Sanna-Gouin, RD, CNSC

Laboratory and other diagnostic tests are tools used by clinicians to gain valuable, objective information about their patients. When used in conjunction with additional patient information, such as anthropometric data, a thorough history, and a physical examination, laboratory tests can provide valuable information about a patient's nutritional status and his or her response to medical nutrition therapy.

This appendix contains an alphabetical list of common laboratory (lab) measurements that are relevant to nutrition assessment. This list is not meant to be comprehensive; rather, it is a quick reference to the lab tests most commonly used by dietitians in the clinical setting.

Normal values are listed, but it must be noted that normal ranges of lab test results vary significantly, depending on the lab and their methods of testing. It is important to always check the normal values at the facility where the test is performed. This information is almost always given directly adjacent to the patient-specific lab result. In this book, Reference Ranges for blood tests are reported in the conventional US system first, then in the SI system (International System of Units or Système Internationale d'Unités), if available. Critical values are also listed, if applicable. All values given are for adults. Conditions that may cause test results to be increased or decreased are listed under the heading "Clinical Implications."

TYPICAL LAB CHARTING

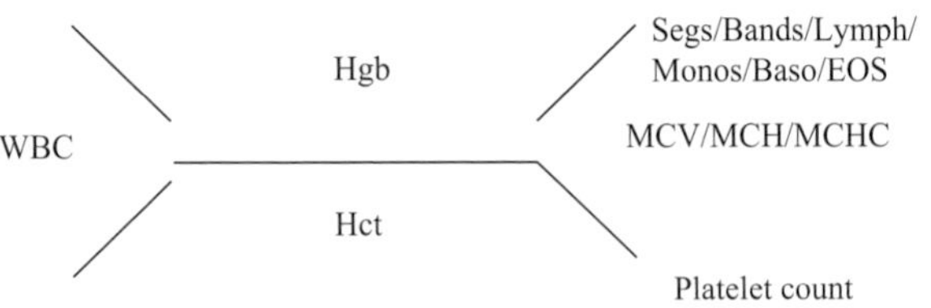

Figure A-1. Complete blood count.

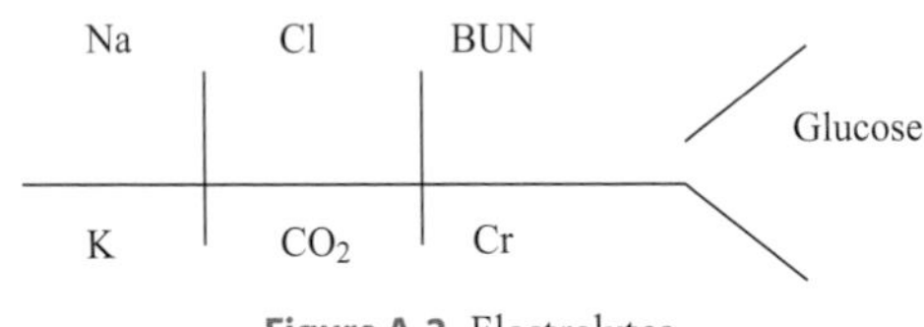

Figure A-2. Electrolytes.

LABORATORY VALUES FOR ASSESSING NUTRITIONAL STATUS

ALBUMIN

Reference Range

3.5–5.0 g/dL or 35–50 g/L

Clinical Implications

Increased Levels

Dehydration

Decreased Levels

Malnutrition; pregnancy; acute and chronic inflammation and infections; cirrhosis, liver disease, alcoholism; nephrotic syndrome, renal disease; burns; third-space losses; protein-losing enteropathies, such as Crohn disease; overhydration

ARTERIAL BLOOD GASES (ABGs; BLOOD GASES)

Reference Range

pH: 7.35–7.45 (critical values: <7.25 or >7.55)

P_{CO_2}: 35–45 mm Hg (critical values: <20 or >60 mm Hg)

HCO_3: 21–28 mEq/L (critical values: <15 or >40)

P_{O_2}: 80–100 mm Hg (critical values: <40)

O_2 saturation: 95%–100% (critical values: 75% or lower)

Clinical Implications: pH

Increased Levels (Alkalosis)

Metabolic: hypokalemia; hypochloremia; chronic vomiting; aldosteronism; chronic and high-volume gastric suctioning; sodium bicarbonate administration

Respiratory: hypoxemic states (e.g., congestive heart failure [CHF], cystic fibrosis [CF], carbon monoxide poisoning, pulmonary emboli, shock, acute pulmonary diseases); anxiety, neuroses, psychoses; pain; pregnancy

Decreased Levels (Acidosis)

Metabolic: ketoacidosis (diabetes and starvation); lactic acidosis; severe diarrhea; renal failure; strenuous exercise

Respiratory: respiratory failure; neuromuscular depression; pulmonary edema

Clinical Implications: P_{CO_2}

Increased Levels

Chronic obstructive pulmonary disease (COPD; bronchitis, emphysema); oversedation; head trauma; other causes of hypoventilation (e.g., Pickwickian syndrome)

Decreased Levels

Hypoxemia; pulmonary emboli; anxiety; pain; pregnancy; other causes of hyperventilation

Clinical Implications: HCO_3

Increased Levels

Chronic vomiting or high-volume gastric suction; aldosteronism; COPD; use of mercurial diuretics

Decreased Levels

Chronic or severe diarrhea; chronic use of loop diuretics; starvation; acute renal failure; diabetic ketoacidosis

Clinical Implications: Po_2

Increased Levels

Polycythemia; increased inspired O_2; hyperventilation

Decreased Levels

Anemias; mucous plug; bronchospasm; atelectasis

BLOOD UREA NITROGEN (BUN)

Reference Range

10–20 mg/dL or 3.6–7.1 mmol/L
(Critical values: >100 mg/dL indicates serious impairment of renal function.)

Clinical Implications

Increased Levels

Prerenal (hypovolemia, shock, burns, dehydration, CHF, myocardial infarction [MI], gastrointestinal [GI] bleeding, excessive protein ingestion, catabolism, starvation, or sepsis); renal (renal disease or failure, nephrotoxic drugs); postrenal (urethral obstruction from stones/tumors/congenital anomalies, bladder outlet obstruction from prostatic hypertrophy, cancer, or congenital anomalies)

Decreased Levels

Liver failure; acromegaly; malnutrition; overhydration; negative nitrogen balance; syndrome of inappropriate secretion of antidiuretic hormone (SIADH); pregnancy; nephrotic syndrome; anabolic steroid use; impaired absorption (celiac disease)

CALCIUM (Ca)—TOTAL AND IONIZED CALCIUM

Reference Range

Total Ca: 9.0–10.5 mg/dL or 2.25–2.75 mmol/L
(Critical values: <6 or >13 mg/dL or <1.5 or >3.25 mmol/L)
Ionized Ca: 4.5–5.6 mg/dL or 1.05–1.30 mmol/L
(Critical values: <2.2 or >7 mg/dL or <0.78 or >1.58 mmol/L)

Clinical Implications

Increased Levels (Hypercalcemia)

Hyperparathyroidism; cancer with parathyroid hormone (PTH)-producing tumors (metastatic bone cancers, Hodgkin lymphoma, leukemia, and non-Hodgkin lymphoma); Paget disease of the bone; prolonged immobilization; milk–alkali syndrome; excessive intake of vitamin D, milk, antacids; Addison disease; granulomatous infections (e.g., sarcoidosis, tuberculosis)

Decreased Levels (Hypocalcemia)

Pseudohypocalcemia caused by low albumin levels[1]; hypoparathyroidism; renal failure; hyperphosphatemia secondary to renal failure; rickets; vitamin D deficiency; osteomalacia; malabsorption; pancreatitis; malnutrition; alkalosis

CHLORIDE (Cl)

Reference Range

98–106 mEq/L or 98–106 mmol/L
(Critical values: <80 or >115 mEq/L)

[1]Because about one-half of blood calcium is bound to albumin, when albumin levels are low, the serum calcium will also be low. Calcium levels can be adjusted with the following equation, when serum albumin is low: Corrected calcium = total calcium mg/dL + 0.8 [4 – serum albumin g/dL].

Implications

Increased Levels (Hyperchloremia)

Dehydration; Cushing syndrome; hyperparathyroidism; renal tubular acidosis; metabolic acidosis; eclampsia; hyperventilation, which causes respiratory alkalosis

Decreased Levels

Overhydration; prolonged vomiting or gastric suctioning; CHF; chronic diarrhea or high-output GI fistula; metabolic alkalosis; burns; Addison disease; salt-losing nephritis; SIADH; fever; ulcerative colitis

CHOLESTEROL[2]

Reference Range

Desirable: 140–199 mg/dL or 3.63–5.17 mmol/L

Borderline high: 200–239 mg/dL or 5.18–6.21 mmol/L

High: >240 mg/dL or >6.22 mmol/L

Clinical Implications

Increased Levels (Hypercholesterolemia)

Familial hypercholesterolemia and/or hyperlipidemia; hypothyroidism; poorly controlled diabetes mellitus (DM); nephrotic syndrome; cholestasis; pregnancy (third trimester); obesity; high dietary intake; Werner syndrome; acute MI; atherosclerosis; biliary cirrhosis; pancreatectomy

Decreased Levels

Malabsorption; malnutrition; advanced cancer; hyperparathyroidism; chronic anemias; severe burns; sepsis/ stress; liver disease

[2]Note: See Chapter 8 for more information on lipoprotein values.

CREATININE (SERUM CREATININE)

Reference Range

Female: 0.5–1.1 mg/dL or 44–97 μmol/L

Male: 0.6–1.2 mg/dL or 53–106 μmol/L

(Critical values for female and male: >4 mg/dL)[3]

Clinical Implications

Increased Levels

Impaired renal function (e.g., glomerulonephritis, pyelonephritis, acute tubular necrosis, urinary tract obstruction); muscle disease (gigantism, acromegaly); rhabdomyolysis; shock (prolonged); diabetic nephropathy; CHF

Decreased Levels

Debilitation; decreased muscle mass (e.g., muscular dystrophy, myasthenia gravis); advanced and severe liver disease, with age proportional to decrease in muscle mass

ERYTHROPOIETIN (EPO)

Reference Range

5–35 IU/L

Clinical Implications

Increased Levels

Anemia (iron deficiency, megaloblastic, hemolytic); myelodysplasia; chemotherapy; AIDS; renal cell carcinoma; adrenal carcinoma; pregnancy

Decreased Levels

Polycythemia vera; rheumatoid arthritis (RA); multiple myeloma

[3]Note: Reduced muscle mass in elderly and young patients may cause decreased values, which may mask renal disease in these age groups.

FOLIC ACID (FOLATE)

Reference Range

5–25 mg/mL or 11–57 mmol/L

Clinical Implications

Increased Levels

Pernicious anemia, vitamin B_{12} deficiency; vegetarianism; recent massive blood transfusion; blind loop syndrome

Decreased Levels

Inadequate intake (malnutrition, chronic disease, alcoholism, anorexia, diet devoid of fresh vegetables); malabsorption (e.g., small bowel disease); pregnancy; megaloblastic anemia; hemolytic anemia; malignancy; chronic renal disease; drugs that are folic antagonists (phenytoin, aminopterin, methotrexate, antimalarials, alcohol, oral contraceptives)

GLUCOSE (BLOOD SUGAR, FASTING BLOOD SUGAR [FBS])

Reference Range

<110 mg/dL or <6.1 mmol/L
(Critical values: <40 and >400 mg/dL)

Clinical Implications

Increased Levels (Hyperglycemia)

DM; Cushing syndrome; acute stress response (MI, cerebrovascular accident [CVA], burns, infection, surgery); pheochromocytoma, acromegaly, gigantism; chronic renal failure; glucagonoma; acute pancreatitis; pregnancy; corticosteroid therapy

Decreased Levels (Hypoglycemia)

Pancreatic islet cell carcinoma; Addison disease; hypothyroidism; hypopituitarism; liver disease; starvation; insulin overdose

GLUCOSE, POSTPRANDIAL (2-HOUR POSTPRANDIAL GLUCOSE [2-HOUR PPG])[4]

Reference Range

0–50 years: 40 mg/dL or <7.8 mmol/L

50–60 years: <150 mg/dL

>60 years: <160 mg/dL

Clinical Implications

Increased Levels

DM; gestational diabetes mellitus (GDM); malnutrition; hyperthyroidism; acute stress response (MI, CVA, burns, infection, surgery); Cushing syndrome; pheochromocytoma; chronic renal failure; glucagonoma; diuretic therapy; corticosteroid therapy; liver disease

Decreased Levels

Insulinoma; hypothyroidism; hypopituitarism; insulin overdose; Addison disease

GLUCOSE TOLERANCE (GT; ORAL GLUCOSE TOLERANCE TEST [OGTT])

Reference Range

Fasting: <110 mg/dL or <6.1 mmol/L

30 minutes: <200 mg/dL or <11.1 mmol/L

1 hour: <200 mg/dL or <11.1 mmol/L

2 hours: <140 mg/dL or <7.8 mmol/L

3 hours: 70–115 mg/dL or <6.4 mmol/L

---

[4]Note: See Chapter 2, Table 2.9, for detailed information on glucose screening for gestational diabetes.

Clinical Implications

Increased Levels

DM; acute stress response (MI, CVA, burns, infection, surgery); Cushing syndrome; pheochromocytoma; chronic renal failure; glucagonoma; diuretic therapy; corticosteroid therapy; liver disease; acute pancreatitis; myxedema; Somogyi response to hypoglycemia

GLYCOSYLATED HEMOGLOBIN (GHB; GLYCOHEMOGLOBIN [GHb], HEMOGLOBIN A1C [HbA1C] OR [A1C])

Reference Range

Nondiabetic adult: 2.2%–4.8%

Good diabetic control: 2.5%–5.9%

Fair diabetic control: 6%–8%

Poor diabetic control: >8%

Clinical Implications

Increased Levels

Newly diagnosed DM; pregnancy; nondiabetic hyperglycemia (acute stress response, Cushing syndrome, pheochromocytoma, glucagonoma, corticosteroid therapy)

Decreased Levels

Hemolytic anemia or other diseases with shortened red blood cell life span such as sickle cell disease and glucose-6-dehydrogenase deficiency; chronic blood loss; chronic renal failure

HEMATOCRIT (Hct; PACKED CELL VOLUME [PCV])

Reference Range[5]

Male: 42%–52% or 0.42–0.52 volume fraction

Female: 37%–47% or 0.37–0.47 volume fraction

[5]Note: Values may be slightly decreased in the elderly.

Clinical Implications

Increased Levels

Erythrocytosis; congenital heart disease; polycythemia vera; severe dehydration; severe COPD; diabetic acidosis; transient cerebral ischemia (TIA); trauma; burns

Decreased Levels

Anemia; hemoglobinopathy; cirrhosis; hemolytic anemia; hemorrhage; dietary deficiency; renal disease; pregnancy; leukemias, lymphomas, Hodgkin lymphoma; peptic ulcer disease; RA

HEMOGLOBIN (Hgb, Hb)

Reference Range[6]

Male: 14–18 g/dL or 8.7–11.2 mmol/L

Female: 12–16 g/dL or 7.4–9.9 mmol/L

(Critical values: <5 g/dL or >20 g/dL)

Clinical Implications

Increased Levels

Erythrocytosis; congenital heart disease; polycythemia vera; severe dehydration; severe COPD; high altitudes; severe burns

Decreased Levels

Anemia; hemoglobinopathy; cirrhosis; hemolytic anemia; hemorrhage; dietary deficiency; bone marrow failure; renal disease; pregnancy; leukemias, lymphomas, Hodgkin lymphoma

HOMOCYSTEINE (HCY)

Reference Range

4–14 μmol/L

[6]Note: Values may be slightly decreased in the elderly.

Clinical Implications

Increased Levels

Vascular diseases (cardiac, cerebral, peripheral); cystinuria; vitamin B_6 or B_{12} deficiency; folate deficiency; malnutrition

IRON LEVEL (Fe)

Reference Range

Male: 80–100 μg/dL or 14–32 μmol/L

Female: 60–60 μg/dL or 11–29 μmol/L

Clinical Implications

Increased Levels

Hemosiderosis or hemochromatosis; iron poisoning; hemolytic anemia; multiple or massive blood transfusions; hepatitis; lead poisoning; nephritis

Decreased Levels

Iron-deficiency anemia; chronic blood loss; insufficient dietary iron intake; third trimester pregnancy; inadequate intestinal absorption of iron

MAGNESIUM (Mg)

Reference Range

1.3–2.1 mEq/L or 0.65–1.05 mmol/L
(Critical values: <0.5 or >3 mEq/L)

Clinical Implications

Increased Levels

Renal insufficiency; Addison disease; hypothyroidism; dehydration; use of magnesium-containing antacids or salts

Decreased Levels

Malnutrition; malabsorption; hypoparathyroidism; alcoholism; chronic renal tubular disease; diabetic acidosis; excessive loss of body fluids (sweating, lactation, diuretic abuse, chronic diarrhea); cirrhosis of the liver; hypokalemia

OSMOLALITY (SERUM OSMOLALITY)

Reference Range

285–295 mOsm/kg H_2O or 285–295 mmol/kg
(Critical values: <265 mOsm/kg or >320 mOsm/kg)

Clinical Implications

Increased Levels

Dehydration; hypernatremia; hypercalcemia; DM, hyperglycemia, diabetic ketoacidosis; azotemia; mannitol therapy; alcohol ingestion (ethanol, methanol, ethylene glycol); uremia; diabetes insipidus

Decreased Levels

Overhydration; SIADH; hyponatremia; acute kidney injury; continuous IV D5W

PHOSPHATE (PO_4), PHOSPHORUS (P)

Reference Range

3.0–4.5 mg/dL or 0.97–1.45 mmol/L
(Critical values: <1 mg/dL)

Clinical Implications

Increased Levels

Renal failure; hypoparathyroidism; acromegaly; bone metastasis; sarcoidosis; hypocalcemia; Addison disease; rhabdomyolysis; healing fractures, hypervitaminosis D

Decreased Levels

Hyperparathyroidism; hypercalcemia; rickets; malnutrition; gram-negative sepsis; hyperinsulinism; alkalosis; IV glucose administration (phosphorus follows glucose into cells); starvation; malabsorption syndrome; hypomagnesemia; chronic alcoholism; vitamin D deficiency; nasogastric suctioning; vomiting

POTASSIUM (K)

Reference Range

3.5–5.0 mEq/L or 3.5–5.0 mmol/L
(Critical values: <2.5 or >6.5 mEq/L)

Clinical Implications

Increased Levels (Hyperkalemia)

Excessive dietary or IV intake; acute or chronic renal failure; Addison disease; hypoaldosteronism; aldosterone-inhibiting diuretics (spironolactone, triamterene); crush or cell damaging injuries (accidents, burns, surgery, chemotherapy); hemolysis; acidosis; dehydration

Decreased Levels (Hypokalemia)

Deficient dietary or IV intake; burns/trauma/surgery; diarrhea/vomiting/sweating; diuretics; hyperaldosteronism; Cushing syndrome; licorice ingestion; alkalosis; glucose administration; CF

PREALBUMIN (PAB; THYROXINE-BINDING PREALBUMIN [TBPA], THYRETIN, TRANSTHYRETIN)

Reference Range

15–36 mg/dL or 150–360 mg/L
(Critical values: <10.7 mg/dL indicates severe nutritional deficiency.)

Clinical Implications

Increased Levels

Hodgkin lymphoma; pregnancy

Decreased Levels

Malnutrition; liver damage; burns; inflammation

PROTHROMBIN TIME (PRO-TIME, INTERNATIONAL NORMALIZED RATIO [INR])

Reference Range

11.0–13.0 seconds; 85%–100% of control
Full anticoagulant therapy: <1.5–2 times control value; 20%–30% of control
(Critical values: >20 seconds; full anticoagulant therapy: 3 times control values)

Clinical Implications

Increased Levels (Prolonged PT)

Liver disease (hepatitis, cirrhosis); hereditary factor deficiency (factors II, V, VII, X); vitamin K deficiency; bile duct obstruction; coumarin ingestion; massive blood transfusion; salicylate intoxication

Decreased Levels

Thrombophlebitis, MI, pulmonary embolism

RED BLOOD CELL COUNT (RBC COUNT; ERYTHROCYTE COUNT)

Reference Range

RBC $\times$ $10^6/\mu L$ or RBC $\times$ $10^{12}/L$
Male: 4.7–6.1; female: 4.2–5.4

Clinical Implications

Increased Levels

Erythrocytosis; congenital heart disease; severe COPD; polycythemia vera; severe dehydration; hemoglobinopathies; high altitude

Decreased Levels

Anemia; cirrhosis; hemorrhage; Addison disease; renal disease; bone marrow failure; pregnancy; rheumatoid/collagen vascular diseases (RA, systemic lupus erythematosus [SLE], sarcoidosis); lymphoma/leukemia/Hodgkin lymphoma; chronic infections, excessive IV fluids

SODIUM (Na)

Reference Range

136–145 mEq/L or 136–145 mmol/L
(Critical values: <120 or >160 mEq/L)

Clinical Implications

Increased Levels (Hypernatremia)

Increased sodium intake (dietary or IV); decreased sodium loss (Cushing syndrome, hyperaldosteronism); excessive free body water loss (GI, excessive sweating, extensive burns, diabetes insipidus, osmotic diuresis)

Decreased Levels (Hyponatremia)

Decreased sodium intake (deficient dietary or IV sodium); increased sodium loss (Addison disease, diarrhea/vomiting, intraluminal bowel loss, diuretic administration, chronic renal insufficiency, gastric suctioning); increased free body water (excessive oral or IV water intake, hyperglycemia, CHF, peripheral edema, pleural effusion, SIADH)

TOTAL IRON-BINDING CAPACITY (TIBC)

Reference Range

250–460 μg/dL or 45–82 μmol/L

Clinical Implications

Increased Levels

Estrogen therapy; polycythemia vera; pregnancy (late); iron-deficiency anemia; acute and chronic blood loss; acute hepatitis

Decreased Levels

Hypoproteinemia (malnutrition or burns); inflammatory diseases; cirrhosis; hemolytic, pernicious, and sickle cell anemias; thalassemia

TRANSFERRIN

Reference Range

Male: 215–365 mg/L or 2.15–3.65 g/L

Female: 250–380 mg/dL or 2.50–3.80 g/L

Clinical Implications

Increased Levels

Estrogen therapy; polycythemia vera; pregnancy (late); iron-deficiency anemia

Decreased Levels

Hypoproteinemia (malnutrition or burns); inflammatory diseases; cirrhosis; hemolytic, pernicious, and sickle cell anemias; renal disease; acute liver disease

TRANSFERRIN SATURATION

Reference Range

Male: 20%–50%

Female: 15%–50%

Clinical Implications

Increased Levels

Hemochromatosis; increased iron intake; hemolytic anemia; thalassemia; acute liver disease

Decreased Levels

Iron-deficiency anemia; anemia of infection and chronic diseases; malignancy

VITAMIN B_{12} (CYANOCOBALAMIN)

Reference Range

160–950 pg/mL or 118–701 mmol/L

Clinical Implications

Increased Levels

Leukemia, polycythemia vera; severe liver dysfunction; diabetes; myeloproliferative disease

Decreased Levels

Pernicious anemia; malabsorption syndromes and inflammatory bowel disease (IBD); intestinal worm infestation; Zollinger–Ellison syndrome; folic acid deficiency; vitamin C deficiency; achlorhydria; large proximal gastrectomy

WHITE BLOOD COUNT AND DIFFERENTIAL COUNT (WBC WITH DIFFERENTIAL)

Reference Range

Total WBCs: 5,000–10,000/mm^3 or 5–10 (10^9/L)
(Critical values: <2,500 or >30,000/mm^3)
Lymphocytes: 1,000–4,000/mm^3 (comprise 20%–40% of the total WBC; and in malnutrition, lymphocyte count is reduced)

Clinical Implications

Increased WBC Count (Leukocytosis)

Infection; leukemic neoplasia or other myeloproliferative disorders; trauma/stress/hemorrhage; tissue necrosis; inflammation; thyroid storm; steroid use

Decreased WBC Count (Leukopenia)

Drug toxicity; bone marrow failure; dietary deficiency of vitamin B_{12} or iron; autoimmune disease; hypersplenism

LABORATORY TEST PANELS

Laboratory tests are often ordered as panels that are disease or organ specific. Next are some common test panels that have significance to the registered dietitian (RD). Note that panels may be modified or expanded at different clinical facilities.

Anemia Panel

Complete blood cell (CBC); RBC indices; reticulocyte count:

Microcytic: erythrocyte sedimentation rate (ESR); iron panel

Normocytic: ESR; hemolysis profile

Macrocytic: vitamin B_{12}; folate; thyroid-stimulating hormone (TSH)

Basic Metabolic Panel (7 Channel/Chem 7/SMA-7)

Carbon dioxide content; chloride, blood; creatinine, blood; glucose, blood; potassium, blood; sodium, blood; urea nitrogen, blood (BUN)

Complete Blood Cell Count with Differential (Diff)

RBC; Hgb; Ht; red blood cell indices (mean corpuscular volume [MCV], mean corpuscular hemoglobin [MCH], mean corpuscular hemoglobin concentration [MCHC], red blood cell distribution width [RDW]); WBC and Diff count (neutrophils, lymphocytes, monocytes, eosinophils, basophils); blood smear; platelet count; mean platelet volume (MPV)

Comprehensive Metabolic Panel (12 Channel/Chem 12)

Albumin; alkaline phosphatase; aspartate aminotransferase (AST) (serum glutamic oxaloacetic transaminase [SGOT]);

bilirubin-total; BUN; calcium; chloride; creatinine; glucose; potassium; protein-total; sodium

The old Comprehensive Metabolic Panel or "Chem 20" includes all the above labs plus:

Alanine aminotransferase (ALT; serum glutamic pyruvic transaminase [SGPT]); bilirubin-direct; carbon dioxide; cholesterol; Gamma glutamyl transpeptidase (GGT); lactase dehydrogenase (LDH); phosphorus; uric acid.

Diabetes Mellitus Management

Anion gap; basic metabolic panel; hemoglobin A1C; lipid profile

Hepatic Function

ALT; albumin; alkaline phosphatase; AST; bilirubin-direct; bilirubin-total; GGT; protein-total; prothrombin time (PT)

Lipid Panel

Cholesterol-total; high-density lipoprotein (HDL); triglyceride; low-density lipoprotein (LDL); very-low-density lipoprotein (VLDL)

Pancreatic Panel

Amylase; calcium; glucose; lipase; triglyceride

Renal Panel

Albumin; basic metabolic panel; calcium; CBC; creatinine clearance; magnesium; phosphorus; protein-total; protein-urine; protein-24-hour urine

References

1. Mayo Clinic. Tests and Procedures. Available at: http://www.mayoclinic.org/tests-procedures. Accessed February 10, 2016.
2. The Science and Practice of Nutrition Support: A Case Based Approach—The Adult Patient. The American Society for Parenteral and Enteral Nutrition; 2007.
3. U.S. National Library of Medicine, Medline Plus. Laboratory Tests. Available at: https://www.nlm.nih.gov/medlineplus/laboratorytests.html. Accessed February 10, 2016.

Appendix B
Food–Drug Interactions

Kelly Sanna-Gouin, RD, CNSC

The following table of medications is not meant to be comprehensive, but instead lists common medications that have significant nutritional implications. The list is alphabetical by generic name (in italics) and cross-referenced by brand or trade name.

Medication	Class and Action	Side Effects	Nutritional Implications
Adalat	See *nifedipine*		
Aldactone	See *spironolactone*		
Apresoline	See *hydralazine*		
Atenolol Tenormin	β-Blocker, antiadrenergic, antiarrhythmic	Diarrhea, constipation, nausea, and vomiting. Possible hypoglycemia. Signs of sympathetic response to hypoglycemia may be masked. May have a decreased insulin release in response to hyperglycemia. Concurrent use of β-adrenergic blockers and St. John's wort or yohimbine may result in a decrease in β-adrenergic blocker effectiveness. Concurrent use of β-adrenergic blockers and ma huang may result in reduced hypotensive effect of β-adrenergic blockers.	Adherence necessary for those following diabetic diet. Monitor blood glucose levels. Be cautious of nonsympathetic signs of hypoglycemia. Consider fluid and electrolyte replacement for diarrhea and vomiting.

Atorvastatin Lipitor	Inhibitor of HMG-CoA reductase	Constipation, diarrhea, gas, upset stomach, and upper right stomach pain. Coenzyme Q10 may be significantly reduced. Concurrent use of atorvastatin and: • Niacin may result in an increased risk of myopathy or rhabdomyolysis. • St. John's wort may result in reduced effectiveness of atorvastatin. • Black cohosh may result in elevated liver enzymes. • Grapefruit juice or grapefruit-containing foods may cause increased bioavailability of atorvastatin, resulting in an increased risk of myopathy or rhabdomyolysis.	Avoid intake of large quantities of grapefruit juice or grapefruit-containing foods, for it increases the absorption of statins (>1 qt/d). Eat a low-cholesterol, low-fat diet for best results. Gastrointestinal (GI) problems are generally transient.
Azithromycin Zithromax	Antibiotic Bacteriostatic or bacteriocidal	Occasional nausea, vomiting, diarrhea, abdominal pain, anorexia, stomatitis, bad taste in mouth.	Take with food to avoid GI disturbances. Azithromycin oral suspension should be taken 1 hr before or 2 hr after meals. Eat small, frequent meals to avoid anorexia. Consider fluid and electrolyte replacement for diarrhea. Avoid alcohol.

(*continued*)

Medication	Class and Action	Side Effects	Nutritional Implications
Bactrim, Bactrim DS	See *sulfamethoxazole*		
Benazepril	Antihypertensive	May increase serum potassium.	Caution with foods high in potassium or potassium supplements. Avoid salt substitutes. Maintain adequate hydration.
Lotensin	ACE inhibitor	May decrease serum sodium.	
		Nausea, salty or metallic taste, mouth sores.	
		Concurrent use of angiotensin-converting enzyme inhibitors and yohimbine or ma huang may result in reduced effectiveness of angiotensin-converting enzyme inhibitors.	
Betaloc	See *metoprolol*		
Biaxin	See *clarithromycin*		
Bumetanide	Diuretic	Ginkgo biloba may cause increased blood pressure. Licorice can increase the risk of hypokalemia. May increase blood glucose, uric acid, cholesterol, LDL, calcium, and triglycerides. May decrease urinary excretion of calcium and increase excretion of magnesium, sodium, and potassium levels.	Consume foods high in potassium and magnesium. Avoid consumption of natural licorice. Monitor electrolyte levels and consider supplementation. Caution with calcium supplements.
Bumex	Loop diuretic		

Bupropion Wellbutrin, Zyban	Antidepressant Serotonin and norepinephrine reuptake inhibitor	Dry mouth, upset stomach, vomiting, weight loss, and constipation. Alcohol may increase side effects.	Monitor weight. Use ice chips or chew gum for dry mouth. Avoid alcohol.
Bumex	See *bumetanide*		
Calan	See *verapamil*		
Calcijex	See *calcitriol*		
Calcium salts PhosLo, Caltrate, Dicarbosil, OsCal, Titralac, Tums, Citracal, Calcitrate	Calcium-based phosphorus binder	Hypercalcemia, stomach pains, nausea, vomiting, constipation, dry mouth, thirst, and frequent urination. Concurrent use of calcium and oxalic acid foods (spinach, rhubarb, beet greens, asparagus, etc.) may result in decreased calcium exposure. Concurrent use of calcium and phytic acid foods (beans, seeds, nuts, whole grains, etc.) may result in decreased calcium effectiveness.	Maintain adequate hydration, serum magnesium, phosphate, potassium levels, and urine calcium levels.

(continued)

Medication	Class and Action	Side Effects	Nutritional Implications
Calcitrate	See *calcium salts*		
Calcitriol	Vitamin D	May increase aluminum concentration, hypercalcemia, serum cholesterol, serum phosphorous, and magnesium concentration. Upset stomach, vomiting, dry mouth, constipation, metallic taste in mouth, increased thirst, decreased appetite, weight loss, and fatty stools.	Avoid use of antacids. Only works in conjunction with appropriate intake of calcium. Consider low-phosphate diet if on dialysis.
Calcijex, Rocaltrol			
Caltrate	See *calcium salts*		
Capoten	See *captopril*		
Capozide	See *captopril*		
Captopril	Antihypertensive	May increase serum potassium.	Caution with foods high in potassium or potassium supplements. Avoid salt substitutes. Maintain adequate hydration.
	ACE inhibitor	May decrease serum sodium.	
		Nausea, salty or metallic taste, mouth sores.	
		Concurrent use of angiotensin-converting inhibitors and yohimbine or ma huang may result in reduced effectiveness of angiotensin-converting enzyme inhibitors.	

Catapres	See *clonidine*		
Celexa	See *citalopram*		
Cholestyramine Questran, Prevalite	Bile acid sequestrant	May decrease serum potassium and calcium. Binds fat-soluble vitamins A, D, E, and K; folic acid; and β-carotene. Constipation, nausea, vomiting, abdominal pain, indigestion. Occasional diarrhea.	Mix with 3 to 6 oz of liquid, such as juice, milk, or water for powdered form. Irritating to GI tract. Take before meals. Take fat-soluble vitamins in a water-miscible form or take a supplement prior to initial daily dose of drug. Monitor nutrient levels if long-term use of drug is indicated. Consider high-fiber diet for constipation.
Cinacalcet Sensipar	Calcimimetic	High fat intake may increase cinacalcet concentration of plasma. Nausea, vomiting, and diarrhea. Concurrent use of cinacalcet and food may result in increased bioavailability of cinacalcet. Concurrent use of cinacalcet and grapefruit juice or grapefruit-containing foods may increase the effects of cinacalcet.	Avoid taking with grapefruit juice or grapefruit-containing foods.

(*continued*)

Medication	Class and Action	Side Effects	Nutritional Implications
Ciprofloxacin	Antibacterial	Upset stomach, vomiting, stomach pain, indigestion. Inflammation of the stomach leading to possible diarrhea. Aluminum, magnesium, calcium, ferrous sulfate, and zinc are thought to form chelation complexes, preventing the drugs from being absorbed. Concurrent use of fluoroquinolones and dandelion may result in decreased fluoroquinolone effectiveness. Concurrent use of ciprofloxacin and: • Iron may result in decreased ciprofloxacin effectiveness. • Fennel may result in decreased bioavailability of ciprofloxacin and possible antibiotic treatment failure. • Zinc may result in decreased ciprofloxacin effectiveness. • Caffeine may result in increased caffeine concentrations and enhanced central nervous system stimulation.	Take with 8 oz of water. Ensure adequate fluid intake. Consider fluid and electrolyte replacement for vomiting and diarrhea. Should not be taken with dairy products or calcium-containing fluids. Do not need to avoid foods containing these products.

Cisplatin Platinol, Platinol-AQ	Alkylating agent	Loss of appetite, weight loss, diarrhea, nausea, vomiting, and altered taste.	Drink plenty of fluids for drug; irritates the kidney. Vomiting is severe. May consider antiemetic therapy. Monitor weight. Encourage food intake when patient feels best (e.g., morning).
Citalopram Celexa	Antidepressant Selective serotonin reuptake inhibitor (SSRI)	Nausea, diarrhea, vomiting, anorexia, dry mouth, and dyspepsia. May decrease serum sodium. Concurrent use of SSRIs and St John's wort or Ginkgo biloba may result in an increased risk of serotonin syndrome (hypertension, hyperthermia, myoclonus, mental status changes).	Consider fluid and electrolyte replacement for diarrhea and vomiting. Use ice chips or chew gum for dry mouth. Avoid alcohol.
Citracal	See *calcium salts*		
Clarithromycin Biaxin	Antibiotic Bacteriostatic or bacteriocidal	Occasional nausea, vomiting, diarrhea, abdominal pain, anorexia, stomatitis, bad taste in mouth.	Take with food to avoid GI disturbances. Eat small, frequent meals to avoid anorexia. Consider fluid and electrolyte replacement for diarrhea. Avoid alcohol.

(*continued*)

Medication	Class and Action	Side Effects	Nutritional Implications
Clonidine Catapres, Duraclon	α-Antiadrenergic	Constipation, nausea, vomiting, dry mouth, and drowsiness. Concurrent use of clonidine and yohimbine may result in reduced clonidine effectiveness. Concurrent use of clonidine and ma huang may result in increased blood pressure.	Avoid alcohol intake, for it can exacerbate drowsiness. Use ice chips or chew gum for dry mouth.
Clopidogrel Plavix	Antiplatelet	Upset stomach, stomach pain, diarrhea, and constipation. Ginger may increase the possibility of bleeding. Concurrent use of clopidogrel and Ginkgo biloba, chaparral (also known as creosote bush), bladderwrack (type of seaweed), vitamin A, kava, licorice, clove oil, garlic, anise, boldo, motherwort, cat's claw, bilberry, bogbean, curcumin, celery, evening primrose, black currant, borage, feverfew, dandelion, angelica, meadowsweet, astragalus, tan-shen (red sage), skullcap, guggul, hawthorn, arnica, and ginger may result in an increased risk of bleeding.	Consider small, frequent meals for anorexia. Consider fluid and electrolyte replacement for diarrhea. Consistency in dietary and supplemental intake must be consistent to achieve steady level of anticoagulation. Those on long-term use should be monitored for bone density. Avoid taking with grapefruit juice or grapefruit-containing foods.

		Concurrent use of clopidogrel and grapefruit juice or grapefruit-containing foods may result in reduced exposure of the active clopidogrel metabolite.	
Co-trimoxazole/ trimethoprim/ Sulfamethoxazole Bactrim, Bactrim DS	Bactericidal	May cause anorexia, nausea, vomiting, diarrhea, abdominal pain, or stomatitis. May hinder folate metabolism.	Take with 8 oz of water on an empty stomach. Eat small, frequent meals to avoid anorexia. Take a folate supplement. Consider fluid and electrolyte replacement for diarrhea.
Coumadin	See *warfarin*		
Covera-HS	See *verapamil*		
Cyclophosphamide Cytoxan	Alkylating agent, nitrogen mustard	Nausea, vomiting, loss of appetite, and weight loss. Concurrent use of cyclophosphamide and St. John's wort may result in reduced cyclophosphamide effectiveness.	Drink plenty of fluids for drug; irritates bladder and kidneys. Encourage food intake when patient feels best (e.g., morning).
Cytoxan	See *cyclophosphamide*		

(*continued*)

Medication	Class and Action	Side Effects	Nutritional Implications
Dialyvite Diatx, Nephrocaps, Nephrovite	B-complex with vitamin C and biotin	Abdominal pain, cramps, dyspepsia, and nausea.	Taken when vitamins inadequate, usually after dialysis when fluid is removed. Used to replace water-soluble vitamin losses.
Diatx	See *Dialyvite*		
Dicarbosil	See *calcium salts*		
Digoxin Lanoxin	Antiarrhythmic, cardiac glycoside	Occasional diarrhea, loss of appetite, lower stomach pain, nausea, and/or vomiting. May reduce potassium levels and increase urinary excretion of magnesium. Concurrent use of digoxin and St. John's wort, khella, charcoal, and kaolin may result in reduced digoxin efficacy. Concurrent use of digoxin and calcium may result in a serious risk of arrhythmia and cardiovascular collapse. Concurrent use of digoxin and oleander, sea cucumber, carob, licorice, lily of the valley, Pheasant's eye, Chan-Su, cascara sagrada	Hypomagnesemia, hypokalemia, and hypercalcemia elevate drug toxicity. Ensure adequate consumption of potassium and magnesium. Care should be taken with calcium supplements and antacids.

		(buckthorn), aloe, or senna may result in increased risk of digoxin toxicity. The use of Siberian ginseng, tan-shen, or ashwagandha may result in falsely elevated digoxin levels.	
Doxercalciferol	See *calcitriol*		
Hectorol			
Duraclon	See *clonidine*		
Dyrenium	See *triamterene*		
Effexor, Effexor XR	See *venlafaxine*		
Enalapril	Antihypertensive	May increase serum potassium.	Caution with foods high in potassium or potassium supplements. Avoid salt substitutes. Maintain adequate hydration.
Vasotec	ACE inhibitor	May decrease serum sodium. Nausea, salty or metallic taste, mouth sores. Concurrent use of angiotensin-converting enzyme inhibitors and yohimbine or ma huang may result in reduced effectiveness of angiotensin-converting enzyme inhibitors.	

(continued)

Medication	Class and Action	Side Effects	Nutritional Implications
Ery-Tab	See *erythromycin*		
Erythromycin Ery-Tab	Antibiotic Bacteriostatic or bacteriocidal	Occasional nausea, vomiting, diarrhea, abdominal pain, anorexia, stomatitis, bad taste in mouth. Concurrent use of erythromycin and autumn crocus (colchicine) may result in increased plasma levels of colchicine and increased risk of toxicity. Concurrent use of erythromycin and grapefruit juice or grapefruit-containing foods may result in increased erythromycin bioavailability.	Take with food to avoid GI disturbances. Eat small, frequent meals to avoid anorexia. Consider fluid and electrolyte replacement for diarrhea. Avoid alcohol. Avoid taking with grapefruit or grapefruit-containing foods.
Effexor	See *venlafaxine*		
Eskalith, Eskalith CR	See *lithium*		
Extentabs	See *quinidine*		
Feostat	See *ferrous fumarate*		
Femiron	See *ferrous fumarate*		

Fenofibrate	See *gemfibrozil*		
Tricor			
Feosol	See *ferrous sulfate*		
Feratab	See *ferrous sulfate*		
Fergon	See *ferrous sulfate*		
Ferrex	See *ferrous sulfate*		
Ferrlecit	See *sodium ferric gluconate*		
Ferrous fumarate Femiron, Feostat	Iron supplement	Constipation, diarrhea, and abdominal discomfort, dark stools.	Emphasize iron-rich food in a well-balanced diet.
Ferrous sulfate Feosol, Feratab, Fergon, Ferrex, Hemocyte, Nephro-Fer, Niferex	Iron supplement	Constipation and stomach upset. Concurrent use of iron and zinc may result in decreased gastrointestinal absorption of iron and/or zinc. Concurrent use of iron and dairy foods may result in decreased iron bioavailability. Concurrent use of iron and phytic acid foods (beans, seeds, nuts, some whole grains) may result in reduced iron absorption.	Emphasize iron-rich food in a well-balanced diet.

(continued)

Medication	Class and Action	Side Effects	Nutritional Implications
Ferrous gluconate	See ferrous sulfate		
Flagyl	See *metronidazole*		
Fluoxetine	Antidepressant	Alcohol may increase depression.	Avoid alcohol. Consider fluid and electrolyte replacement for diarrhea and vomiting. Use ice chips or chew gum for dry mouth. Consider small, frequent meals for decreased appetite.
Prozac	Selective serotonin reuptake inhibitor (SSRI)	Nausea, diarrhea, decreased appetite, dry mouth, vomiting, constipation, and abdominal pain. Concurrent use of SSRIs and St. John's wort or Ginkgo biloba may result in increased risk of serotonin syndrome (hypertension, hyperthermia, myoclonus, mental status changes).	
Fluvastatin	See *atorvastatin*		
Lescol	Diuretic		
Furosemide	Loop diuretic	Ginkgo biloba may cause increased blood pressure. Licorice can increase the risk of hypokalemia. May increase blood glucose, uric acid, cholesterol, LDL, calcium, and triglycerides. May decrease urinary excretion of calcium and increase excretion of magnesium, sodium, and potassium levels.	Consume foods high in potassium and magnesium. Avoid consumption of natural licorice. Monitor electrolyte levels and consider supplementation. Caution with calcium supplements.
Lasix			

		Loss of appetite. Concurrent use of loop diuretics and ginseng or geranium may result in increased risk of diuretic resistance. Concurrent use of loop diuretics and yohimbine may result in reduced diuretic effectiveness.	
Gemfibrozil Lopid	Fibric acid derivative	Stomach pain, diarrhea, constipation, vomiting, and gas.	Eat a low-cholesterol, low-fat, low-sucrose diet for best results. Avoid alcohol. Consider fluid and electrolyte replacement for diarrhea and vomiting.
Hectorol	See d*oxercalciferol*		
Hydralazine Apresoline	Antiarrhythmic Antiprotozoal	Nausea, vomiting, diarrhea, fluid retention, and edema. Impedes metabolism of pyridoxine (vitamin B_6). Concurrent use of hydralazine and yohimbine or ma huang may result in reduced hydralazine effectiveness.	Doctor may prescribe a low-salt or low-sodium diet. Take with food. Monitor for pyridoxine deficiency. Consume diet high in pyridoxine. Consider supplementation.

(*continued*)

Medication	Class and Action	Side Effects	Nutritional Implications
Hemocyte	See *ferrous sulfate*		
Imfed	See *iron dextran*		
Iron dextran Imfed	IV iron, hematinic	Nausea, vomiting, and metallic taste. Concurrent use of iron and zinc may result in decreased GI absorption of iron and/or zinc. Concurrent use of iron and phytic acid foods (beans, seeds, nuts, some whole grains) may result in reduced iron absorption.	Avoid taking oral iron. Emphasize iron-rich food in a well-balanced diet.
Iron sucrose Venofer	IV iron, hematinic	Diarrhea.	Avoid taking oral iron. Emphasize iron-rich food in a well-balanced diet.
Isocarboxazid Marplan	Antidepressant Monoamine oxidase inhibitor (MAOI)	Sudden high blood pressure may occur with ingestion of certain foods. Alcohol may increase depressant effect. Caffeine may increase blood pressure and cardiac arrhythmias. Concurrent use of MAOIs and: • Yerba mate, guarana, or bitter orange may result in acute headache and increased blood pressure.	Avoid foods high in tyramine: cheeses, fava, or broad bean pods; yeast or meat extracts, smoked or pickled meat, poultry, or fish; fermented sausage such as bologna, pepperoni, salami, or other fermented meat; avocados; bananas; beer; wine; and raisins. Avoid excess amounts of caffeine, tea, or chocolate. Avoid alcohol.

		• Kava, ma huang, licorice, Ginkgo biloba, or nutmeg may result in increased risk of adverse effects from excessive monoamine oxidase inhibition. • St. John's wort may result in an increased risk of serotonin syndrome (hypertension, hyperthermia, myoclonus, mental status changes) and/or an increased risk of hypertensive crisis. • Ginseng may result in insomnia, tremor, headache, agitation, and worsening of depression.
Isoptin, Isoptin SR	See *verapamil*	
Keflex	See *cephalexin*	
Kinidine	See *quinidine*	
Lanoxin	See *digoxin*	
Lasix	See *furosemide*	
Lescol	See *fluvastatin*	
Lipitor	See *atorvastatin*	

(*continued*)

Medication	Class and Action	Side Effects	Nutritional Implications
Lisinopril	Antihypertensive	May increase serum potassium.	Caution with foods high in potassium or potassium supplements. Avoid salt substitutes. Maintain adequate hydration.
Prinivil, Zestril	ACE inhibitor	May decrease serum sodium.	
		Nausea, salty or metallic taste, mouth sores.	
Lithane	See *lithium*		
Lithium	Antimanic agent	Drug interferes with the regulation of sodium and water levels in the body and may lead to dehydration. Toxicity may result from sodium depletion. Caffeine appears to reduce serum lithium concentrations and increase side effects. Loss of appetite, stomach pain or bloating, gas, indigestion, weight gain or loss, dry mouth, excessive saliva in the mouth, tongue pain, change in the ability to taste food, swollen lips, and constipation.	Maintain steady salt and fluid intake. Avoid salt-free diet or sodium depletion. Avoid caffeine.
Eskalith, Eskalith CR, Lithobid, Lithane, Lithonate, Lithotabs		Concurrent use of lithium and: • Yohimbine may result in increased risk of manic episodes.	

		• Psyllium may result in decreased plasma levels and effectiveness of lithium. • Guarana or yerba mate may result in alterations in serum lithium levels.	
Lithobid	See *lithium*		
Lithonate	See *lithium*		
Lithotabs	See *lithium*		
Lopid	See *gemfibrozil*		
Lopressor	See *metoprolol*		
Marplan	See *isocarboxazid*		
Methotrexate	Antimetabolite, folate antagonist	Nausea, vomiting, diarrhea, stomach pain, mouth sores, and loss of appetite. Inhibitor of dihydrofolate reductase, thus decreasing availability of active folate. Concurrent use of methotrexate and cola may result in increased methotrexate serum levels and increased risk of toxicity.	Consume high-vitamin B_{12} diet. Consider fluid and electrolyte replacement for diarrhea and vomiting. Encourage food intake when patient feels best (e.g., morning). Drink extra fluids to pass more drug through the urine. Leucovorin should be considered to reverse toxic effect of folic acid antagonists.

(*continued*)

Medication	Class and Action	Side Effects	Nutritional Implications
Metoprolol Betaloc, Lopressor, Toprol XL	β-Blocker, antiadrenergic, antiarrhythmic	Diarrhea, constipation, nausea, and vomiting. Possible hypoglycemia. Signs of sympathetic response to hypoglycemia may be masked. May have a decreased insulin release in response to hyperglycemia. Concurrent use of β-adrenergic blockers and: • St. John's wort or yohimbine may result in decreased effectiveness of β-adrenergic blockers. • Dong quai may result in low blood pressure. • Ma huang may result in reduced hypotensive effect of β-adrenergic blockers.	Adherence necessary for those following diabetic diet. Monitor blood glucose levels. Be cautious of nonsympathetic signs of hypoglycemia. Consider fluid and electrolyte replacement for diarrhea and vomiting.
Metronidazole Flagyl	Antibacterial, antiprotozoal	Anorexia, nausea, dry mouth, stomatitis, diarrhea or constipation, vomiting, and metallic taste. Concurrent use of metronidazole and milk thistle may result in reduced metronidazole and active metabolite exposure.	Avoid alcohol and alcohol-containing products during and at least 5 days after treatment. Avoid hot and spicy foods. Consider fluid and electrolyte replacement for diarrhea. Take with food to prevent GI distress. Consider small, frequent meals for anorexia. Use ice chips or chew gum for dry mouth.

Nardil	See *phenelzine*		
Nephrocaps	See *dialyvite*		
Nephro-Fer	See *ferrous sulfate*		
Nephrovite	See *dialyvite*		
Niacin Niacor, Niaspan, Nicotinex, Slo-Niacin	Nicotinic acid derivative	Alcohol may increase side effects of niacin. Occasional gas, nausea, vomiting, and diarrhea. May increase blood uric acid and glucose levels.	Caution with diabetes. Ensure adherence to diabetic diet if necessary. May consider low-purine diet if necessary. Consider fluid and electrolyte replacement for diarrhea and vomiting.
Niacor	See *niacin*		
Niaspan	See *niacin*		
Nicotinex	See *niacin*		
Nifedical	See *nifedipine*		
Nifedipine Adalat, Nifedical, Procardia	Calcium channel blocker	Upset stomach, heartburn, nausea, and constipation. Concurrent use of nifedipine and: • Ginseng or Ginkgo biloba may result in an increased risk of nifedipine side effects.	Avoid drinking grapefruit juice or eating grapefruit 1 hr before or for 2 hr after taking nifedipine.

(*continued*)

Medication	Class and Action	Side Effects	Nutritional Implications
		• Dong quai may result in low blood pressure. • Ma huang may result in reduced hypotensive effect of calcium channel blockers. • Yohimbine may result in reduced calcium channel blocker effectiveness. • Grapefruit juice or grapefruit-containing foods may result in severe hypotension, myocardial ischemia, and increased vasodilator side effects.	
Niferex	See *ferrous sulfate*		
Oncovin	See *vincristine*		
Orlistat Xenical	Lipase inhibitor	Flatulence, fatty stools, nausea, diarrhea. Decreased absorption vitamins A and E.	Side effects are transient. Monitor nutrient levels.
OsCal	See *calcium salts*		
Parnate	See *tranylcypromine*		

Paroxetine Pexeva, Paxil, Paxil CR	Antidepressant Selective serotonin reuptake inhibitor (SSRI)	Nausea, dry mouth, constipation, diarrhea, and decreased appetite. Concurrent use of SSRIs and St. John's wort or Ginkgo biloba may result in an increased risk of serotonin syndrome (hypertension, hyperthermia, myoclonus, mental status changes).	Consider fluid and electrolyte replacement for diarrhea. Use ice chips or chew gum for dry mouth. Consider small, frequent meals for decreased appetite.
Pecxeva	See *paroxetine*		
Paxil, Paxil CR	See *paroxetine*		
Penicillin	Antibiotic Kill or prevent growth of bacteria	GI disturbances including mild diarrhea, nausea, or vomiting (stomatitis, black or hairy tongue has been reported). Some may contain high amounts of sodium or potassium.	Should be taken 1 hr before or 2 hr after food to facilitate absorption. Consider fluid and electrolyte replacement for diarrhea. Caution if on low-sodium diet. Some strengths of amoxicillin may contain phenylalanine.
Paricalcitol Zemplar	See *calcitriol*		

(*continued*)

Medication	Class and Action	Side Effects	Nutritional Implications
Phenelzine Nardil	Antidepressant Monoamine oxidase inhibitor (MAOI)	Sudden high blood pressure may occur with ingestion of certain foods. Alcohol may increase depressant effect. Caffeine may increase blood pressure and cardiac arrhythmias. Concurrent use of MAOIs and: • Yerba mate, guarana, or bitter orange may result in acute headache and increased blood pressure. • Kava, ma huang, licorice, Ginkgo biloba, or nutmeg may result in increased risk of adverse effects from excessive monoamine oxidase inhibition. • St. John's wort may result in an increased risk of serotonin syndrome (hypertension, hyperthermia, myoclonus, mental status changes) and/or an increased risk of hypertensive crisis.	Avoid foods high in tyramine: cheeses, fava, or broad bean pods; yeast or meat extracts, smoked or pickled meat, poultry, or fish; fermented sausage such as bologna, pepperoni, salami, or other fermented meat; avocados; bananas; beer; wine; and raisins. Avoid excess amounts of caffeine, tea, or chocolate. Avoid alcohol.

		• Ginseng may result in insomnia, tremor, headache, agitation, and worsening of depression. • Avocado may result in hypertensive crisis (headache, palpitation, neck stiffness).	
PhosLo	See *calcium salts*		
Platinol, Platinol-AQ	See *cisplatin*		
Plavix	See *clopidogrel*		
Pravachol	See *pravastatin*		
Pravastatin Pravachol	Inhibitor of HMG-CoA reductase	Constipation, diarrhea, gas, upset stomach, and upper right stomach pain. Coenzyme Q10 may be significantly reduced. Concurrent use of HMG-CoA reductase inhibitors and oat bran may result in reduced effectiveness of HMG-CoA reductase inhibitors. Concurrent use of pravastatin and St. John's wort may result in reduced effectiveness of pravastatin.	Avoid intake of large quantities of grapefruit juice or grapefruit-containing foods, for it increases the absorption of statins (>1 quart/d). Eat a low-cholesterol, low-fat diet for best results. GI problems are generally transient.

(*continued*)

Medication	Class and Action	Side Effects	Nutritional Implications
Prevalite	See *cholestyramine*		
Prinivil	See *lisinopril*		
Procardia	See *nifedipine*		
Propanolol	See *atenolol*		
Inderal			
Prozac	See *fluoxetine*		
Questran	See *cholestyramine*		
Quinidex	See *quinidine*		
Quinidine Kinidine, Quinidex, Extentabs	Antiarrhythmic, antiprotozoal	Abdominal pain and cramps, diarrhea, nausea, and vomiting. May cause hypokalemia, hypomagnesemia, and/or hypocalcemia. Concurrent use of quinidine and grapefruit juice may result in decreased metabolic conversion of quinidine to 3-hydroxyquinidine.	Consider fluid and electrolyte replacement for diarrhea and vomiting. Consume diet adequate in potassium, magnesium, and calcium. Supplementation maybe necessary.
Renagel	See *sevelamer*		
Rocaltrol	See *calcitriol*		
Sensipar	See *cinacalcet*		

Sertraline	Antidepressant		
Zoloft	Selective serotonin reuptake inhibitor (SSRI)	May increase serum triglyceride and total cholesterol. May decrease uric acid levels. St. John's wort may increase adverse side effects. Nausea, diarrhea, dry mouth, constipation, altered taste, and dyspepsia. Concurrent use of SSRIs and St. John's wort or Ginkgo biloba may result in an increased risk of serotonin syndrome (hypertension, hyperthermia, myoclonus, mental status changes). Concurrent use of sertraline and grapefruit juice or grapefruit-containing foods may result in elevated sertraline serum concentrations and an increased risk of adverse side effects.	Monitor blood lipid levels. Consider fluid and electrolyte replacement for diarrhea and vomiting. Use ice chips or chew gum for dry mouth. Avoid alcohol. Avoid grapefruit or grapefruit-containing foods.
Sevelamer Renagel	Non–calcium-based phosphorus binder	Diarrhea, dyspepsia, gas, constipation, nausea, and vomiting.	Take with food. Use of aluminum should be limited to <14 days. Monitor bicarbonate, chloride, calcium, and phosphorous levels.

(continued)

Medication	Class and Action	Side Effects	Nutritional Implications
Simvastatin Zocor	Inhibitor of HMG-CoA reductase	Constipation, diarrhea, gas, upset stomach, and upper right stomach pain. Coenzyme Q10 may be significantly reduced. Concurrent use of HMG-CoA reductase inhibitors and oat bran may result in reduced effectiveness of HMG-CoA reductase inhibitors. Concurrent use of simvastatin and cranberry juice may result in increased risk of hepatitis and myopathy/rhabdomyolysis. Concurrent use of HMG-CoA reductase inhibitors and pectin may result in reduced effectiveness of HMG-CoA reductase inhibitors.	Avoid intake of large quantities of grapefruit juice, for it increases the absorption of statins (>1 quart/d). Eat a low-cholesterol, low-fat diet for best results. GI problems are generally transient.
Slo-Niacin	See *niacin*		
Sodium ferric Gluconate complex	See *iron sucrose*		

Ferrlecit			
Spironolactone	Diuretic	Hyperkalemia, dehydration, hyponatremia, nausea, vomiting, anorexia, abdominal cramps, and diarrhea.	Avoid foods high in potassium, potassium supplements, and salt substitutes.
Aldactone	Potassium-sparing diuretic	Concurrent use of diuretics and licorice may result in increased risk of hypokalemia and/or reduced effectiveness of the diuretic.	
		Concurrent use of potassium-sparing diuretics and ma huang may result in reduced hypotensive effect of potassium-sparing diuretics.	
		Concurrent use of diuretics and yohimbine may result in reduced diuretic effectiveness.	
Tenormin	See *atenolol*		
Titralac	See *calcium salts*		
Toprol XL	See *metoprolol*		

(*continued*)

Medication	Class and Action	Side Effects	Nutritional Implications
Tranylcypromine Parnate	Antidepressant Monoamine oxidase inhibitor (MAOI)	Sudden high blood pressure or increased MAOI activity may occur with ingestion of certain foods and herbals (avocado, yerba mate, guarana, kava, liquorice, ma huang, St. John's wort, bitter orange, ginseng, ginkgo, nutmeg, caffeine). Alcohol may increase depressant effect. Caffeine may increase blood pressure and cardiac arrhythmias. GI upset.	Avoid foods high in tyramine: cheeses, fava, or broad bean pods; yeast or meat extracts, smoked or pickled meat, poultry, or fish; fermented sausage such as bologna, pepperoni, salami, or other fermented meat; avocados; bananas; beer; wine; and raisins. Avoid excess amounts of caffeine, tea, or chocolate. Avoid alcohol.
Triamterene Dyrenium	Diuretic Potassium-sparing diuretic	Hyperkalemia, dehydration, hyponatremia, nausea, vomiting, anorexia, abdominal cramps, and diarrhea. Concurrent use of diuretics and yohimbine may result in reduced diuretic effectiveness. Concurrent use of potassium-sparing diuretics and ma huang may result in reduced hypotensive effect of potassium-sparing diuretics. Concurrent use of triamterene and potassium foods may result in hyperkalemia.	Avoid foods high in potassium, potassium supplements, and salt substitutes.

Tricor	See *fenofibrate*		
Trovafloxacin Trovan	Quinolone	Iron preparations may increase drug absorption. Dandelion may increase drug effect. Fennel seed may decrease drug effect, resulting in treatment failure. Diarrhea.	Consider fluid and electrolyte replacement for diarrhea.
Trovan	See *trovafloxacin*		
Tums	See *calcium salts*		
Vasotec	See *enalapril*		
Velban	See *vinblastine*		
Velsar	See *vinblastine*		
Venlafaxine Effexor, Effexor XR	Antidepressant	Nausea, dry mouth, anorexia, and constipation. St. John's wort may increase sedative effect. Concurrent use of venlafaxine and St. John's wort may result in an increased risk of serotonin syndrome (hypertension, hyperthermia, myoclonus, mental status changes).	Use ice chips or chew gum for dry mouth. Monitor weight.
Venofer	See *iron sucrose*		

(continued)

Medication	Class and Action	Side Effects	Nutritional Implications
Verapamil Calan, Verelan, Verelan PM, Isoptin, Isoptin SR, Covera-HS	Calcium channel blocker	Constipation, upset stomach, heartburn. Concurrent use of verapamil and caffeine may result in increased caffeine serum concentrations and enhanced CNS stimulation.	Avoid drinking grapefruit juice or eating grapefruit 1 hr before or for 2 hr after taking nifedipine.
Verelan, Verelan PM	See *verapamil*		
Vinblastine Velban, Velsar, vinblastine sulfate, VBL	Plant alkaloid	Nausea, vomiting, stomach pain, constipation, and diarrhea.	Drink plenty of fluids to decrease constipation.
Vincristine Oncovin	Plant alkaloid	Nausea, vomiting, stomach pain, stomach cramps, constipation, and diarrhea. Concurrent use of vincristine and grapefruit juice or grapefruit-containing foods may result in increased plasma concentrations of vincristine.	Consider fluid and electrolyte replacement for diarrhea and vomiting. May consider laxatives for constipation. Mild vomiting remedied with antiemetic. Avoid grapefruit or grapefruit-containing foods.

Warfarin Coumadin	Anticoagulant	Anorexia, nausea, abdominal cramping, and diarrhea. Prevents the conversion of vitamin K to its active form. Garlic may increase the risk of bleeding. Mineralization of newly formed bone may be deterred.	Consider small, frequent meals for anorexia. Consider fluid and electrolyte replacement for diarrhea. Dietary and supplemental intake, particularly vitamin K, must be consistent to achieve steady level of anticoagulation. Those on long-term use should be monitored for bone density.
Wellbutrin	See *bupropion*		
Xenical	See *orlistat*		
Zemplar	See *paricalcitol*		
Zestril	See *lisinopril*		
Zithromax	See *azithromycin*		
Zocor	See *simvastatin*		
Zoloft	See *sertraline*		
Zyban	See *bupropion*		

REFERENCES

1. Micromedex by Truven Health Analytics—Micromedex drug, disease and toxicology management. Available at: https://www.micromedexsolutions.com/home/dispatch/ssl/true.

Appendix C
Vitamins, Minerals, and Dietary Supplement Facts

LISTING OF CONTENTS

1. Conversion Tables
2. Vitamin Facts and Nutrient Lists
3. Mineral Facts
4. Dietary Supplements

TABLE C.1. Conversion Tables

A. Length

1 m = 39 in.

1 cm = 0.4 in.

1 in. = 2.5 cm

1 ft = 30 cm

B. Temperature

	Celsius	*Fahrenheit*
Steam	100°C	212°F
Body temp.	37°C	98.6°F
Ice	0°C	32°F

°C = (°F − 32) × 5/9

°F = (°C × 9/5) + 32

(continued)

TABLE C.1. Conversion Tables (*continued*)

C. Volume

1 L	= 1,000 mL	0.26 gal	1.06 qt	2.1 pt
1 mL	= 1/1,000 L	0.03 fluid oz		
1 gal	= 128 oz	8 cups	3.8 L	
1 qt	= 32 oz	4 cups	0.95 L	
1 pt	= 16 oz	2 cups	0.47 L	
1 cup	= 8 oz	16 Tbsp	~250 mL	0.25 L
1 oz	= 30 mL			
1 tablespoon (Tbsp)	= 3 tsp	15 mL		
1 teaspoon (tsp)	= 5 mL			

D. Weight

1 kg	= 1,000 g	2.2 lb	
1 g	= 1/1,000 kg	1,000 mg	0.035 oz
1 mg	= 1/1,000 g	1,000 μg	
1 μg	= 1/1,000 mg		
1 lb	= 16 oz	454 g	0.45 kg
1 oz	= ~28 g		

E. Energy

1 kJ	= 0.24 kcal	
1 mJ	= 240 kcal	
1 kcal	= 4.2 kJ	
1 g carbohydrate	= 4 kcal	17 kJ
1 g fat	= 9 kcal	17 kJ
1 g protein	= 4 kcal	17 kJ
1 g alcohol	= 7 kcal	29 kJ

TABLE C.2. Vitamin Facts and Nutrient Lists

A. Vitamins

Vitamin	Functions	Deficiency	Toxicity
A	Maintains integrity of cornea, epithelial cells, and mucous membranes; skin and bone and teeth growth; regulates synthesis of reproductive hormones and immune system; cancer protection	Anemia Blindness, night blindness Bone growth deficit Corneal breakdown Diarrhea Joint pain Kidney stones Infection susceptibility	Amenorrhea Anorexia Bone pain Fatigue Headache Nosebleeds Skin rash
D	Maintains bone tissue by regulating the absorption and excretion of calcium and phosphorus	Defective bone growth (bowed legs, joint pain) Muscle spasms	Anorexia Headaches Excessive thirst hypercalcemia Kidney stones Nausea Weakness
E	Maintains cell membranes; acts as an antioxidant in fighting disease-causing free radicals and in protecting other important compounds from oxidation	Anemia Breast cysts Leg cramps Weakness	Enhances action of anticoagulants Gastrointestinal distress

(*continued*)

TABLE C.2. Vitamin Facts and Nutrient Lists (*continued*)

Vitamin	Functions	Deficiency	Toxicity
K	Synthesis of blood clotting compounds; regulation of calcium levels in blood	Excessive bleeding	Jaundice Interference of anticoagulant drugs
B_1 Thiamin	Coenzyme in energy metabolism; maintenance of appetite and nervous system function	Abnormal heart beat Cardiomegaly/ heart failure Fluid retention Mental confusion Muscle pain, weakness, wasting paralysis	None documented
B_2 Riboflavin	Coenzyme in energy metabolism; maintenance of skin and visual function	Corneal abnormalities Dry, cracking at corners of mouth Sensitivity to light Skin rash Tongue abnormalities	None documented
B_3 Niacin, Nicotinamide	Coenzyme in energy metabolism; maintenance of skin, and nervous and digestive systems	Anorexia Diarrhea Skin rash Tongue abnormalities Weakness and dizziness	Diarrhea Dizziness Liver dysfunction Low blood pressure Sweating, flushing

Vitamin	Functions	Deficiency	Toxicity
B_6 Pyridoxine	Coenzyme in protein and fat metabolism; synthesis of red blood cells; synthesis of niacin	Anemia Kidney stones Dermatitis Spastic muscles, convulsions Tongue abnormalities	Fluid retention Depression, memory loss Fatigue Weakness
Folate	Coenzyme in cellular synthesis	Anemia Depression, mental confusion Diarrhea, constipation Infection susceptibility Tongue abnormalities	Mask B_{12} deficiency
B_{12} Cobalamine	Cellular synthesis; maintenance of nervous system function	Anemia Fatigue Paralysis Skin abnormalities Tongue abnormalities	None documented
Pantothenic Acid	Coenzyme in energy metabolism	Fatigue Insomnia Vomiting, other intestinal problems	Fluid retention
Biotin	Coenzyme in energy metabolism; synthesis of fat and glycogen	Alopecia Anorexia Depression Fatigue	None documented

(*continued*)

TABLE C.2. Vitamin Facts and Nutrient Lists (*continued*)

Vitamin	Functions	Deficiency	Toxicity
		Heartbeat abnormalities Nausea Skin rash	
Choline	Coenzyme in energy metabolism; synthesis of phospholipids and neurotransmitters	Growth failure Kidney failure Liver dysfunction (fat accumulation) Memory abnormalities	Fishy body odor Low blood pressure
C **Ascorbic Acid**	Collagen synthesis; antioxidant; immune function; enhancement of iron absorption; synthesis of thyroid hormone; protein metabolism	Anemia Bleeding gums, loose teeth Bone fracture susceptibility Depression Infection susceptibility	Abdominal cramps, diarrhea Headache Nausea Skin rash
		Joint pain Muscle pain and wasting Skin problems Wound healing delayed	Interferes with interpretation of some laboratory values

B. Vitamin C

Food	Portion Size	Vitamin C (mg)	% Daily Value (DV)
Papaya	1, whole fresh	188	313
Orange juice	1 cup, fresh	124	207
Brussel sprouts	1 cup, cooked	96	160
Grapefruit juice	1 cup, fresh	94	157
Green pepper	1, whole	90	150
Strawberries	1 cup, fresh	85	142
Orange	1, medium fresh	80	133
Broccoli	1 cup, cooked	74	123
Cauliflower	1 cup, cooked	72	120
Cantaloupe	1 cup, fresh	68	113
Mango	1, fresh	57	95
Pink grapefruit	½, fresh	47	78
Honeydew melon	1 cup, fresh	42	70
Turnip greens	1 cup, cooked	40	67%
Parsley	½ cup, chopped	40	67
Mustard greens	1 cup, cooked	36	60
Tomatoes	1, whole canned	36	60
Cabbage	1 cup, raw	34	57
Sauerkraut	1 cup, canned	34	57

(continued)

TABLE C.2. Vitamin Facts and Nutrient Lists (*continued*)

Food	Portion Size	Vitamin C (mg)	% Daily Value (DV)
Tomato juice	6 oz, canned	33	55
Raspberries	1 cup, fresh	31	52
Butternut squash	1 cup, boiled	30	50
Sweet potato	1, baked w/skin	28	47
Baked potato	1, whole	26	43
Pineapple chunks	1 cup, fresh	24	40
Asparagus	1 cup, cooked	20	33
Watermelon	1 cup, fresh	15	25
Apple	1, medium fresh	8	13
Milk, 2%	8 oz	2	3

Quick Reference Diet Integration

- Snacks: orange, tomato, and grapefruit juices
- Entree: fried broccoli, brussel sprouts, green pepper, and cauliflower
- Mashed, baked, or boiled potatoes
- Fruit salad of strawberries, papaya, mango, watermelon in places of sweets
- Kabob of green peppers, cherry tomatoes, strawberries, and pineapples

C. Riboflavin

			% Dietary Reference Intake (DRI)	
Food	Portion Size	Riboflavin	Women	Men
Brewer's yeast	1 Tbsp	1.21	110	93
Yogurt	1 cup, low fat	0.51	46	39

Food	Portion Size	Riboflavin	% Dietary Reference Intake (DRI)	
			Women	Men
Mushrooms	1 cup, cooked	0.46	42	35
Ricotta cheese	1 cup, part skim	0.46	42	35
Corn flakes	1 cup	0.43	39	33
Cottage cheese	1 cup, low fat	0.42	38	32
Milk, 2%	8 oz	0.4	36	31
Buttermilk	1 cup	0.38	35	29
Sirloin steak	3.5 oz, broiled	0.29	26	22
Peach halves	10, dried	0.28	25	22
Pork chop	3.5 oz, roasted	0.26	24	20
Ground beef	3.5 oz, lean baked	0.24	22	18
Black-eyed peas	1 cup, cooked	0.24	22	18
Kidney beans	1 cup, canned	0.23	21	18
Asparagus	1 cup, cooked	0.22	20	17
Almonds	1 oz, whole dried	0.22	20	17
Oysters	3 oz, raw	0.2	18	15
Ham	3.5 oz, cooked	0.19	17	15
Turkey	3.5 oz, w/o skin	0.18	16	14
Broccoli	1 cup, cooked	0.16	15	12
Green beans	1 cup, cooked	0.14	13	11

(*continued*)

TABLE C.2. Vitamin Facts and Nutrient Lists (*continued*)

Food	Portion Size	Riboflavin	% Dietary Reference Intake (DRI)	
			Women	Men
Cheddar cheese	1 oz	0.11	10	8
Spinach	1 cup, cooked	0.1	9	8
Strawberries	1 cup, fresh	0.1	9	8
Chicken breast	1/2 breast, roasted	0.1	9	8
Sole/ flounder	3 oz baked	0.07	6	5
Orange	1, medium fresh	0.06	5	5
Bread	Whole wheat, 1 slice	0.05	5	4
Bean sprouts	1 cup, stir fried	0.04	4	3
Cantaloupe	1 cup, fresh	0.03	3	2
Apple	1, medium fresh	0.02	2	2

Quick Reference Diet Integration

- A bowl of corn flakes with 8 oz milk provides 75% of DRI for women.
- Yogurt as a snack and as a dip for fruits and vegetables
- Mushrooms in pizza, salads, or stir frys
- Low-fat cottage or ricotta cheeses in lasagna, ravioli, or other main dish

D. Vitamin B_6

Food	Portion Size	B_6 (mg)	% DRI
Beef liver	3.5 oz, braised	0.91	70
Baked potato	1, whole	0.7	54

Food	Portion Size	B_6 (mg)	% DRI
Salmon	3 oz, cooked	0.7	54
Banana	1, peeled	0.66	51
Chicken breast	½ breast, w/o skin	0.51	39
Corn flakes	1 cup	0.5	38
Avocado	½ average	0.48	37
Trout	3 oz, broiled	0.46	35
Turkey	3.5 oz, w/o skin	0.46	35
Brewer's yeast	1 oz	0.45	35
Sirloin steak	3.5 oz, broiled	0.45	35
Pork chop	3.5 oz, roasted	0.45	35
Spinach	1 cup, cooked	0.44	34
Soybeans	1 cup, cooked	0.4	31
Wheat germ	¼ cup	0.38	29
Tuna, in water	3 oz, canned	0.3	23
Navy beans	1 cup, cooked	0.3	23
Sunflower seeds	¼ cup, dry	0.3	23
Turnip greens	1 cup, cooked	0.26	20
Cauliflower	1 cup, cooked	0.26	20
Broccoli	1 cup, cooked	0.24	18
Green pepper	1, whole	0.24	18
Watermelon	1 cup, fresh	0.23	18
Ground beef	3.5 oz, lean baked	0.22	17
Asparagus	1 cup, cooked	0.22	17
Figs	5, dried	0.21	16
Cantaloupe	1 cup, fresh	0.18	14
Sole/ flounder	3 oz, cooked	0.18	14

(*continued*)

TABLE C.2. Vitamin Facts and Nutrient Lists (*continued*)

Food	Portion Size	B_6 (mg)	% DRI
Mustard greens	1 cup, cooked	0.16	12
Zucchini	1 cup, cooked	0.14	11
Milk	2%, 8 oz	0.11	8

Quick Reference Diet Integration

- Baked potato for lunch with fat-free sour cream or dressing
- Banana with corn flakes for breakfast
- Poach, grill, or broil salmon for a quick meal

E. Vitamin B_{12}

Food	Portion Size	B_{12} (µg)	% DRI
Clams	3 oz, cooked	84.1	3,500
Beef liver	3.5 oz, braised	71	3,000
Oysters	3 oz, cooked	32.5	1,350
Clam chowder	1 cup	10.3	427
Rabbit	3.5 oz, roasted	8.3	346
Braunschweiger	1 oz, tube type	5.2	216
Sirloin steak	3.5 oz, broiled	2.9	119
Salmon	3 oz, cooked	2.7	113
Tuna, in water	3 oz, canned	2.5	106
Lamb chop	3.5 oz, braised	2.3	95
Vegetarian burger	½ cup	2	83
Raisin bran	¾ cup	2	83
Ground beef	3.5 oz, lean baked	1.7	71
Cottage cheese	1 cup, 1% fat	1.4	58
Sole/flounder	3 oz, cooked	1.3	54
Shrimp	3 oz, cooked	1.3	54

Food	Portion Size	B_{12} (μg)	% DRI
Halibut	3 oz, broiled	1.2	50
Milk	2%, 8 oz	0.89	37
Frankfurter	1 beef, 2 oz	0.88	37
Ham	3.5 oz, cooked	0.74	29
Tempeh	½ cup	0.7	29
Pork chop	3.5 oz, roasted	0.6	25
Buttermilk	8 oz, cultured	0.54	23
Egg	1, whole fresh	0.5	21
Turkey	3.5 oz, w/o skin	0.37	15
Canadian bacon	2 slices, cooked	0.36	15
Miso	½ cup	0.29	12
Chicken breast	½ breast, w/o skin	0.29	12
Yogurt	8 oz, low fat	0.24	10
Cheddar cheese	1 oz	0.23	10
Goat's milk	8 oz	0.16	7

Quick Reference Diet Integration

- Raisin bran with low-fat milk for breakfast
- Low-fat cottage cheese with fruit as a snack
- 3 oz of salmon, tuna, or rabbit provides 100% DRI of B_{12}.
- Oysters or clams served steamed or in stews and chowders

F. Biotin

Food	Portion Size	Biotin (μg)	% DRI
Egg	1, whole fresh	10	33
Wheat germ	¼ cup, toasted	7	23
Ry-Krisp	½ oz	6.8	23
Granola	¼ cup w/raisins	5	17
Egg noodles	1 cup, cooked	4	13
Almonds	1 oz, whole natural	1	3

(continued)

TABLE C.2. Vitamin Facts and Nutrient Lists (*continued*)

Food	Portion Size	Biotin (μg)	% DRI
Pistachios	1 oz, red	1	3
Corn meal	1 oz, yellow	1	3

Quick Reference Diet Integration

- Granola as a cereal or snack, or mixed into yogurt
- Wheat germ in casseroles and breads or on cereal
- Ry-Krisp with peanut butter and jelly for a snack
- Egg noodles with veggies, fat-free Italian dressing
- Scrambled, poached, or hardboiled eggs

G. Choline

			% DRI	
Food	Portion Size	Choline (μg)	Women	Men
Beef liver	3.5 oz	583.1	137	106
Cauliflower	1 cup, cooked	162	38	29
Peanuts	1 oz, dried	127.3	30	23
Peanut butter	2 Tbsp	124.6	29	23
Grape juice	8 oz, canned	120	28	22
Potato	1, whole baked	103.2	24	19
Iceberg lettuce	1 leaf, raw	58.6	14	11
Tomato	1, whole raw	52.9	12	10
Milk	Whole 8 oz	36.6	9	7
Orange	1, fresh medium	28	7	5
Banana	1, whole peeled	27.4	6	5
Bread	Whole wheat 1 slice	24.2	6	4
Cucumber	½ cup, raw	11.3	3	2
Beef steak	3.5 oz	7.5	2	1
Apple	1, fresh medium	3.7	<1	<1

			% DRI	
Food	Portion Size	Choline (µg)	Women	Men
Egg	1, fresh whole	2.1	<1	<1
Ginger ale	12 oz	0.73	<1	<1
Butter	1 tsp	0.21	<1	<1
Margarine	1 tsp, tub type	0.15	<1	<1
Corn oil	1 Tbsp	0.04	<1	<1

Quick Reference Diet Integration Guide

- Dinner: 3.5 oz beef liver, 1 cup cauliflower, baked potato, 8 oz grape juice, banana
- Add iceberg lettuce to a sandwich
- Swap straight soda for a "Choline Cocktail"—8 oz grape juice, 12 oz ginger ale
- Snack: 1 oz peanuts and 8 oz milk
- Lunch: peanut butter and jelly sandwich with 8 oz grape juice

H. Folate

Food	Portion Size	Folate (µg)	% DRI
Pinto beans	1 cup, cooked	294	74
Asparagus	1 cup, cooked	264	66
Spinach	1 cup, cooked	262	66
Navy beans	1 cup, cooked	255	64
Beef liver	3.5 oz, braised	217	54
Black-eyed peas	1 cup, cooked	209	52
Great northern beans	1 cup, cooked	181	45
Turnip greens	1 cup, cooked	170	43
Lima beans	1 cup, cooked	156	39
Kidney beans	1 cup, canned	129	32
Broccoli	1 cup, cooked	104	26
Corn flakes	1 cup	100	25
Parsley	1 cup, chopped	92	23
Beets	1 cup, cooked	90	23

(continued)

TABLE C.2. Vitamin Facts and Nutrient Lists (*continued*)

Food	Portion Size	Folate (µg)	% DRI
Wheat germ	1/4 cup	82	21
Romaine lettuce	1 cup, chopped	76	19
Cauliflower	1 cup, cooked	64	16
Pineapple juice	8 oz, canned	58	15
Orange	1, fresh medium	47	12
Zucchini	1 cup, cooked	30	8
Peanuts	1 oz, dried	29	7
Cantaloupe	1 cup, fresh	27	7
Winter squash	1 cup, cooked	26	7
Strawberries	1 cup, fresh	26	7
Grapefruit juice	1 cup, canned	26	7
Egg	1, whole fresh	23	6
Green beans	1 cup, cooked	22	6
Tofu	1/2 cup, raw	19	5
Tomato	1, whole raw	18	5
Bread, whole wheat	1 slice	14	4

Quick Reference Diet Integration

- Use dry beans in soups or as a main dish salad
- Add spinach to lasagna or serve cooked with lemon juice
- Salad of spinach, romaine, tomato, broccoli, cauliflower, and beets
- Dinner: 3.5 oz beef liver, 1 cup asparagus, 1 cup lima beans
- Breakfast: cornflakes in milk; fruit salad of cantaloupe, strawberries, orange

I. Niacin

Food	Portion Size	Niacin (mg)	% DRI Women	% DRI Men
Chicken breast	½ roasted w/o skin	11.8	84	74
Tuna, in water	3 oz, canned	11.3	81	71

Food	Portion Size	Niacin (mg)	% DRI Women	% DRI Men
Beef liver	3.5 oz, braised	10.7	76	67
Brewer's yeast	1 oz	10.7	76	67
Salmon	3 oz, broiled	8.6	61	54
Mushrooms	1 cup, cooked	7	50	44
Halibut	3 oz, broiled	6.1	44	38
Peach halves	10, dried	5.7	41	36
Pink salmon	3 oz, canned	5.6	40	35
Pork chop	3.5 oz, roasted	5.5	39	34
Lamb chop	3.5 oz, braised	5.5	39	34
Turkey	3.5 oz w/o skin	5.4	39	34
Sirloin steak	3.5 oz, broiled	4.3	31	27
Ground beef	3.5 oz, lean baked	4.2	30	26
Peanuts	1 oz, dried unsalted	4	29	25
Baked potato	1, whole	3.3	24	21
Sole/flounder	3 oz, baked	2.5	18	16
Kidney beans	1 cup, canned	2.4	17	15
Braunschweiger	1 oz, tube type	2.3	16	14
Shrimp	3 oz, boiled	2.2	16	14
Wheat bran	¼ cup	2	14	13
Asparagus	1 cup, cooked	2	14	13
Oysters	3 oz, raw	1.7	12	11
Sardines	2, sardines in oil	1.3	9	8

(continued)

TABLE C.2. Vitamin Facts and Nutrient Lists (*continued*)

Food	Portion Size	Niacin (mg)	% DRI Women	% DRI Men
Crab meat	3 oz, canned	1.2	9	8
Bread, whole wheat	1 slice	1	8	6
Summer squash	1 cup, cooked	1	8	6
Cantaloupe	1 cup, fresh	0.9	6	6
Peach	1, fresh medium	0.9	6	6
Spinach	1 cup, cooked	0.9	6	6
Broccoli	1 cup, cooked	0.8	6	5

Quick Reference Diet Integration

- Choose tuna, halibut, and salmon instead of red meat
- Add mushrooms to soups and salads, and stir fry
- Dinner: half chicken breast, baked potato, 1 cup asparagus
- Fortified breakfast cereals contain 25% of the DRI for niacin per serving.

J. Pantothenic Acid

Food	Serving Size	Pantothenic Acid (mg)	% DRI
Beef liver	3.5 oz, braised	4.6	91
Mushrooms	½ cup, boiled	1.7	34
Avocado	1, medium	1.7	34
Salmon	3 oz, cooked	1.4	28
Lentils	1 cup, boiled	1.3	25
Split peas	1 cup, boiled	1.2	23
Potato	1, whole baked	1.1	22
Turkey	3.5 oz w/o skin	0.94	19
Pomegranate	1, medium raw	0.92	18

Food	Serving Size	Pantothenic Acid (mg)	% DRI
Chicken breast	½, roasted w/o skin	0.83	17
Peanuts	1 oz, dried	0.79	16
Milk, 2%	8 oz	0.78	16
Sweet potato	1, whole baked	0.74	15
Chickpeas	1 cup, canned	0.72	14
Wheat germ	¼ cup	0.66	13
Pork chop	3.5 oz, roasted	0.65	13
Egg	1, whole fresh	0.63	13
Broccoli	1 cup, cooked	0.5	10
Ham	3.5 oz, cooked	0.47	9
Sole/flounder	3 oz, cooked	0.43	9
Kidney beans	1 cup, canned	0.38	8
Sirloin steak	3.5 oz, broiled	0.37	7
Corn	1 cup, boiled	0.36	7
Orange	1, fresh medium	0.35	7
Watermelon	1 cup, fresh	0.34	7
Ground beef	3.5 oz, baked lean	0.27	5
Spinach	1 cup, cooked	0.26	5
Bread, whole wheat	1 slice	0.18	4
Tuna, in water	3 oz, canned	0.18	4
Macaroni	1 cup, cooked, enriched	0.16	3
Cheddar cheese	1 oz	0.12	2

Quick Reference Diet Integration

- Avocado sliced in a salad or in a dip (guacamole)
- Dinner: 3 oz salmon, 1 baked potato, 8 oz milk, 1 cup broccoli
- Soups with lentils or split peas
- Salad: chicken breast, avocado, spinach, mushrooms, broccoli

(continued)

TABLE C.2. Vitamin Facts and Nutrient Lists (*continued*)

K. Thiamin

Food	Portion Size	Thiamin (mg)	% DRI	
			Women	Men
Brewer's yeast	1 oz	4.43	403	369
Pork chop	3.5 oz, roasted	0.91	83	76
Ham	3.5 oz, cooked	0.78	71	65
Green peas	1 cup, cooked	0.42	38	35
Canadian bacon	2 pieces, cooked	0.38	35	32
Corn flakes	1 cup	0.38	35	32
Split peas	1 cup, cooked	0.37	34	31
Macaroni, enriched	1 cup, cooked	0.29	26	24
Kidney beans	1 cup, canned	0.27	25	23
Oatmeal	1 cup, cooked	0.26	24	22
Millet	1 cup, cooked	0.25	23	21
Acorn squash	1 cup, boiled	0.24	22	20
Baked potato	1, whole	0.22	20	18
Asparagus	1 cup, cooked	0.22	20	18
Peanuts	1 oz, dry, unsalted	0.19	17	16
Black eyed peas	1 cup, cooked	0.17	15	14
Watermelon	1 cup, fresh	0.13	12	11
Sirloin steak	3.5 oz, broiled	0.13	12	11
Honeydew melon	1 cup, fresh	0.13	12	11
Orange	1, fresh medium	0.12	11	10

Food	Portion Size	Thiamin (mg)	% DRI	
			Women	Men
Tofu	½ cup	0.1	9	8
Milk, 2%	8 oz	0.1	9	8
Green beans	1 cup, cooked	0.1	9	8
Broccoli	1 cup, cooked	0.1	9	8
Bread, whole wheat	1 slice	0.09	8	8
Sole/ flounder	3 oz, cooked	0.08	7	7
Cauliflower	1 cup, cooked	0.08	7	7
Tomato	1, whole raw	0.07	6	6

Quick Reference Diet Integration

- Include lean pork in weekly menus
- Use green peas, split peas, black peas, black-eyed peas, kidney beans in soups
- Choose enriched pasta and bread products
- Breakfast: oatmeal or fortified cereal
- Side dish: boiled or baked squash

L. Vitamin A

Food	Portion Size	Vitamin A (RE)	% DRI
Beef liver	3 oz, fried	9,123	1,042
Pumpkin	1 cup, canned	5,424	620
Sweet potato	1, whole baked	2,486	284
Carrot	1, whole fresh	2,024	231
Spinach	1 cup, cooked	1,474	168
Butternut squash	1 cup, baked	1,435	164
Mango	1, medium fresh	806	92
Papaya	1, medium fresh	612	70
Cantaloupe	1 cup, fresh	516	59
Turnip greens	½ cup, chopped	396	45

(*continued*)

TABLE C.2. Vitamin Facts and Nutrient Lists (*continued*)

Food	Portion Size	Vitamin A (RE)	% DRI
Collard greens	1 cup, chopped	349	40
Apricot halves	10 halves	253	29
Winter squash	½ cup, cubes	235	27
Mustard greens	½ cup, chopped	212	24
Broccoli	½ cup, frozen	174	20
Parsley	½ cup, chopped	156	18
Milk, 2%	8 oz	140	16
Egg	1, whole fresh	95	11
Cheddar cheese	1 oz	86	10
Watermelon	1 cup, fresh	58	7
Margarine	1 tsp, tub-type	47	5
Sole/flounder	3 oz, cooked	28	3
Orange	1, medium fresh	26	3
Green beans	½ cup, canned	24	3
Corn	½ cup, canned	13	2
Apple	1, medium fresh	7	1
Chicken breast	½, roasted w/o skin	5	0.5
Sirloin steak	3.5 oz, broiled	0	0
Brewer's yeast	1 oz	0	0
Bread, whole wheat	1 slice	0	0

Quick Reference Diet Integration

- Use fresh spinach, romaine lettuce, carrots, and tomatoes in salads
- Use canned pumpkin in cookies, pies, and desserts
- Serve baked sweet potatoes in place of baked potatoes
- Breakfast: fruit salad of mango, papaya, and cantaloupe
- Snack: dried peaches and apricots

M. Vitamin D

Food	Portion Size	Vitamin D (μg)	% DRI
Milk, 2%	8 oz	1.6	33
Corn flakes	1 cup	0.81	16
Cod liver oil	1 Tbsp	0.55	11
Egg	1, whole fresh	0.41	8
Margarine	1 tsp, tub type	0.34	7
Frankfurter	1 beef, frank	0.18	4
Braunschweiger	1 oz, tube type	0.15	3
Rice, wild	⅔ cup, instant	0.07	1
Rice, white	⅔ cup, instant	0.03	<1
Cheddar cheese	1 oz	0.02	<1

Quick Reference Diet Integration

- Drink 2–3 eight-oz glasses of milk per day
- 10–15 minutes of sunlight exposure 3 times per week
- Breakfast: vitamin D-fortified cereals with milk
- Snack: pudding made with low-fat milk
- Use vitamin D-fortified margarine instead of butter

N. Vitamin E

Food	Portion Size	Vitamin E (mg)	% DRI
Wheat germ oil	1 Tbsp	20.3	102
Sunflower seeds	1 oz, dry roasted	14.2	71
Mayonnaise	1 Tbsp	11	55
Almonds	1 oz, dried	6.7	34
Dried filberts	1 oz	6.7	34
Sunflower seed oil	1 Tbsp	6.3	32
Sweet potato	1, medium raw	5.9	30
Almond oil	1 Tbsp	5.3	27
Cottonseed oil	1 Tbsp	4.8	24
Safflower oil	1 Tbsp	4.6	23
Wheat germ	¼ cup, toasted	4.1	20
Peanut butter	2 Tbsp	3	15

(*continued*)

TABLE C.2. Vitamin Facts and Nutrient Lists (*continued*)

Food	Portion Size	Vitamin E (mg)	% DRI
Shrimp	3 oz, boiled	3	15
Canola oil	1 Tbsp	2.5	13
Asparagus	1 cup, cooked	2.4	12
Mango	1, medium raw	2.3	12
Avocado	½ cup	2.3	12
Peanuts	1 oz, dry roasted	2.2	11
Brazil nuts	1 oz, dried	2.1	11
Salmon	3 oz, baked	2	10
Corn oil	1 Tbsp	1.9	10
Olive oil	1 Tbsp	1.7	8
Peanut oil	1 Tbsp	1.6	8
Soybean oil	1 Tbsp	1.5	8
Apple	1, medium fresh	1.5	8
Brussel sprouts	1 cup, cooked	1.3	7
Spinach	1 cup, raw	1.1	5
Macaroni	1 cup, cooked	1	5
Parsley	1 Tbsp	1	5
Pear	1, medium fresh	0.83	4
Cheddar cheese	1 oz	0.5	3

Quick Reference Diet Integration

- Use wheat germ or sunflower oil in salad dressings or baked goods
- Serve sweet potato chips instead of regular chips—slice thin and bake
- Replace cream cheese with peanut butter on bagels
- Add wheat germ to cereal or yogurt
- Snack: sunflower seeds, peanuts, or almonds

O. Vitamin K

Food	Portion Size	Vitamin K (μg)	% DRI
Turnip greens	1 cup, chopped raw	364	455
Green tea	1 oz, dry	199	249
Spinach	1 cup, raw	148	185

Food	Portion Size	Vitamin K (μg)	% DRI
Broccoli	1 cup, cooked	126	158
Beef liver	3.5 oz, raw	104	104
Cauliflower	1 cup, raw	96	120
Soybean oil	1 Tbsp	76	95
Chickpeas	1 oz, dry	74	93
Asparagus	1 cup, cooked	69	86
Lentils	1 oz, dry	62	78
Soybeans	1 oz	53	66
Cabbage	1 cup, raw shredded	52	65
Mung beans	1 oz, dry	48	60
Green beans	1 cup, boiled	44	55
Wheat flour	Whole wheat, 1 cup	36	45
Tomato	1, whole fresh	28	35
Egg	1, whole fresh	25	31
Peas	1 oz, dry	23	29
Wheat bran	1 oz	23	29
Lettuce	1 leaf iceberg	22	28
Strawberries	1 cup, raw	21	26
Watercress	1 cup, chopped	20	25
Oats	1 oz, dry	18	23
Wheat germ	1 oz	10	13
Carrot	1, medium raw	9	11
Corn oil	1 Tbsp	8	10
Orange	1, medium fresh	7	9
Potato	1, whole baked	6	8
Cucumber	1 cup, raw	6	8

Quick Reference Diet Integration

- Add turnip greens to soup or eat as a side dish
- Entree: stir fry of broccoli, cauliflower, spinach, carrots, and asparagus
- Add spinach, watercress, and tomatoes to sandwiches
- Use soybean oil to make salad dressing
- Salad: spinach and lettuce with tomatoes and chickpeas
- Appetizer: coleslaw with low-fat or fat-free dressing

TABLE C.3. Mineral Facts

Mineral/Symbol	Functions	Deficiency	Toxicity
Calcium, Ca	Bone/teeth structure; nerve transmission; blood clotting; muscle contraction	Osteoporosis; osteomalacia; neuromuscular excitability; cramps, tetany; hypoparathyroidism; convulsion	Kidney stones, constipation
Sources Canned sardines, cheese, milk, tofu made with calcium sulfate, yogurt			
Chromium, Cr	Glucose metabolism, an insulin cofactor	Weight loss; diabetes; abnormal glucose metabolism; neuropathy	None known
Sources Broccoli, grape juice, grain products			
Copper, Cu	Iron absorption; component of several metalloenzymes	Menkes disease; microcytic anemia; cognitive deficits; hypothermia; hair depigmentation	Wilson disease; cirrhosis
Sources Liver, clams, oysters, crab meat, cashews, hazelnuts, sunflower seeds, lentils, mushrooms			
Fluoride, F	Dental caries prevention	Dental caries	Dental mottling
Sources Fluoridated water, crab, rice, fish			

Iodine, I	Constituent of thyroid hormones	Hypothyroidism; goiter	Goiter
Sources Iodized salt, cod, milk, potatoes, turkey breast, shrimp			
Iron, Fe	Component of hemoglobin and myoglobin; electron transport	Microcytic anemia; fatigue; skin pallor; glossitis; tachycardia	Hemosiderosis; hemochromatosis
Sources Oysters, beef, chicken (dark meat), blackstrap molasses, prune juice, lentils			
Magnesium, Mg	Component of several enzymes involved in metabolism (including nutrient); muscle contraction; nerve transmission	Muscle spasms, tetany, and seizures; hypocalcemia; hypokalemia; paresthesias	Diarrhea; cardiorespiratory failure and abnormal nerve transmission in kidney patients
Sources Bran cereal, brown rice, almonds, spinach, Swiss chard, peanuts, blackstrap molasses, hazelnuts			
Manganese, Mn	Cofactor in several enzymes; gluconeogenesis, metabolism of lipids and mucopolysaccharides; antioxidant as Mn superoxide dismutase	Limited evidence for increased bone remodelling; reduction of serum cholesterol; skin rash; abnormal glucose tolerance	Neurologic damage if inhaled in certain occupations; limited evidence for oral toxicity of neurologic and cognitive problems
Sources Pecans, pineapple, almonds, peanuts, bran cereal brown rice			

(*continued*)

TABLE C.3. Mineral Facts (*continued*)

Mineral/Symbol	Functions	Deficiency	Toxicity
Molybdenum, Mo	Cofactor in enzymes	Tachycardia; coma	Limited evidence for gout-like symptoms
Sources Legumes, lentils, grain products, nuts			
Phosphorus, P	Cell membrane and nucleic acid component; glycolysis; component of ATP in all energy reactions; regulation of acid–base balance	Muscular weakness; glucose intolerance; abnormal cellular function; growth deficit and bone deformation in children	Diarrhea; hyperparathyroidism; soft tissue calcification
Sources Dairy products, cereal products, meat, fish, food additives (phosphates)			
Potassium, K	Intracellular cation; nerve transmission; muscle contraction; blood pressure regulation	Muscular weakness; hypotension; ileus; cardiac arrhythmias; respiratory failure	Cardiac arrhythmia; heart failure
Sources Potatoes, prunes/prune juice, bananas, tomatoes/tomato juice, raisins, lima beans, acorn squash			

Selenium, Se	Antioxidant as glutathione peroxidases and part of other enzymes; part of amino acid selenocysteine	Susceptibility to physiologic stresses; prolonged deficiency linked to Keshan and Kashin–Beck diseases	Hair and nail brittleness and loss; gastrointestinal distress; skin rash; garlic breath odor; fatigue; irritability; neurologic disorders
Sources Brazil nuts, tuna, oysters, salmon, shrimp, halibut, crab, beef, chicken, rice, sunflower seeds			
Sodium, Na; chloride, Cl	Na and Cl principle extracellular ions; maintenance of membrane potential; nutrient absorption and transport; regulation of blood volume and pressure	Headache; nausea; vomiting; muscle cramps; fatigue; disorientation; dizziness; seizure and coma	Nausea; vomiting; diarrhea; abdominal cramps; edema; coma
Sources Snack foods, processed meats, breads, cereals, canned tomato/vegetable juice, soup, pickles, olives			
Zinc, Zn	Enzyme cofactor in reactions related to growth, sexual maturation, reproduction, immunity, night vision, taste acuity	Hypogonadism; growth failure; impaired taste and smell; impaired wound healing; infection; fatigue; diminished appetite, dry and hyperpigmented skin, acrodermatitis	Interference with copper and iron metabolism; impaired immunity
Sources Oysters, crab, beef, poultry (dark meat), yogurt, cashews			

TABLE C.4. Dietary Supplements

—*Virginia Uhley, PhD, RDN*

Name	Use	Contraindications/Potential Side Effects
α-Lipoic acid	**Diabetes**, neuropathy, alcoholic liver disease, HIV, kidney disease, pancreatic cancer, wound healing	**Adverse effects:** nausea, vomiting, dizziness **Potential drug interactions:** diabetic medications, thyroid medications, Doxorubicin, Adriamycin, NSAIDs
Ascorbic acid (vitamin C)	**Cold prevention**, scurvy, iron absorption, cancer prevention	**Adverse effects:** nausea, vomiting, heartburn, abdominal pain, flushing, dizziness, headache **Potential drug interactions:** acetaminophen, aluminum antacids, aspirin, barbiturates, fluphenazine, indinavir, levodopa, tetracycline, antibiotics, oral estrogens, anticoagulants, nicotine
β-Carotene	**Cancer**, photosensitivity, age-related macular degeneration, oral leukoplakia, scleroderma, metabolic syndrome, heart disease, asthma, COPD	**Adverse effects:** skin discoloration, loose stools, bruising, joint pain **Potential drug interactions:** statins, cholesterol-lowering medications, orlistat, niacin Patients who smoke or drink heavily or have a history of asbestos exposure should avoid β-carotene supplements because of a possible increase of the risk of heart disease and cancer.

Bitter orange	**Obesity/weight loss**	**Adverse effects:** tachycardia, hypertension, fainting, heart attack, stroke, nervousness **Potential drug interactions:** MAOIs, midazolam (Versed), caffeine, dextromethorphan, felodipine (Plendil), indinavir (Crixivan), CYP450 agents, amiodarone (Cordarone), disopyramide (Norpace), dofetilide (Tikosyn), ibutilide (Corvert), procainamide (Pronestyl), quinidine, sotalol (Betapace), thioridazine (Mellaril), stimulant drugs
Black cohosh	**Postmenopausal symptoms**, arthritis pain, breast cancer, infertility, migraines	**Adverse effects:** gastric discomfort, hepatotoxicity, fatigue, arrhythmia **Potential drug interactions:** anticoagulants, SSRIs, NSAIDs, CYP450 agents, antineoplastics, Antabuse, hormonal agents, antifungals ,alcohol, tamoxifen, raloxifene
Chondroitin sulfate	**Osteoarthritis**, urinary incontinence, interstitial cystitis, muscle aches, knee pain	**Adverse effects:** rash, photosensitivity, diarrhea, constipation, dyspepsia, hair loss **Potential drug interactions:** anticoagulants, NSAIDs, photosensitizing agents Patients with prostate cancer (family history) and patients with shellfish allergies should avoid.

(continued)

TABLE C.4. Dietary Supplements (*continued*)

Name	Use	Contraindications/Potential Side Effects
Chromium	**Diabetes**, hypoglycemia, PCOS, hyperlipidemia, bipolar disorder, depression, Parkinson disease, obesity/weight loss	**Adverse effects:** glucose/insulin metabolism, nausea, vomiting, anemia, headache, insomnia, mood changes, renal failure **Potential drug interactions:** antacids, NSAIDs, SSRI medications, MAOI medications, antidiabetic agents, antihypertensive agents, antilipemic drugs, steroids, immunomodulators
CoQ10	**CoQ10 deficiency**, hypertension, cancer, chronic fatigue syndrome, **CHF, adjunct to statin medication**, migraine headache, diabetes, tinnitus, enhance exercise performance	**Adverse effects:** nausea, rash, flu-like symptoms, headache, photosensitivity, elevated liver enzymes **Potential drug interactions:** antihypertensive medications, antilipidemic medications, TCAs, Coumadin, antineoplastics, immunosuppressants
Echinacea	**Colds/URIs**, cancer, immune system stimulation, radiation-associated leukopenia, herpes simplex virus	**Adverse effects:** urticaria, rash, nausea, vomiting, leukopenia, dry eyes **Potential drug interactions:** amoxicillin, anesthetics, CYP450 agents, antifungals, immunosuppressants, steroids, antineoplastics, caffeine Patients with tuberculosis, leukemia, diabetes, connective tissue disorders, multiple sclerosis, HIV or AIDS, any autoimmune diseases, or, possibly liver disorders should [illegible]

Evening primrose oil	**Postmenopausal symptoms (PMS),** diabetic neuropathy, allergies, rheumatoid arthritis, ADHD, breast cancer, hypertension, osteoporosis	**Adverse effects:** headache, abdominal pain, nausea, and loose stools **Potential drug interactions:** anticoagulants, cyclosporine, phenothiazines, chemotherapy agents Patients with seizure disorders should avoid.
5-HTP (5-hydroxytryptophan)	**Depression**, fibromyalgia, cerebellar ataxia, headache, anxiety, sleep disorders	**Adverse effects:** rash, nausea, diarrhea, heartburn, abdominal pain, irritability, heart palpitations, allergic reactions, hypomania, eosinophilia **Potential drug interactions:** angiotensin receptor blockers, antidepressants, antiepileptics, antipsychotics, CNS depressants, Ultram, lithium, CYP450 agents, β-blockers
Garlic	**Heart disease,** cancer, hypertension, cold/flu	**Adverse effects:** upset stomach, bloating, bad breath, body odor, headache, fatigue, loss of appetite, muscle aches, dizziness, asthmatic reaction, skin rash, skin lesions (topical exposure) **Potential drug interactions:** oral contraceptives, isoniazid, cyclosporine, anticoagulants, HIV/AIDS medications(protease inhibitors), NSAIDs

(*continued*)

TABLE C.4. Dietary Supplements (*continued*)

Name	Use	Contraindications/Potential Side Effects
Ginger	**Pregnancy-related nausea and vomiting, chemotherapy nausea, nausea and vomiting after surgery,** motion sickness, osteoarthritis	**Adverse effects:** mild heartburn, diarrhea, irritation of the mouth **Potential drug interactions:** anticoagulants, antidiabetic medications, hypertensives Patients who have a bleeding disorder or are taking blood-thinning medications, including aspirin, should avoid.
Ginkgo biloba	**Dementia and Alzheimer disease**, intermittent claudication, anxiety, glaucoma, macular degeneration, PMS, Raynaud's	**Adverse effects:** stomach upset, headaches, skin reactions, dizziness, internal bleeding **Potential drug interactions:** NSAIDs, medications broken down by the liver, anticonvulsants, antidepressants, antihypertensives, anticoagulants, alprazolam, cyclosporine, antidiabetic medication, thiazide diuretics Patients who have epilepsy should not take ginkgo, because it might cause seizures.
Ginseng (American)	**Postmenopausal symptoms,** boost the immune system, reduce the risk of cancer, improve cognition, well-being, diabetes, colds/flu, ADHD	**Adverse effects:** hypoglycemia, hypertension, bipolar disorder mania, insomnia, restlessness, anxiety, euphoria, diarrhea, vomiting, headache, nosebleeds, breast pain, vaginal bleeding **Potential drug interactions:** antidiabetics, anticoagulants, antipsychotics, MAOIs, stimulants, morphine

Glucosamine sulfate	**Osteoarthritis, rheumatoid arthritis**, leg pain, inflammatory bowel disease	**Adverse effects:** tachycardia, photosensitivity, rash, GI upset, drowsiness, asthma exacerbation **Potential drug interactions:** acetaminophen, antineoplastics, anticoagulants, diabetic agents, diuretics Patients with shellfish allergies should avoid.
Hawthorn	**CHF**, anxiety, hypertension, **CAD/angina**	**Adverse effects:** nausea, agitation, headache, dizziness, fatigue, dyspnea, rash, insomnia, diaphoresis, tachycardia **Potential drug interactions:** antihypertensives, metronidazole, Antabuse, ephedrine, anticoagulants
Kava Kava	**Anxiety**, insomnia, Parkinson disease, stress, pain	**Adverse effects:** GI distress, rash, tachycardia, headache, sedation **Potential drug interactions:** opioids, ACE inhibitors, anxiolytics, anesthetics, MAOIs, SSRIs, anticoagulants, benzodiazepines, β-blockers, CYP450 agents, CNS depressants, diuretics, contraceptives, hepatotoxic agents
Lycopene	**Cancer, enlarged prostate (benign prostatic hypertrophy)**, atherosclerosis, asthma, menopausal symptoms, oral mucositis	**Adverse effects:** none reported **Potential drug interactions:** none known Patients with a prostate cancer diagnosis should avoid.

(*continued*)

TABLE C.4. Dietary Supplements (*continued*)

Name	Use	Contraindications/Potential Side Effects
Melatonin	**Insomnia,** jet lag, anti-inflammatory, age-related macular degeneration, anxiety, chronic fatigue syndrome, hypertension, menopausal symptoms, seasonal affective disorder, tinnitus, heart disease, fibromyalgia, IBS, ADHD, breast/prostate cancer, benzodiazepine withdrawal, epilepsy, sarcoidosis, PCOS	**Adverse effects:** disorientation, hypotension, hormonal levels, hyperglycemia, nausea, vomiting, diarrhea, fatigue, dizziness, headache, irritability, drowsiness, seizure, mood changes **Potential drug interactions:** anticonvulsants, anesthesia, anxiolytics, antidiabetic medication, antihypertensives, SSRIs, CYP450 agents, CNS depressants, Haldol, HRT, INH, propofol, valproic acid, zolpidem, venlafaxine, antipsychotic medications, benzodiazepines, contraceptives, β-blockers, NSAIDs, interleukin-2, anticoagulants, immunosuppressants, tamoxifen
Milk thistle	**Alcoholic hepatitis/cirrhosis, viral hepatitis**, mushroom poisoning, cancer	**Adverse effects:** stomach upset, diarrhea, nausea and vomiting, rash (topical) **Potential drug interactions:** allergy medications, statins, antianxiety medications, antipsychotics, oral contraceptives, phenytoin (Dilantin), anesthesia, antiplatelet/anticoagulant drugs, CYP450 agents, therapeutic cancer drugs Patients with a history of hormone-related cancers, including breast, uterine, and prostate cancer, should avoid.

		Patients with allergies to ragweed, chrysanthemums, marigolds, chamomile, yarrow, or daisies should avoid.
Omega-3 fish oil	**CAD**, hyperlipidemia, hypertension, stroke	**Adverse effects:** nausea, diarrhea, fishy breath/taste, rash, nose bleeds **Potential drug interactions:** anticoagulants, antihypertensives, antilipidemics, contraceptive drugs Patients with fish/shellfish allergies should avoid. Patients with HIV or other lowered immune response should avoid.
Red clover	**Postmenopausal symptoms** (PMS), cancer prevention, indigestion, high cholesterol, whooping cough, cough, asthma, bronchitis, osteoporosis	**Adverse effects:** estrogenic effects, reduction of blood clotting **Potential drug interactions:** contraceptives, estrogens, CYP450 agents, anticoagulants, aspirin, antidiabetics, tamoxifen
Red yeast rice	**CAD**, hyperlipidemia, diabetes	**Adverse effects:** headache, heartburn, abdominal bloating, myopathy, increased liver enzymes, dizziness, rhabdomyolysis **Potential drug interactions:** NSAIDs, anticoagulants, alcohol, antifungals, antilipidemics, antihypertensives, antidiabetic meds, CYP450 agents, digoxin, thyroid hormones, antibiotics Patients who have allergies to yeast or molds should avoid.

(*continued*)

TABLE C.4. Dietary Supplements (*continued*)

Name	Use	Contraindications/Potential Side Effects
Saw palmetto	**BPH (benign prostatic hyperplasia),** alopecia, hypotonic neurogenic bladder, prostatitis, prostate cancer	**Adverse effects:** abdominal pain, diarrhea, fatigue, nausea, headache, decreases libido, rhinitis, hypertension, tachycardia, increased risk of bleeding **Potential drug interactions:** oral contraceptives and hormone replacement therapy, Proscar, Lupron, Casodex, NSAIDs, Antabuse, immunomodulators, antiplatelet and anticoagulant drugs
St John's wort	**Depression**, anxiety, ADHD, OCD, pain, PMS	**Adverse effects:** anxiety, fatigue, restlessness, dizziness, photosensitivity, sexual dysfunction, headache, dry mouth, HTN, tachycardia, rash, nausea, diarrhea, vomiting, constipation **Potential drug interactions:** anxiolytics, anesthetics, anticoagulants, MAOIs, SSRIs, TCAs, fexofenadine, digoxin, antifungals, immunosuppressants, opiates, statins, theophylline, antineoplastics, contraceptives, omeprazole, Imodium, P450 agents
Turmeric	**Cancer**, ulcerative colitis, indigestion/dyspepsia, heart disease, neurodegenerative conditions, osteoarthritis, pruritus	**Adverse effects:** stomach upset, hypoglycemia, bleeding, ulcers, GERD, iron deficiency **Potential drug interactions:** anticoagulants, antacids, diabetic medications

Valerian	**Insomnia,** postmenopausal symptoms, joint pain, ADHD	**Adverse effects:** feeling anxious, restlessness, headache, excitability, sluggish in the morning if taken the previous night **Potential drug interactions:** CYP450 agents, sedatives, antihistamines, statins, antifungals, anesthesia , alprazolam (Xanax), alcohol
Vitamin D	**Osteoporosis**, hypothyroid, hypocalcemia, hypothyroidism, osteomalacia, psoriasis, rickets, muscle pain/weakness, cancer prevention, diabetes, hypertension, multiple sclerosis	**Adverse effects:** hypercalcemia, increased thirst, metal taste in mouth, poor appetite, weight loss, bone pain, tiredness, sore eyes, itchy skin, vomiting, diarrhea, constipation, frequent need to urinate, muscle problems **Potential drug interactions:** antacids, cholestyramine, orlistat, mineral oil, laxatives, thiazide, diuretics, atorvastatin, calcipotriene, calcium channel blockers, corticosteroids, digoxin, antiseizure medications, rifampin Patients with high blood calcium or phosphorus levels, heart problems, kidney disease, sarcoidosis, and tuberculosis should be careful when considering taking vitamin D supplements.

NSAID, nonsteroidal anti-inflammatory drug; COPD, chronic obstructive pulmonary disease; SSRI, selective serotonin reuptake inhibitor; PCOS, polycystic ovary syndrome; MAOI, monoamine oxidase inhibitor; CHF, congestive heart failure; URI, upper respiratory infection; TCA, tricyclic antidepressant; ADHD, Attention-deficit/hyperactivity disorder; CAD, coronary artery disease; CNS, central nervous system; ACE, angiotensin converting enzyme; OCD, obsessive-compulsive disorder; GERD, gastroesophageal reflux disease.

Appendix D
Dietary Reference Intakes

TABLE D.1. Dietary Reference Intakes (DRIs): Recommended Dietary Allowances and Adequate Intakes, Vitamins
Food and Nutrition Board, Institute of Medicine, National Academies

Life Stage Group	Vitamin A (μg/d)[a]	Vitamin C (mg/d)	Vitamin D (μg /d)[b,c]	Vitamin E (mg/d)[d]	Vitamin K (μg/d)	Thiamin (mg/d)	Riboflavin (mg/d)	Niacin (mg/d)[e]	Vitamin B_6 (mg/d)	Folate (μg/d)[f]	Vitamin B_{12} (μg/d)	Pantothenic Acid (mg/d)	Biotin (μg/d)	Choline (mg/d)[g]
Infants														
0 to 6 mo	400*	40*	10	4*	2.0*	0.2*	0.3*	2*	0.1*	65*	0.4*	1.7*	5*	125*
6 to 12 mo	500*	50*	10	5*	2.5*	0.3*	0.4*	4*	0.3*	80*	0.5*	1.8*	6*	150*
Children														
1–3 yr	300	15	15	6	30*	0.5	0.5	6	0.5	150	0.9	2*	8*	200*
4–8 yr	400	25	15	7	55*	0.6	0.6	8	0.6	200	1.2	3*	12*	250*
Males														
9–13 yr	600	45	15	11	60*	0.9	0.9	12	1.0	300	1.8	4*	20*	375*
14–18 yr	900	75	15	15	75*	1.2	1.3	16	1.3	400	2.4	5*	25*	550*
19–30 yr	900	90	15	15	120*	1.2	1.3	16	1.3	400	2.4	5*	30*	550*
31–50 yr	900	90	15	15	120*	1.2	1.3	16	1.3	400	2.4	5*	30*	550*
51–70 yr	900	90	15	15	120*	1.2	1.3	16	1.7	400	2.4[h]	5*	30*	550*
> 70 yr	900	90	20	15	120*	1.2	1.3	16	1.7	400	2.4[h]	5*	30*	550*

Females														
9–13 yr	600	45	15	11	60*	0.9	0.9	12	1.0	300	1.8	4*	20*	375*
14–18 yr	700	65	15	15	75*	1.0	1.0	14	1.2	400[i]	2.4	5*	25*	400*
19–30 yr	700	75	15	15	90*	1.1	1.1	14	1.3	400[i]	2.4	5*	30*	425*
31–50 yr	700	75	15	15	90*	1.1	1.1	14	1.3	400[i]	2.4	5*	30*	425*
51–70 yr	700	75	15	15	90*	1.1	1.1	14	1.5	400	2.4[h]	5*	30*	425*
> 70 yr	700	75	20	15	90*	1.1	1.1	14	1.5	400	2.4[h]	5*	30*	425*
Pregnancy														
14–18 yr	750	80	15	15	75*	1.4	1.4	18	1.9	600[j]	2.6	6*	30*	450*
19–30 yr	770	85	15	15	90*	1.4	1.4	18	1.9	600[j]	2.6	6*	30*	450*
31–50 yr	770	85	15	15	90*	1.4	1.4	18	1.9	600[j]	2.6	6*	30*	450*
Lactation														
14–18 yr	1,200	115	15	19	75*	1.4	1.6	17	2.0	500	2.8	7*	35*	550*
19–30 yr	1,300	120	15	19	90*	1.4	1.6	17	2.0	500	2.8	7*	35*	550*
31–50 yr	1,300	120	15	19	90*	1.4	1.6	17	2.0	500	2.8	7*	35*	550*

NOTE: This table (taken from the DRI reports, see www.nap.edu) presents Recommended Dietary Allowances (RDAs) in **bold type** and Adequate Intakes (AIs) in ordinary type followed by an asterisk (*). An RDA is the average daily dietary intake level; sufficient to meet the nutrient requirements of nearly all (97–98 percent) healthy individuals in a group. It is calculated from an Estimated Average Requirement (EAR). If sufficient scientific evidence is not available to establish an EAR, and thus calculate an RDA, an AI is usually developed. For healthy breastfed infants, an AI is the mean intake. The AI for other life stage and gender groups is believed to cover the needs of all healthy individuals in the groups, but lack of data or uncertainty in the data prevent being able to specify with confidence the percentage of individuals covered by this intake.

(*continued*)

TABLE D.1. Dietary Reference Intakes (DRIs): Recommended Dietary Allowances and Adequate Intakes, Vitamins
Food and Nutrition Board, Institute of Medicine, National Academies (*continued*)

[a]As retinol activity equivalents (RAEs). 1 RAE = 1 μg retinol, 12 μg β-carotene, 24 μg α-carotene, or 24 μg β-cryptoxanthin. The RAE for dietary provitamin A carotenoids is two-fold greater than retinol equivalents (RE), whereas the RAE for preformed vitamin A is the same as RE.

[b]As cholecalciferol. 1 μg cholecalciferol = 40 IU vitamin D.

[c]Under the assumption of minimal sunlight.

[d]As α-tocopherol. α-Tocopherol includes *RRR*-α-tocopherol, the only form of α-tocopherol that occurs naturally in foods, and the *2R*-stereoisomeric forms of α-tocopherol (*RRR*-, *RSR*-, *RRS*-, and *RSS*-α-tocopherol) that occur in fortified foods and supplements. It does not include the *2S*-stereoisomeric forms of α-tocopherol (*SRR*-, *SSR*-, *SRS*-, and *SSS*-α-tocopherol), also found in fortified foods and supplements.

[e]As niacin equivalents (NE). 1 mg of niacin = 60 mg of tryptophan; 0–6 months = preformed niacin (not NE).

[f]As dietary folate equivalents (DFE). 1 DFE = 1 μg food folate = 0.6 μg of folic acid from fortified food or as a supplement consumed with food = 0.5 μg of a supplement taken on an empty stomach.

[g]Although AIs have been set for choline, there are few data to assess whether a dietary supply of choline is needed at all stages of the life cycle, and it may be that the choline requirement can be met by endogenous synthesis at some of these stages.

[h]Because 10 to 30 percent of older people may malabsorb food-bound B_{12}, it is advisable for those older than 50 years to meet their RDA mainly by consuming foods fortified with B_{12} or a supplement containing B_{12}.

[i]In view of evidence linking folate intake with neural tube defects in the fetus, it is recommended that all women capable of becoming pregnant consume 400 μg from supplements or fortified foods in addition to intake of food folate from a varied diet.

[j]It is assumed that women will continue consuming 400 μg from supplements or fortified food until their pregnancy is confirmed and they enter prenatal care, which ordinarily occurs after the end of the periconceptional period—the critical time for formation of the neural tube.

SOURCES: *Dietary Reference Intakes for Calcium, Phosphorous, Magnesium, Vitamin D, and Fluoride* (1997); *Dietary Reference Intakes for Thiamin, Riboflavin, Niacin, Vitamin* B_6 *Folate, Vitamin* B_{12}*, Pantothenic Acid, Biotin, and* Choline (1998); *Dietary Reference Intakes for Vitamin* C, *Vitamin E, Selenium, and Carotenoids* (2000); *Dietary Reference Intakes for Vitamin A, Vitamin K, Arsenic, Boron, Chromium, Copper, Iodine, Iron, Manganese, Molybdenum, Nickel, Silicon, Vanadium, and Zinc* (2001); *Dietary Reference Intakes for Water, Potassium, Sodium, Chloride, and* Sulfate (2005); and *Dietary Reference Intakes for Calcium and Vitamin D* (2011). These reports may be accessed via www.nap.edu.

TABLE D.2. Dietary Reference Intakes (DRIs): Recommended Dietary Allowances and Adequate Intakes, Elements
Food and Nutrition Board, Institute of Medicine, National Academies

Life Stage Group	Calcium (mg/d)	Chromium (µg/d)	Copper (µg/d)	Fluoride (mg/d)	Iodine (µg/d)	Iron (mg/d)	Magnesium (mg/d)	Manganese (mg/d)	Molybdenum (µg/d)	Phosphorus (mg/d)	Selenium (µg/d)	Zinc (mg/d)	Potassium (g/d)	Sodium (g/d)	Chloride (g/d)
Infants															
0 to 6 mo	200*	0.2*	200*	0.01*	110*	0.27*	30*	0.003*	2*	100*	15*	2*	0.4*	0.12*	0.18*
6 to 12 mo	260*	5.5*	220*	0.5*	130*	**11**	75*	0.6*	3*	275*	20*	**3**	0.7*	0.37*	0.57*
Children															
1–3 yr	**700**	11*	**340**	0.7*	**90**	**7**	**80**	1.2*	**17**	**460**	**20**	**3**	3.0*	1.0*	1.5*
4–8 yr	**1,000**	15*	**440**	1*	**90**	**10**	**130**	1.5*	**22**	**500**	**30**	**5**	3.8*	1.2*	1.9*
Males															
9–13 yr	**1,300**	25*	**700**	2*	**120**	**8**	**240**	1.9*	**34**	**1,250**	**40**	**8**	4.5*	1.5*	2.3*
14–18 yr	**1,300**	35*	**890**	3*	**150**	**11**	**410**	2.2*	**43**	**1,250**	**55**	**11**	4.7*	1.5*	2.3*
19–30 yr	**1,000**	35*	**900**	4*	**150**	**8**	**400**	2.3*	**45**	**700**	**55**	**11**	4.7*	1.5*	2.3*
31–50 yr	**1,000**	35*	**900**	4*	**150**	**8**	**420**	2.3*	**45**	**700**	**55**	**11**	4.7*	1.5*	2.3*
51–70 yr	**1,000**	30*	**900**	4*	**150**	**8**	**420**	2.3*	**45**	**700**	**55**	**11**	4.7*	1.3*	2.0*
> 70 yr	**1,200**	30*	**900**	4*	**150**	**8**	**420**	2.3*	**45**	**700**	**55**	**11**	4.7*	1.2*	1.8*

(continued)

TABLE D.2. Dietary Reference Intakes (DRIs): Recommended Dietary Allowances and Adequate Intakes, Elements
Food and Nutrition Board, Institute of Medicine, National Academies (*continued*)

Life Stage Group	Calcium (mg/d)	Chromium (μg/d)	Copper (μg/d)	Fluoride (mg/d)	Iodine (μg/d)	Iron (mg/d)	Magnesium (mg/d)	Manganese (mg/d)	Molybdenum (μg/d)	Phosphorus (mg/d)	Selenium (μg/d)	Zinc (mg/d)	Potassium (g/d)	Sodium (g/d)	Chloride (g/d)
Females															
9–13 yr	1,300	21*	700	2*	120	8	240	1.6*	34	1,250	40	8	4.5*	1.5*	2.3*
14–18 yr	1,300	24*	890	3*	150	15	360	1.6*	43	1,250	55	9	4.7*	1.5*	2.3*
19–30 yr	1,000	25*	900	3*	150	18	310	1.8*	45	700	55	8	4.7*	1.5*	2.3*
31–50 yr	1,000	25*	900	3*	150	18	320	1.8*	45	700	55	8	4.7*	1.5*	2.3*
51–70 yr	1,200	20*	900	3*	150	8	320	1.8*	45	700	55	8	4.7*	1.3*	2.0*
> 70 yr	1,200	20*	900	3*	150	8	320	1.8*	45	700	55	8	4.7*	1.2*	1.8*
Pregnancy															
14–18 yr	1,300	29*	1,000	3*	220	27	400	2.0*	50	1,250	60	12	4.7*	1.5*	2.3*
19–30 yr	1,000	30*	1,000	3*	220	27	350	2.0*	50	700	60	11	4.7*	1.5*	2.3*
31–50 yr	1,000	30*	1,000	3*	220	27	360	2.0*	50	700	60	11	4.7*	1.5*	2.3*

Lactation															
14–18 yr	**1,300**	44*	**1,300**	3*	**290**	**10**	**360**	2.6*	**50**	**1,250**	**70**	**13**	5.1*	1.5*	2.3*
19–30 yr	**1,000**	45*	**1,300**	3*	**290**	**9**	**310**	2.6*	**50**	**700**	**70**	**12**	5.1*	1.5*	2.3*
31–50 yr	**1,000**	45*	**1,300**	3*	**290**	**9**	**320**	2.6*	**50**	**700**	**70**	**12**	5.1*	1.5*	2.3*

NOTE: This table (taken from the DRI reports, see www.nap.edu) presents Recommended Dietary Allowances (RDAs) in **bold type** and Adequate Intakes (AIs) in ordinary type followed by an asterisk (*). An RDA is the average daily dietary intake level; sufficient to meet the nutrient requirements of nearly all (97–98 percent) healthy individuals in a group. It is calculated from an Estimated Average Requirement (EAR). If sufficient scientific evidence is not available to establish an EAR, and thus calculate an RDA, an AI is usually developed. For healthy breastfed infants, an AI is the mean intake. The AI for other life stage and gender groups is believed to cover the needs of all healthy individuals in the groups, but lack of data or uncertainty in the data prevent being able to specify with confidence the percentage of individuals covered by this intake.

SOURCES: *Dietary Reference Intakes for Calcium, Phosphorous, Magnesium, Vitamin D, and Fluoride* (1997); *Dietary Reference Intakes for Thiamin, Riboflavin, Niacin, Vitamin* B_6 *Folate, Vitamin* B_{12}*, Pantothenic Acid, Biotin, and Choline* (1998); *Dietary Reference Intakes for Vitamin C, Vitamin E, Selenium, and Carotenoids* (2000); and *Dietary Reference Intakes for Vitamin A, Vitamin K, Arsenic, Boron, Chromium, Copper, Iodine, Iron, Manganese, Molybdenum, Nickel, Silicon, Vanadium, and Zinc* (2001); *Dietary Reference Intakes for Water, Potassium, Sodium, Chloride, and* Sulfate (2005); and *Dietary Reference Intakes for Calcium and Vitamin D* (2011). These reports may be accessed via www.nap.edu.

TABLE D.3. **Dietary Reference Intakes (DRIs): Recommended Dietary Allowances and Adequate Intakes, Total Water and Macronutrients**

Food and Nutrition Board, Institute of Medicine, National Academies

Life Stage Group	*Total* Water[a] (L/d)	Carbohydrate (g/d)	Total Fiber (g/d)	Fat (g/d)	Linoleic Acid (g/d)	α-Linolenic Acid (g/d)	Protein[b] (g/d)
Infants							
0 to 6 mo	0.7*	60*	ND	31*	4.4*	0.5*	9.1*
6 to 12 mo	0.8*	95*	ND	30*	4.6*	0.5*	**11.0**
Children							
1–3 yr	1.3*	**130**	19*	ND[c]	7*	0.7*	**13**
4–8 yr	1.7*	**130**	25*	ND	10*	0.9*	**19**
Males							
9–13 yr	2.4*	**130**	31*	ND	12*	1.2*	**34**
14–18 yr	3.3*	**130**	38*	ND	16*	1.6*	**52**
19–30 yr	3.7*	**130**	38*	ND	17*	1.6*	**56**
31–50 yr	3.7*	**130**	38*	ND	17*	1.6*	**56**
51–70 yr	3.7*	**130**	30*	ND	14*	1.6*	**56**
> 70 yr	3.7*	**130**	30*	ND	14*	1.6*	**56**
Females							
9–13 yr	2.1*	**130**	26*	ND	10*	1.0*	**34**
14–18 yr	2.3*	**130**	26*	ND	11*	1.1*	**46**
19–30 yr	2.7*	**130**	25*	ND	12*	1.1*	**46**

31–50 yr	2.7*	**130**	25*	ND	12*	1.1*	**46**
51–70 yr	2.7*	**130**	21*	ND	11*	1.1*	**46**
> 70 yr	2.7*	**130**	21*	ND	11*	1.1*	**46**
Pregnancy							
14–18 yr	3.0*	**175**	28*	ND	13*	1.4*	**71**
19–30 yr	3.0*	**175**	28*	ND	13*	1.4*	**71**
31–50 yr	3.0*	**175**	28*	ND	13*	1.4*	**71**
Lactation							
14–18 yr	3.8*	**210**	29*	ND	13*	1.3*	**71**
19–30 yr	3.8*	**210**	29*	ND	13*	1.3*	**71**
31–50 yr	3.8*	**210**	29*	ND	13*	1.3*	**71**

NOTE: This table (take from the DRI reports, see www.nap.edu) presents Recommended Dietary Allowances (RDA) in **bold type** and Adequate Intakes (AI) in ordinary type followed by an asterisk (*). An RDA is the average daily dietary intake level; sufficient to meet the nutrient requirements of nearly all (97–98 percent) healthy individuals in a group. It is calculated from an Estimated Average Requirement (EAR). If sufficient scientific evidence is not available to establish an EAR, and thus calculate an RDA, an AI is usually developed. For healthy breastfed infants, an AI is the mean intake. The AI for other life stage and gender groups is believed to cover the needs of all healthy individuals in the groups, but lack of data or uncertainty in the data prevent being able to specify with confidence the percentage of individuals covered by this intake.

[a]*Total* water includes all water contained in food, beverages, and drinking water.

[b]Based on g protein per kg of body weight for the reference body weight, e.g., for adults 0.8 g/kg body weight for the reference body weight.

[c]Not determined.

SOURCES: *Dietary Reference Intakes for Energy, Carbohydrate, Fiber, Fat, Fatty Acids, Cholesterol, Protein, and Amino Acids* (2002/2005) and *Dietary Reference Intakes for Water, Potassium, Sodium, Chloride, and Sulfate* (2005). The report may be accessed via www.nap.edu.

TABLE D.4. Dietary Reference Intakes (DRIs): Acceptable Macronutrient Distribution Ranges
Food and Nutrition Board, Institute of Medicine, National Academies

	Range (Percent of Energy)		
Macronutrient	Children, 1–3 yr	Children, 4–18 yr	Adults
Fat	30–40	25–35	20–35
n-6 polyunsaturated fatty acids[a] (linoleic acid)	5–10	5–10	5–10
n-3 polyunsaturated fatty acids[a] (α-linolenic acid)	0.6–1.2	0.6–1.2	0.6–1.2
Carbohydrate	45–65	45–65	45–65
Protein	5–20	10–30	10–35

[a]Approximately 10 percent of the total can come from longer-chain *n*-3 or *n*-6 fatty acids.

SOURCE: *Dietary Reference Intakes for Energy, Carbohydrate, Fiber, Fat, Fatty Acids, Cholesterol, Protein, and Amino Acids* (2002/2005). The report may be accessed via www.nap.edu.

TABLE D.5. Dietary Reference Intakes (DRIs): Acceptable Macronutrient Distribution Ranges
Food and Nutrition Board, Institute of Medicine, National Academies

Macronutrient	Recommendation
Dietary cholesterol	As low as possible while consuming a nutritionally adequate diet
Trans fatty Acids	As low as possible while consuming a nutritionally adequate diet
Saturated fatty acids	As low as possible while consuming a nutritionally adequate diet
Added sugars[a]	Limit to no more than 25% of total energy

[a]Not a recommended intake. A daily intake of added sugars that individuals should aim for to achieve a healthful diet was not set.

SOURCE: *Dietary Reference Intakes for Energy, Carbohydrate, Fiber, Fat, Fatty Acids, Cholesterol, Protein, and Amino Acids* (2002/2005). The report may be accessed via www.nap.edu.

TABLE D.6. Dietary Reference Intakes (DRIs): Tolerable Upper Intake Levels, Vitamins
Food and Nutrition Board, Institute of Medicine, National Academies

Life Stage Group	Vitamin A (µg/d)[a]	Vitamin C (mg/d)	Vitamin D (µg/d)	Vitamin E (mg/d)[b,c]	Vitamin K	Thiamin	Ribo-flavin	Niacin (mg/d)[c]	Vitamin B_6 (mg/d)	Folate (µg/d)[c]	Vitamin B_{12}	Panto-thenic Acid	Biotin	Choline (g/d)	Carote-noids[d]
Infants															
0 to 6 mo	600	ND[e]	25	ND	ND	ND	ND	ND	ND	ND	ND	ND	ND	ND	ND
6 to 12 mo	600	ND	38	ND	ND	ND	ND	ND	ND	ND	ND	ND	ND	ND	ND
Children															
1–3 yr	600	400	63	200	ND	ND	ND	10	30	300	ND	ND	ND	1.0	ND
4–8 yr	900	650	75	300	ND	ND	ND	15	40	400	ND	ND	ND	1.0	ND
Males															
9–13 yr	1,700	1,200	100	600	ND	ND	ND	20	60	600	ND	ND	ND	2.0	ND
14–18 yr	2,800	1,800	100	800	ND	ND	ND	30	80	800	ND	ND	ND	3.0	ND
19–30 yr	3,000	2,000	100	1,000	ND	ND	ND	35	100	1,000	ND	ND	ND	3.5	ND
31–50 yr	3,000	2,000	100	1,000	ND	ND	ND	35	100	1,000	ND	ND	ND	3.5	ND
51–70 yr	3,000	2,000	100	1,000	ND	ND	ND	35	100	1,000	ND	ND	ND	3.5	ND
> 70 yr	3,000	2,000	100	1,000	ND	ND	ND	35	100	1,000	ND	ND	ND	3.5	ND

(continued)

TABLE D.6. Dietary Reference Intakes (DRIs): Tolerable Upper Intake Levels, Vitamins
Food and Nutrition Board, Institute of Medicine, National Academies (*continued*)

Life Stage Group	Vitamin A (µg/d)[a]	Vitamin C (mg/d)	Vitamin D (µg/d)	Vitamin E (mg/d)[b,c]	Vitamin K	Thiamin	Riboflavin	Niacin (mg/d)[c]	Vitamin B_6 (mg/d)	Folate (µg/d)[c]	Vitamin B_{12}	Pantothenic Acid	Biotin	Choline (g/d)	Carotenoids[d]
Females															
9–13 yr	1,700	1,200	100	600	ND	ND	ND	20	60	600	ND	ND	ND	2.0	ND
14–18 yr	2,800	1,800	100	800	ND	ND	ND	30	80	800	ND	ND	ND	3.0	ND
19–30 yr	3,000	2,000	100	1,000	ND	ND	ND	35	100	1,000	ND	ND	ND	3.5	ND
31–50 yr	3,000	2,000	100	1,000	ND	ND	ND	35	100	1,000	ND	ND	ND	3.5	ND
51–70 yr	3,000	2,000	100	1,000	ND	ND	ND	35	100	1,000	ND	ND	ND	3.5	ND
> 70 yr	3,000	2,000	100	1,000	ND	ND	ND	35	100	1,000	ND	ND	ND	3.5	ND
Pregnancy															
14–18 yr	2,800	1,800	100	800	ND	ND	ND	30	80	800	ND	ND	ND	3.0	ND
19–30 yr	3,000	2,000	100	1,000	ND	ND	ND	35	100	1,000	ND	ND	ND	3.5	ND
31–50 yr	3,000	2,000	100	1,000	ND	ND	ND	35	100	1,000	ND	ND	ND	3.5	ND

Lactation															
14–18 yr	2,800	1,800	100	800	ND	ND	ND	30	80	800	ND	ND	ND	3.0	ND
19–30 yr	3,000	2,000	100	1,000	ND	ND	ND	35	100	1,000	ND	ND	ND	3.5	ND
31–50 yr	3,000	2,000	100	1,000	ND	ND	ND	35	100	1,000	ND	ND	ND	3.5	ND

NOTE: A Tolerable Upper Intake Level (UL) is the highest level of daily nutrient intake that is likely to pose no risk of adverse health effects to almost all individuals in the general population. Unless otherwise specified, the UL represents total intake from food, water, and supplements. Due to a lack of suitable data, ULs could not be established for vitamin K, thiamin, riboflavin, vitamin B_{12}, pantothenic acid, biotin, and carotenoids. In the absence of a UL, extra caution may be warranted in consuming levels above recommended intakes. Members of the general population should be advised not to routinely exceed the UL. The UL is not meant to apply to individuals who are treated with the nutrient under medical supervision or to individuals with predisposing conditions that modify their sensitivity to the nutrient.

[a]As preformed vitamin A only.

[b]As α-tocopherol; applies to any form of supplemental α-tocopherol.

[c]The ULs for vitamin E, niacin, and folate apply to synthetic forms obtained from supplements, fortified foods, or a combination of the two.

[d]β-Carotene supplements are advised only to serve as a provitamin A source for individuals at risk of vitamin A deficiency.

[e]ND = Not determinable due to lack of data of adverse effects in this age group and concern with regard to lack of ability to handle excess amounts. Source of intake should be from food only to prevent high levels of intake.

SOURCES: *Dietary Reference Intakes for Calcium, Phosphorous, Magnesium, Vitamin D, and Fluoride* (1997); *Dietary Reference Intakes for Thiamin, Riboflavin, Niacin, Vitamin B_6 Folate, Vitamin B_{12}, Pantothenic Acid, Biotin, and Choline* (1998); *Dietary Reference Intakes for Vitamin C, Vitamine E, Selenium, and Carotenoids* (2000); *Dietary Reference Intakes for Vitamin A, Vitamin K, Arsenic, Boron, Chromium, Copper, Iodine, Iron, Manganese, Molybdenum, Nickel, Silicon, Vanadium, and Zinc* (2001); and *Dietary Reference Intakes for Calcium and Vitamin D* (2011). These reports may be accessed via www.nap.edu.

TABLE D.7. Dietary Reference Intakes (DRIs): Tolerable Upper Intake Levels, Elements
Food and Nutrition Board, Institute of Medicine, National Academies

Life Stage Group	Arsenic[a]	Boron (mg/d)	Calcium (mg/d)	Chromium	Copper (μg/d)	Fluoride (mg/d)	Iodine (μg/d)	Iron (mg/d)	Maesium (mg/d)[b]	Manganese (mg/d)	Molybdenum (μg/d)	Nickel (mg/d)	Phos-Plums (g/d)	Selenium (μg/d)	Silicon[c]	Vanadium (mg/d)[d]	Zinc (mg/d)	Sodium (g/d)	Chloride (g/d)
Infants																			
0 to 6 mo	ND[e]	ND	1,000	ND	ND	0.7	ND	40	ND	ND	ND	ND	ND	45	ND	ND	4	ND	ND
6 to 12 mo	ND	ND	1,500	ND	ND	0.9	ND	40	ND	ND	ND	ND	ND	60	ND	ND	5	ND	ND
Children																			
1–3 yr	ND	3	2,500	ND	1,000	1.3	200	40	65	2	300	0.2	3	90	ND	ND	7	1.5	2.3
4–8 yr	ND	6	2,500	ND	3,000	2.2	300	40	110	3	600	0.3	3	150	ND	ND	12	1.9	2.9
Males																			
9–13 yr	ND	11	3,000	ND	5,000	10	600	40	350	6	1,100	0.6	4	280	ND	ND	23	2.2	3.4
14–18 yr	ND	17	3,000	ND	8,000	10	900	45	350	9	1,700	1.0	4	400	ND	ND	34	2.3	3.6
19–30 yr	ND	20	2,500	ND	10,000	10	1,100	45	350	11	2,000	1.0	4	400	ND	1.8	40	2.3	3.6
31–50 yr	ND	20	2,500	ND	10,000	10	1,100	45	350	11	2,000	1.0	4	400	ND	1.8	40	2.3	3.6
51–70 yr	ND	20	2,000	ND	10,000	10	1,100	45	350	11	2,000	1.0	4	400	ND	1.8	40	2.3	3.6
> 70 yr	ND	20	2,000	ND	10,000	10	1,100	45	350	11	2,000	1.0	3	400	ND	1.8	40	2.3	3.6

Females																			
9–13 yr	ND	11	3,000	ND	5,000	10	600	40	350	6	1,100	0.6	4	280	ND	ND	23	2.2	3.4
14–18 yr	ND	17	3,000	ND	8,000	10	900	45	350	9	1,700	1.0	4	400	ND	ND	34	2.3	3.6
19–30 yr	ND	20	2,500	ND	10,000	10	1,100	45	350	11	2,000	1.0	4	400	ND	1.8	40	2.3	3.6
31–50 yr	ND	20	2,500	ND	10,000	10	1,100	45	350	11	2,000	1.0	4	400	ND	1.8	40	2.3	3.6
51–70 yr	ND	20	2,000	ND	10,000	10	1,100	45	350	11	2,000	1.0	4	400	ND	1.8	40	2.3	3.6
> 70 yr	ND	20	2,000	ND	10,000	10	1,100	45	350	11	2,000	1.0	3	400	ND	1.8	40	2.3	3.6
Pregnancy																			
14–18 yr	ND	17	3,000	ND	8,000	10	900	45	350	9	1,700	1.0	3.5	400	ND	ND	34	2.3	3.6
19–30 yr	ND	20	2,500	ND	10,000	10	1,100	45	350	11	2,000	1.0	3.5	400	ND	ND	40	2.3	3.6
61–50 yr	ND	20	2,500	ND	10,000	10	1,100	45	350	11	2,000	1.0	3.5	400	ND	ND	40	2.3	3.6
Lactation																			
14–18 yr	ND	17	3,000	ND	8,000	10	900	45	350	9	1,700	1.0	4	400	ND	ND	34	2.3	3.6
19–30 yr	ND	20	2,500	ND	10,000	10	1,100	45	350	11	2,000	1.0	4	400	ND	ND	40	2.3	3.6
31–50 yr	ND	20	2,500	ND	10,000	10	1,100	45	350	11	2,000	1.0	4	400	ND	ND	40	2.3	3.6

NOTE: A Tolerable Upper Intake Level (UL) is the highest level of daily nutrient intake that is likely to pose no risk of adverse health effects to almost all individuals in the general population. Unless otherwise specified, the UL represents total intake from food, water, and supplements. Due to a lack of suitable data, ULs could not be established for vitamin K, thiamin, riboflavin, vitamin B_{12}, pantothenic acid, biotin, and carotenoids. In the absence of a UL, extra caution may be warranted in consuming levels above recommended intakes. Members of the general population should be advised not to routinely exceed the UL. The UL is not meant to apply to individuals who are treated with the nutrient under medical supervision or to individuals with predisposing conditions that modify their sensitivity to the nutrient.

(*continued*)

TABLE D.7. Dietary Reference Intakes (DRIs): Tolerable Upper Intake Levels, Elements
Food and Nutrition Board, Institute of Medicine, National Academies (*continued*)

[a]Although the UL was not determined for arsenic, there is no justification for adding arsenic to food or supplements.

[b]The ULs for magnesium represent intake from a pharmacological agent only and do not include intake from food and water.

[c]Although silicon has not been shown to cause adverse effects in humans, there is no justification for adding silicon to supplements.

[d]Although vanadium in food has not been shown to cause adverse effects in humans, there is no justification for adding vanadium to food and vanadium supplements should be used with caution. The UL is based on adverse effects in laboratory animals and this data could be used to set a UL for adults but not children and adolescents.

[e]ND = Not determinable due to lack of data of adverse effects in this age group and concern with regard to lack of ability to handle excess amounts. Source of intake should be from food only to prevent high levels of intake.

SOURCES: *Dietary Reference Intakes for Calcium, Phosphorous, Magnesium, Vitamin D, and Fluoride* (1997); *Dietary Reference Intakes for Thiamin, Riboflavin, Niacin, Vitamin B_6 Folate, Vitamin B_{12}, Pantothenic Acid, Biotin, and Choline* (1998); *Dietary Reference Intakes for Vitamin C, Vitamin E, Selenium, and Carotenoids* (2000); *Dietary Reference Intakes for Vitamin A, Vitamin K, Arsenic, Boron, Chromium, Copper, Iodine, Iron, Manganese, Molybdenum, Nickel, Silicon, Vanadium, and Zinc* (2001); *Dietary Reference Intakes for Water, Potassium, Sodium, Chloride, and Sulfate* (2005); and *Dietary Reference Intakes for Calcium and Vitamin D* (2011). These reports may be accessed via www.nap.edu.

Index

Note: Page numbers followed by *b*, *f*, and *t* indicate boxes, figures, and tables, respectively.

D

E

G

H

I

K

L

M

N

U

V

W

X

Z